Generic Drug Product Development

Solid Oral Dosage Forms

DRUGS AND THE PHARMACEUTICAL SCIENCES
A Series of Textbooks and Monographs

Generic Drug Product Development
Solid Oral Dosage Forms

Leon Shargel
Eon Labs, Inc.
Wilson, North Carolina

Isadore Kanfer
Rhodes University
Grahamstown, South Africa

MARCEL DEKKER

MARCEL DEKKER

NEW YORK

Library of Congress Cataloging-in-Publication Data
A catalog record for this book is available from the Library of Congress.

ISBN: 0-8247-5460-3

This book is printed on acid-free paper.

Headquarters
Marcel Dekker, Inc., 270 Madison Avenue, New York, NY 10016, U.S.A.
tel: 212-696-9000; fax: 212-685-4540

Distribution and Customer Service
Marcel Dekker, Inc., Cimarron Road, Monticello, New York 12701, U.S.A.
tel: 800-228-1160; fax: 845-796-1772

World Wide Web
http://www.dekker.com

The publisher offers discounts on this book when ordered in bulk quantities. For more information, write to Special Sales/Professional Marketing at the headquarters address above.

Preface

Early development and approval of generic drug products was associated with issues concerning safety, efficacy and therapeutic equivalence of such products compared to the innovator or brand-name drug product. Current development of generic drug products is based on sound scientific principles and processes to ensure that these drug products satisfy accepted standards for quality, safety and efficacy prior to obtaining marketing approval. However, the generic pharmaceutical industry is still challenged by legislative, regulatory and scientific issues that must be addressed to allow for the manufacture, approval and marketing of generic drug products.

The objectives of this textbook are to describe, from concept to market approval, the development of high quality, safe and efficacious solid oral generic drug products and to give a comprehensive account of the temporal and legal/regulatory considerations and associated processes from project initiation to marketing approval. The emphasis of this textbook is on the development of solid oral generic drug products. However, much of the material contained in this book may be applied to the development of other generic drug products.

Drug product development for the generic drug industry is different than that for the brand-name pharmaceutical industry. Generic drug product manufacturers must formulate a drug product that will have the same therapeutic efficacy and clinical performance as their brand-name counterpart. Moreover, generic drug product formulators have certain restraints in generic drug product development as well as regulatory and legal challenges that differ from those relating to the development of innovator or brand-name products.

The book initially explains the economic importance for developing therapeutic equivalent drug products and the various legislative and regulatory issues surrounding the approval process. The reader is guided through the drug development process starting with a discussion on active pharmaceutical ingredients (API's), including their chemistry, patent issues, sourcing and requisite quality specifications and requirements followed by a comprehensive account of analytical method development and validation procedures. Later chapters provide a description of the formulation development process, scale-up, process validation, technology transfer and stability requirements. Quality control and quality assurance requirements for drug products are described along with the importance and utility of in vitro characterization and in vivo performance of solid oral dosage forms.

A comprehensive account of the Abbreviated New Drug Application (ANDA) approval process is discussed, including the organization of the U.S. Food and Drug Administration and ANDA review process. Bioequivalence is discussed in two separate chapters from both a regulatory and statistical perspective, respectively. A brief section of the bioequivalence requirements for generic drug products in Canada, Japan and the European Union is also included.

After market approval, the reader is exposed to issues on scale-up, post-approval changes and post-marketing surveillance. Since most bioequivalence studies are out-sourced, the book gives an account of the services provided by Contract Research Organizations (CRO's) including selection of a CRO, time and cost considerations, project management and the conduct of bioequivalence trials.

Finally, the book discusses legal and legislative hurdles to generic drug development, approval and marketing with an explanation of citizen petitions, exclusivity issues, suitability petitions and other legal matters.

The audiences for this book include undergraduate and graduate pharmacy students, pharmacy faculty, drug manufacturers and regulators in the pharmaceutical industry who are interested in generic drug development and need more information concerning drug product initiation, drug product formulation, biopharmaceutics, drug delivery, bioequivalence, regulatory and legislative issues. Emphasis is on practical information for the development of generic drug products. The text assumes that the reader has basic knowledge in pharmaceutical sciences and is interested in generic drug product development and manufacture.

Leon Shargel, Ph.D.
Vice President, Biopharmaceutics
Eon Labs Inc.
Wilson, NC, U.S.A.

Adjunct Associate Professor
School of Pharmacy
University of Maryland
Baltimore, MD, U.S.A.

Izzy Kanfer, Ph.D.
Professor of Pharmacy
Dean & Head
Faculty of Pharmacy
Rhodes University,
Grahamstown, South Africa

Contents

Contributors

Salah U. Ahmed Research & Development, Barr Laboratories, Inc., Pomona, New York, U.S.A.

Timothy W. Ames Division of Labeling and Program Support, Office of Generic Drugs, Center for Drug Evaluation and Research, U.S. Food and Drug Administration, Rockville, Maryland, U.S.A.

Karen A. Bernard Chemistry Division II, Office of Generic Drugs, Center for Drug Evaluation and Research, U.S. Food and Drug Administration, Rockville, Maryland, U.S.A.

Pranab K. Bhattacharyya Quality Management and Analytical Services, Eon Labs, Inc., Laurelton, New York, U.S.A.

Sanford Bolton University of Arizona, Tuscon, Arizona, U.S.A.

Sadie M. Ciganek Regulatory Affairs, Eon Labs, Inc., Laurelton, New York, U.S.A.

Edward M. Cohen* Business Development, Schein Pharmaceuticals, Inc., Danbury, Connecticut, U.S.A.

Dale P. Conner Division of Bioequivalence, Office of Generic Drugs, Center for Drug Evaluation and Research, U.S. Food and Drug Administration, Rockville, Maryland, U.S.A.

Current affiliation: EMC Consulting Services, Newtown, Connecticut, U.S.A.

Barbara M. Davit   Division of Bioequivalence, Office of Generic Drugs, Center for Drug Evaluation and Research, U.S. Food and Drug Administration, Rockville, Maryland, U.S.A.

Beth Fabian Fritsch   Division of Labeling and Program Support, Office of Generic Drugs, Center for Drug Evaluation and Research, U.S. Food and Drug Administration, Rockville, Maryland, U.S.A.

Quanyin Gao   Watson Laboratories, Inc., Corona, California, U.S.A.

Loren Gelber   Quality and Compliance, Andrx Pharmaceuticals, LIC, Davie, Florida, U.S.A.

Ajaz S. Hussain   Office of Pharmaceutical Sciences, Center for Drug Evaluation and Research, U.S. Food and Drug Administration, Rockville, Maryland, U.S.A.

Joan Janulis   Regulatory Affairs, Able Laboratories, Inc., Cranbury, New Jersey, U.S.A.

Izzy Kanfer   Division of Pharmaceutics, Faculty of Pharmacy, Rhodes University, Grahamstown, South Africa

Koung Lee   Division of Labeling and Program Support, Office of Generic Drugs, Center for Drug Evaluation and Research, U.S. Food and Drug Administration, Rockville, Maryland, U.S.A.

Lih-Yang Lin[†]   Regulatory and Technology Division, ScinoPharm, San Matteo, California, U.S.A.

Aruna J. Mehta   New Products, Eon Labs, Inc., Laurelton, New York, U.S.A.

Frank J. Mellina   Eon Labs, Inc., Laurelton, New York, U.S.A.

Venkatesh Naini   Schering-Plough Research Institute, Kenilworth, New Jersey, U.S.A.

Patrick K. Noonan   PK Noonan & Associates, LLC, Richmond, Virginia, U.S.A.

Larry A. Ouderkirk   Office of Pharmaceutical Sciences, Center for Drug Evaluation and Research, U.S. Food and Drug Administration, Rockville, Maryland, U.S.A.

Peter Persicaner   Arrow Pharmaceuticals, Croydon, Victoria, Australia

---

[†] Deceased.

Andre S. Raw Office of Generic Drugs, Center for Drug Evaluation and Research, U.S. Food and Drug Administration, Rockville, Maryland, U.S.A.

Aida L. Sanchez Division of Bioequivalence, Office of Generic Drugs, Center for Drug Evaluation and Research, U.S. Food and Drug Administration, Rockville, Maryland, U.S.A.

Dilip R. Sanvordeker Watson Laboratories, Inc., Corona, California, U.S.A.

Pradeep M. Sathe Office of Generic Drugs, Center for Drug Evaluation and Research, U.S. Food and Drug Administration, Rockville, Maryland, U.S.A.

Krista M. Scardina Office of Generic Drugs, Center for Drug Evaluation and Research, U.S. Food and Drug Administration, Rockville, Maryland, U.S.A.

Leon Shargel Biopharmaceutics, Eon Labs, Inc., Wilson, North Carolina, U.S.A.

Martin Shimer Regulatory Support Branch, Division of Labeling and Program Support, Office of Generic Drugs, Center for Drug Evaluation and Research, U.S. Food and Drug Administration, Rockville, Maryland, U.S.A.

Arthur Y. Tsien Olsson, Frank and Weeda, PC, Washington, D.C., U.S.A.

Robert Vita Gram Laboratories, Inc, Costa Mesa, California , U.S.A.

Dilip Wadgaonkar Research and Development, Interpharm Inc., Hauppauge, New York, U.S.A.

Roderick B. Walker Division of Pharmaceutics, Faculty of Pharmacy, Rhodes University, Grahamstown, South Africa

Lawrence X. Yu Office of Generic Drugs, Center for Drug Evaluation and Research, U.S. Food and Drug Administration, Rockville, Maryland, U.S.A.

Generic Drug Product Development

Solid Oral Dosage Forms

1

Introduction to Generic Drug Product Development

Leon Shargel

Biopharmaceutics, Eon Labs, Inc., Wilson, North Carolina, and
University of Maryland, Baltimore, Maryland, U.S.A.

Izzy Kanfer

Faculty of Pharmacy, Rhodes University, Grahamstown, South Africa

A generic drug product, also referred to as a multisource pharmaceutical product, is considered to be "essentially similar" (1) or bioequivalent (2) to an innovator (brand name) product. Bioequivalence implies that a generic drug product is essentially identical to the brand name (reference) drug product in terms of active ingredient(s), strength, dosage form, route of administration, quality, safety, efficacy, performance characteristics, and therapeutic indication. Generic drug products are typically sold at substantial discounts from their brand name counterparts.

The 2002 sales of prescription drug products in the United States has been reported to be approximately $192 billion (3). Approximately 47% of all prescription drugs sold in the United States are generic drug products (Fig. 1) (4). Generic drug products account for about 10% of the total dollar expenditure for prescription drugs. The demand for lower cost generic drug products is an increasing trend worldwide. Individuals, particularly the elderly who are on a fixed income, health maintenance organizations (HMOs), health insurance programs, federal and state government health

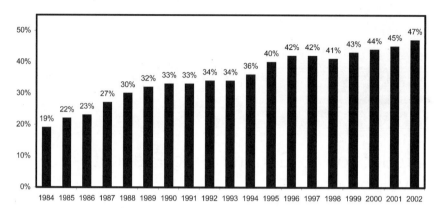

FIGURE 1 U.S. generic share of prescription units (%). *Source*: MS Health, Bank of American Securities LLC Estimates (4).

programs such as Medicaid, hospitals, and other institutions are creating a demand for generic drug products as a means to slow the rising cost of healthcare expenditures. In the next few years, as patents and exclusivities for many important brand name drug products expire (Fig. 2) (4), the value of sales of generic drug products is likely to exceed $10 billion (5).

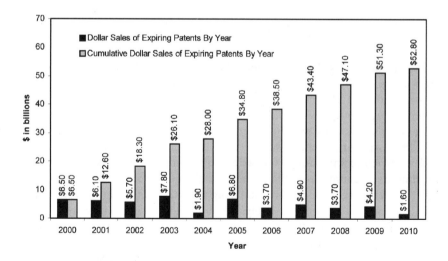

♦ **$35 billion in branded drugs expected to come off patent from 2000 through 2005**

FIGURE 2 Sales of branded drug products vulnerable to generic competition, by year. *Source*: FDA *Orange Book* and Bank of America Securities (4,10).

The manufacture of generic drug products must make provision for market competition and lower prices for the consumer, thereby making medicines more affordable and more accessible to the wider population. Generic drug product availability almost certainly influences the innovator drug product manufacturer to develop new drug products that have improved efficacy and/or safety features.

Generic drug product development uses a different approach and strategy compared to that used to develop a brand name drug product containing a new chemical entity. Generic drug product manufacturers must formulate a drug product that will have the *same* therapeutic efficacy, safety, and performance characteristics as its brand name counterpart. In order to gain market approval, a generic drug product cannot be "*superior*" or "*better*" than the brand name drug product. The key factor is that the generic drug product should meet all the necessary criteria to be therapeutically equivalent and bioequivalent to the brand name (reference) drug product.

The manufacturer of a generic drug product has certain constraints in formulation development that differ from the formulation development of a brand name drug product. For example, a generic drug manufacturer may have to use the same or similar inactive ingredients or excipients as in the brand formulation. Generic drug manufacturers also face a variety of legal challenges from the brand name (innovator) pharmaceutical industry. Many of these issues will be discussed in subsequent chapters.

1. SELECTION OF A GENERIC DRUG PRODUCT FOR MANUFACTURE

The main driving force for the selection of generic drug products for manufacture is the estimated sales volume for the branded product and the potential market share that the firm expects to have once the generic drug product is manufactured and approved for marketing (Table 1). Patent and legal considerations are also very important and are discussed more fully in Chapter 14. In addition to the expiration date of the patent for the active ingredient, the generic firm must consider any other patent claims and exclusivities that the innovator firm has filed. The generic drug manufacturer needs to consider the lead time that is needed to make the product and submission of an Abbreviated New Drug Application (ANDA) to the U.S. Food and Drug Administration(FDA) for approval. Moreover, there is a financial incentive to being the first generic drug product filed and approved by FDA. The Hatch–Waxman Act, as explained below, provides a 180-day exclusivity, under certain conditions, for the generic manufacturer who is first to file.

The availability of technology and the cost of acquiring technology to manufacture the product will also impact on the choice of generic drug. For

TABLE 1 Considerations in the Selection of a Generic Drug Product for Manufacture

Sales and potential market share
Patent expiration and exclusivity issues
Availability of active pharmaceutical ingredient
Timing
Technology
Formulation
Experience

example, if the technology requires a fluidized bed coater, roller compactor, or any other special equipment, then the firm must consider whether this equipment is available or must be acquired. Formulation considerations include the availability of raw materials, chemical purity, polymorphic form, and particle size of the active pharmaceutical ingredient and any patents that the innovator company has filed, including patents for the synthesis of the active pharmaceutical ingredient and composition of the dosage form. Experience with certain drug products will also affect the choice of generic drug product development. For example, some generic drug manufacturers may make a wide variety of dosage forms as well as solid and liquid oral dosage forms including immediate and modified release products. Other generic firms may make specialty drug products such as transdermal or inhalation drug products. Niche drug products, such as transdermal drug products, may be difficult to make and also riskier, but may have a greater financial reward due to less competition from other generic drug firms.

The decision to proceed with the development of a generic drug product should therefore be based on well-researched data that primarily indicate market value together with a sound knowledge of patent expiry dates, predicted market share, and growth rate for the product, amongst others. Government spending trends on medicines, which, in some countries, may be in the region of 40% or even more of the total market, should not be overlooked. The predicted profitability of the new generic product will require strategic planning for the subsequent launch timing, which must take into account the expected generic price and knowledge of anticipated competitors, such as who they are and when they are expected.

2. LEGISLATIVE AND REGULATORY ISSUES

The U.S. Food and Drug Administration was established in 1906 by the Federal Food, Drug, and Cosmetic Act (the "Wiley Act") to prevent the manufacture, sale, or transportation of adulterated or misbranded or poisonous or deleterious foods, drugs, medicines, and liquors, and for regulating traffic therein, amongst others. In 1938, the Act was amended to require drug manufacturers to file a New Drug Application (NDA) for each newly introduced drug and to provide data to establish the safety of the drug product. In 1962, the Kefauver–Harris Amendments to the Act required all drug manufacturers to establish that their products were effective for their claimed indication(s), in addition to adhering to the safety requirements. Consequently, the FDA contracted with the National Academy of Sciences/National Research Council in 1968 to evaluate those drugs first introduced between 1938 and 1962 for effectiveness. This review program was called the Drug Efficacy Study Implementation (DESI) review, and drugs for which effectiveness was determined through the DESI review could be marketed with approval of an NDA. For drugs approved through the DESI review process, manufacturers of brand name products submitted data as a supplement to the existing NDAs, confirming the safety and effectiveness of their products. During the implementation of the DESI review program, more than 3400 products and related generics were reviewed and approximately 900 drug products were removed from the market. Many other products were reformulated or relabeled to limit their uses to selected indications only. One effect of the DESI study was the development of the ANDA in 1970 for reviewed marketed products that required changes in existing labeling to be in compliance. However, manufacturers of any new drug product (brand name or generic) marketed after 1962 were required to prove both the safety and efficacy of such products. The 1962 legislation provided an exemption from the NDA approval process for drugs that had been marketed before 1938, based on the assumption that they were generally recognized as safe and effective— the so-called "*grandfather*" provision. Manufacturers continued to conduct clinical efficacy and safety studies until 1978, when a dispensation was granted to manufacturers whereby the citation of published reports of trials documenting safety and efficacy would suffice (7,8).

In 1984, the Drug Price Competition and Patent Term Restoration Act (Waxman–Hatch Act) extended the ANDA process to generic versions of drugs marketed after 1962 (Table 2). This Act eliminated the requirement that generic drug manufacturers duplicate expensive, time-consuming clinical and nonclinical studies to demonstrate safety and efficacy. Furthermore, this Act expedites the availability of generic drug products provided that the generic drug manufacturer shows that no patent infringement would occur. The Waxman–Hatch Act also compensated the innovator drug manufacturer for perceived losses due to competition from the generic drug products by extending the patent terms of some brand name drug products

TABLE 2   Drug Price Competition and Term Restoration Act of 1984
(Waxman–Hatch Act)

Created a framework for patent term extensions and nonpatent exclusivity periods for
   brand name drug products
Established for the first time an Abbreviated New Drug Application (ANDA) approval
   process specifically for generic manufacturers
Provided for prepatent expiration testing (*Bolar* provision) and generic drug exclusivity

for up to an additional 5 years to make up for time lost while their products
were going through FDA's approval process.

The Drug Price Competition and Patent Term Restoration Act was
subsequently amended to make provision for a pharmaceutical manufacturer (sponsor) to seek approval from the FDA to market a generic drug
before the expiration of a patent relating to the brand name drug upon which
the generic is based. This amendment, known as the "*Bolar* amendment",
allowed the ANDA approval process to begin before the patent on the brand
name drug expired. As part of the ANDA, submission the sponsor must
consider the pertinent patents and provide a *certification* that, in the opinion
of the sponsor and to the best of the sponsor's knowledge with respect to each
patent that claims the listed drug, the patent is invalid or is not infringed by
the generic product (6,7).

The current FDA Federal Food, Drug, and Cosmetic Act, with its
subsequent amendments, is the basic food and drug law of the USA
(http://www.fda.gov/opacom/laws/fdcact/fdctoc.htm) and is intended to
assure consumers that foods are pure and wholesome, safe to eat, and
produced under sanitary conditions; that drugs and devices are safe and
effective for their intended uses; that cosmetics are safe and made from
appropriate ingredients; and that all labeling and packaging is truthful,
informative, and not deceptive. The mission of the FDA is to enforce laws
enacted by the U.S. Congress and regulations established by the Agency to
protect the consumer's health, safety, and pocketbook.

The Federal Register publishes a daily record of proposed rules, final
rules, meeting notices, etc. (http://www.access.gpo.gov/). The final
regulations are collected in the *Code of Federal Regulations*, CFR
(http://www.access.gpo.gov/). The CFR is divided into 50 titles representing broad areas subject to Federal regulations. The FDA's portion of the
CFR interprets the Federal Food, Drug, and Cosmetic Act and related
statutes. Section 21 of the CFR contains most of the regulations pertaining
to food and drugs. The regulations document most actions of all drug
sponsors that are required under Federal law.

3. GENERIC DRUG APPROVAL

The FDA's Office of Generic Drugs is responsible for reviewing the ANDA and approving the drug product for marketing. The FDA's Office of Generic Drugs has a website, *http://www.fda.gov/cder/ogd/*, that provides additional information for manufacturers of generic drug products that includes an interactive flow chart presentation of the ANDA review process (Fig. 3), and describes how FDA determines the quality, safety, and efficacy of generic drug products prior to approval for marketing. Generic drug application reviewers focus on bioequivalence data, chemistry and manufacture quality, microbiology data where relevant, requests for plant inspection, and drug labeling information. The FDA website is designed for individuals from pharmaceutical companies, government agencies, academic institutions, private organizations, or other organizations interested in bringing a generic drug to market. Details of the FDA review and approval process are discussed in Chapter 9.

The ANDA is based on bioequivalence to the brand name product, appropriate chemistry and manufacturing information, and appropriate labeling. Generic drug sponsors do not have to duplicate the nonclinical animal toxicity studies or expensive clinical efficacy and safety studies that are included in the new drug application, NDA, which is submitted to the FDA for market approval of the brand name drug product. The ANDA contains data, which, when submitted to FDA's Center for Drug Evaluation and Research, Office of Generic Drugs, provide for the review and ultimate approval for marketing a generic drug product.

FDA approved generic drugs must meet the same rigid standards as the innovator drug. To obtain FDA approval, a generic drug product must:

- Contain the same active ingredients as an approved *reference listed drug product** (generally, the innovator drug — the inactive ingredients may vary);
- be identical in strength, dosage form, and route of administration;
- have the same use indications;
- be bioequivalent;
- meet the same batch requirements for identity, strength, purity, and quality;
- be manufactured under the same strict standards of FDA's good manufacturing practice regulations as required for innovator products.

---

*The reference listed drug (RLD) may be found in the most current copy of FDA's publication, *Approved Drug Products with Therapeutic Equivalence Evaluations* ("Orange Book"). The *Orange Book* is published on the internet at http://www.fda.gov/cder/ob/default.htm

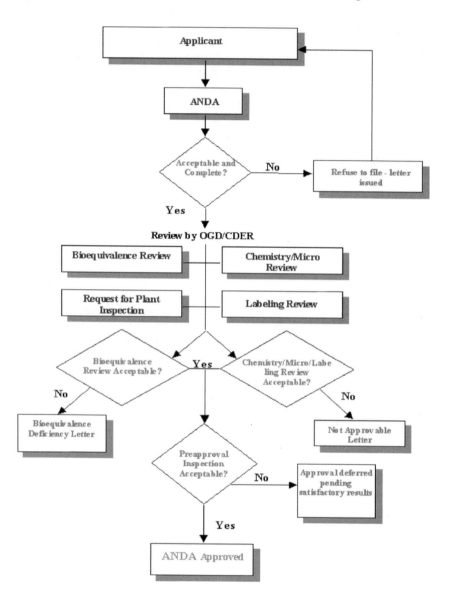

FIGURE 3 Generic drug (ANDA) review process.

An FDA approved generic drug product is considered a therapeutic equivalent to the innovator or brand name drug product in terms of quality and performance characteristics and is expected to have the same safety and efficacy. An ANDA checklist for completeness and acceptability of an application is available on the FDA website at http://www.fda.gov/cder/ogd/anda_checklist.doc.

3.1. Approved Drug Products with Therapeutic Equivalence Evaluations (Orange Book)

The FDA's *Approved Drug Products with Therapeutic Equivalence Evaluations* (*Orange Book*) lists all approved products, both innovator and generic (10). The *Orange Book* is available on the internet at http://www.fda.gov/cder/ob/default.htm and is updated monthly. Therapeutic equivalence or inequivalence for prescription products is determined on the basis of the therapeutic equivalence codes provided within that specific dosage form (Table 3). The coding system for therapeutic equivalence evaluations is constructed to allow users to determine quickly whether the FDA has evaluated a particular approved product as therapeutically equivalent to other pharmaceutically equivalent products (first letter) and to provide additional information on the basis of FDA's evaluations (second letter).

4. PATENTS

New drugs, like most other new products, are developed under patent protection. The patent protects the investment in the drug's development by giving the company the sole right to sell the drug while the patent is in effect. Patents are granted by the U.S. Patent and Trademark Office anytime in the "life" of the drug. A patent expires 20 years from the date of filing. When patents or other periods of exclusivity expire, manufacturers can apply to the FDA to sell generic versions.

The *Orange Book* provides patent and exclusivity information in an Addendum. This Addendum identifies drugs that qualify under the Drug Price Competition and Patent Term Restoration Act (1984 Amendments) for periods of exclusivity, during which ANDAs and applications described in Section 505(b)(2) of the Federal Food, Drug, and Cosmetic Act (the Act) for those drug products may, in some instances, not be submitted or made effective, and provides patent information concerning the listed drug products. Those drugs that have qualified for Orphan Drug Exclusivity pursuant to Section 527 of the Act and those drugs that have qualified for Pediatric Exclusivity pursuant to Section 505A are also included in this Addendum.

TABLE 3 *Orange Book* Codes

A	Drug products that are considered to be therapeutically equivalent to other pharmaceutically equivalent products. "A" products are those for which actual or potential bioequivalence problems have been resolved with adequate in vivo and/or in vitro evidence supporting bioequivalence
AA	Drug products in conventional dosage forms not presenting bioequivalence problems
AB	Drug products meeting necessary bioequivalence requirements
AN	Solutions and powders for aerosolization
AO	Injectable oil solutions
AP	Injectable aqueous solutions and, in certain cases, intravenous non–aqueous solutions
AT	Topical products
B	Drug products that FDA, at this time, considers not to be therapeutically equivalent to other pharmaceutically equivalent products
B*	Drug products requiring further FDA investigation and review to determine therapeutic equivalence
BC	Extended-release dosage forms (capsules, injectables, and tablets)
BD	Active ingredients and dosage forms with documented bioequivalence problems
BE	Delayed-release oral dosage forms
BN	Products in aerosol-nebulizer drug delivery systems
BP	Active ingredients and dosage forms with potential bioequivalence problems
BR	Suppositories or enemas that deliver drugs for systemic absorption
BS	Products associated with drug standard deficiencies
BT	Topical drug products with bioequivalence issues
BX	Drug products for which the data are insufficient to determine therapeutic equivalence

Exclusivity prevents the submission or effective approval of ANDAs or applications described in Section 505(b)(2) of the Act.

Patents that are listed in the *Orange Book* include:

- Patents that claim the active ingredients or ingredients.
- Drug product patents which include formulation/composition patents.
- Use patents for a particular approved indication or method of using the product.

The *Bolar* amendment to the Drug Price Competition and Patent Term Restoration Act allows a pharmaceutical manufacturer (sponsor) to seek approval from FDA to market a generic drug before the expiration of a patent relating to the brand name drug upon which the generic is based.

As part of the ANDA, the sponsor must consider the pertinent patents and provide the results to the FDA. The Act requires patent information to be filed with all newly submitted Section 505 drug applications and that no NDA may be approved after September 24, 1984, without the submission of pertinent patent information to the FDA. The ANDA sponsor must provide a *certification* that, in the opinion of the sponsor and to the best of the sponsor's knowledge with respect to each patent that claims the listed drug, some or all of the following certification may be submitted:

Paragraph I: that such patent information has not been filed;
Paragraph II: that such patent has expired;
Paragraph III: of the date on which such patent will expire, or
Paragraph IV: that such patent is invalid or will not be infringed by the manufacture, use, or sale of the new drug for which the application is submitted.

A certification under Paragraph I or II permits the ANDA to be approved immediately, if it is otherwise eligible. A certification under Paragraph III indicates that the ANDA may be approved on the patent expiration date.

If the *Orange Book* lists one or more unexpired patents, the sponsor of the ANDA who seeks effective approval prior to the patent's expiration must either:

- Challenge the listing of the patent (e.g., file a Paragraph IV Certification that the patent is invalid or will not be infringed by the manufacture, use, or sale of the drug product).
- File a statement that the application for use is not claimed in the listed patent.

4.1. Exclusivity

The generic applicant must notify the patent holder of the submission of the ANDA. Since the patent holder can immediately sue the first generic sponsor company who submits an ANDA with a Paragraph IV statement, a 180-day period of market exclusivity is provided to that generic applicant. This special dispensation is considered as a reward to the generic manufacturer who took a risk in challenging the patent. If the patent holder files an infringement suit against the generic applicant within 45 days of the ANDA notification, FDA approval to market the generic drug is automatically postponed for 30 months, unless, before that time, the patent expires or is judged to be invalid or not infringed. This 30-month

TABLE 4 Types of Exclusivity

Exclusivity	Time for exclusivity	Exclusivity criteria
Orphan drug exclusivity (ODE)	7 years	Upon approval of designated orphan drug—Office of Orphan Products issues letter when exclusivity granted—separate from other types of exclusivity
New chemical entity (NCE)	5 years	Upon first time approval of new chemical entity
"Other" exclusivity	3 years for a "significant change" if criteria are met	For certain "significant changes" approved on an NDA or supplement if new clinical studies essential for approval, conducted or sponsored by applicant, have been done "Changes" may include (but are not limited to): new ester/salt, new dosage form, new route, new indication, new strength, new dosing schedule
Pediatric exclusivity (PED)	6 months added to existing patents or exclusivity	A period of 6 months' exclusivity is added to any existing exclusivity or patents on all applications held by the sponsor for that active moiety pediatric exclusivity does not stand alone

postponement gives the patent holder time to assert its patent rights in court before a generic competitor is permitted to enter the market. Only an application containing a Paragraph IV certification may be eligible for exclusivity, and to earn the period of exclusivity, the ANDA applicant must be sued by the patent holder and successfully defend the suit (see Chapter 14 for more details).

Under certain circumstances, the patent holder may obtain exclusivity for a branded drug product that essentially extends the time on the market without competition from the generic drug product. Exclusivity works similar to patents and is granted by the FDA if statutory provisions are met. Types of exclusivity are listed in Table 4.

5. RESOURCES FOR ANDA SUBMISSIONS

FDA's Center for Drug Evaluation and Research, CDER (http://www.fda.gov/cder/), and the Office of Generic Drugs, OGD (http://www.fda.gov/cder/ogd/), provide assistance to the sponsor of an ANDA to meet the legal and regulatory requirements of an application. FDA provides assistance through its website and publications, guidances, internal ANDA review principles, policies, and procedures.

5.1. Guidance Documents for ANDAs

Guidance documents represent the Agency's current thinking on a particular subject (http://www.fda.gov/cder/regulatory/default.htm). These documents are prepared for FDA review staff and applicants/sponsors to provide guidelines to the processing, content, and evaluation/approval of applications and also to the design, production, manufacturing, and testing of regulated products. They also establish policies intended to achieve consistency in the Agency's regulatory approach and establish inspection and enforcement procedures. Because guidances are not regulations or laws, they are not enforceable, either through administrative actions or through the courts. An alternative approach may be used if such an approach satisfies the requirements of the applicable statute, regulations, or both. The FDA has numerous guidances for industry that relate to ANDA content and format issues (11).

5.2. Manual of Policies and Procedures

Manuals of Policies and Procedures (MaPPs) provide official instructions for internal practices and procedures followed by CDER staff to help standardize the drug review process and other activities, both internal and external (12). MaPPs define external activities as well. All MAPPs are available for the public to review to get a better understanding of office policies, definitions, staff responsibilities, and procedures. MaPP documents to help prepare ANDAs are listed together on CDER's Manual of Policies and Procedures web page (http://www.fda.gov/cder/mapp.htm).

5.3. Freedom of Information (FOI)

The 1996 amendments to the Freedom of Information Act, FOIA, mandate publicly accessible "electronic reading rooms" with FDA FOIA response materials and other information routinely available to the public with electronic search and indexing features. Before submitting an FOIA request, the sponsor should check to see if the information is already available on FDA's website (http://www.fda.gov/foi/foia2.htm). There is a search engine to help find information (13).

5.4. Additional Resources Regarding Drug Development

FDA provides additional resources regarding drug development on its website: http://www.fda.gov/cder/ode4/preind/Gen_Additional_Resources.htm. These resources are summarized in Table 5.

5.5. Drug Master File

The Drug Master File (DMF) is a submission to the FDA that may be used to provide confidential detailed information about facilities, processes, or articles used in the manufacturing, processing, packaging, and storing of one or more human drug substances. The submission of a DMF is not required by law or FDA regulation. Further information regarding DMFs is available in the CDER Guidance Document on Drug Master Files or 21 CFR 314.420.

5.6. United States Pharmacopeia

The U.S. Pharmacopeia, USP (www.usp.org), promotes public health by establishing and disseminating officially recognized standards of quality and authoritative information for the use of medicines and other healthcare technologies by health professionals, patients, and consumers. USP works closely with the FDA, the pharmaceutical industry, and the health professions to establish authoritative drug standards. These standards are enforceable by the FDA and the governments of more than 35 other countries, and are recognized worldwide as a hallmark of quality. More than 3700 standards monographs are published in the USP and National Formula (NF), the official drug standards compendia. USP also provides more than

TABLE 5   General Information Regarding Drug Development

General FDA Information
Resources Within FDA
External Resources—General
External Resources—Education
Review Jurisdiction of Drug Product Classes within ODE IV
Items of General Interest
CDER Guidance Documents/MaPPs
Federal Register
Title 21 Code of Federal Regulations
FDA Forms Distribution Page
International Conference on Harmonisation Documents
IND/NDA Jackets/Submission Covers
Drug Master File (DMF) Information

1600 premier chemical Reference Standards to carry out the tests specified in USP–NF (14).

5.7. International Conference on Harmonisation

The International Conference on Harmonisation of Technical Requirements for Registration of Pharmaceuticals for Human Use (ICH) is composed of the regulatory authorities of Europe, Japan, and the United States and experts from the pharmaceutical industry in the three regions to discuss scientific and technical aspects of product registration (http://www.ifpma.org/ich1.html).

The purpose of ICH is to make recommendations on ways to achieve greater harmonisation in the interpretation and application of technical guidelines and requirements for product registration in order to reduce or obviate the need to duplicate the testing carried out during the research and development of new medicines. The objective of such harmonisation is a more economical use of human, animal, and material resources, and the elimination of unnecessary delay in the global development and availability of new medicines whilst maintaining safeguards on quality, safety, and efficacy, and regulatory obligations to protect public health (15).

6. SUMMARY

The market for generic drug products will increase rapidly in the next decade due to the expiration of patents and exclusivities for major brand name drug products and due to the demand by consumers and governments for less expensive generic alternatives. From a scientific perspective, generic drug product manufacturers must formulate a drug product that will have the same quality, therapeutic efficacy, safety, and performance as its brand name counterpart. Formulation development of an innovator drug product has minimal constraints with respect to choice of excipients, manufacturing methods, and performance characteristics. In contrast, generic drug manufacturers must demonstrate that their formulation is a pharmaceutical equivalent, is bioequivalent, and has the same quality and performance characteristics as the brand name counterpart. Moreover, the generic drug manufacturer will continue to face a variety of legal, regulatory, and patent challenges from the brand name pharmaceutical industry that may delay the entry of the generic drug in the marketplace. The availability of generic drug products will, nevertheless, continue to play an important role, both nationally and internationally, by providing cost-effective medicines to the wider public, which will bring great benefits to consumers as well as to health authorities in nations around the world in their quest to make medicines more available and affordable.

REFERENCES

1. The European Agency for the Evaluation of Medicinal Products Note for Guidance in the Investigation of Bioavailability and Bioequivalence (CPMP/EWP/QWP/1401/98). December 14, 2000. (http://www.emea/eu.int/pdfs/human/ewp/140198en.pdf).
2. United States Code of Federal Regulation (CFR) contains Food and Drug Regulations, 2003. (http://www.access.gpo.gov/). Bioavailability and Bioequivalence Requirements are in 21 CFR Part 320.
3. IMS Health Data. Wall Street Journal, February 21, 2003.
4. Maris DW, Vukhac K-L, Friedrich AM, Lohman DM. The Future of the Generic Industry, Specialty Pharmaceutical Industry Overview. New York, NY: Bank of America Securities, June 2003.
5. Kirking DM, Ascione FJ, Gaither CA, Welage LS. Economics and structure of the generic pharmaceutical industry. J Am Pharm Assoc (Wash) 2001; 41(4):578–584.
6. Federal Food, Drug, and Cosmetic Act., 2003. http://www.fda.gov/opacom/laws/fdcact/fdctoc.htm.
7. Parker RE, Martinez DR, and Covington, TR. Drug product selection—part 1: history and legal overview. American Pharmacy; NS 31, 72–7, (1991).
8. History of the Food and Drug Administration. Center for Drug Evaluation and Research., 2003. http://www.fda.gov/cder/about/history/.
9. Ascione FJ, Kirking DM, Gaither CA, Welage LS. Historical overview of generic medication policy. J Am Pharm Assoc (Wash) 2001; 41(4):567–577.
10. Approved Drug Products with Therapeutic Equivalence Evaluations, "Orange Book", 2003. http://www.fda.gov/cder/ob/default.htm.
11. FDA guidance documents, 2003. www.fda.gov/cder/guidance/index.htm.
12. FDA Center for Drug Evaluation and Research (CDER). Manual of Policies and Procedures, 2003. http://www.fda.gov/cder/mapp.htm.
13. FDA Freedom of Information, 2003. (http://www.fda.gov/foi/foia2.htm). Freedom of Information may be contacted at Freedom of Information Staff, 5600 Fishers Lane, Room 12A-30, Rockville, MD 20857, USA, and at Dockets Management Branch, 5630 Fishers Lane, Room 1061, Mail Stop HFA-305, Rockville, MD 20852, USA.
14. United States Pharmacopeia—National Formulary (USP). United States Pharmacopeia. Published annually, 2003. http://www.usp.org.
15. International Conference on Harmonisation, 2003. http://www.ifpma.org/ich1.html.

2

Active Pharmaceutical Ingredients

Edward M. Cohen[*]

Schein Pharmaceuticals, Danbury, Connecticut, U.S.A.

Lih-Yang Lin[†]

ScinoPharm Taiwan, Ltd., Tainan, Taiwan, R.O.C.

1. INTRODUCTION

Active Pharmaceutical Ingredients are also known in regulatory and pharmacopeial parlance as "Drug Substances". Additional terms frequently employed in commerce and the literature are Bulk Pharmaceutical Compound (BPC), Bulk Actives, and "active ingredient". All terms relate to the same "article". New chemical entities (NCE), also termed new molecular entities (NME) refer to drug substances that are first to enter the drug regulatory arena under the banner of a New Drug Application (NDA). The term "official substance"—"is defined in the USP as an active or inactive ingredient (frequently termed an excipient), a nutrient, a dietary supplement ingredient, and/or a pharmaceutical ingredient, or a component of an official device" (1). Official substances are the subject of formal monographs in the USP or NF. Drug substance (API) monographs grace the USP exclusively. The other official articles noted are in other sections of the compendia. Not surprisingly, the end use of the API is to produce a drug product, which

[*]*Current affiliation*: EMC Consulting Services, Newtown, Connecticut, U.S.A.

[†]Deceased

is the final form of the drug substance administered to patients. Drug products are the subjects of companion monographs in the USP. The ultimate safety and efficacy of the finally administered drug product are dependent on the assurance of the consistency of the physical and chemical properties of the API. This chapter will focus on the plethora of issues involved with the API, which must be considered when developing a generic drug product. In particular, the point of establishing specifications for critical quality attributes of the API that will assure that the generic drug product, employing the API material, will have consistent in vitro/in vivo characteristics, batch after batch. As part of the routine evaluation of the compendial status of an API, in addition to the USP, the EP, JP, BP, IP, and other "recognized" compendia should be checked to verify the presence or absence of published "official monographs" for the API.

A recently published overview of the regulatory oversight for both drug substances and drug products provides an excellent starting point for the particular issues that a firm faces when attempting to file an ANDA for an API (2). The reference provides detailed accounting of all relevant Food and Drug Administration (FDA) documents and guidances covering the areas of concern. Finally, this chapter will not cover ex-USA regulatory issues concerning APIs.

2. SOURCES OF ACTIVE PHARMACEUTICAL INGREDIENTS

The three most commonly recognized categories of APIs are synthetic, semi-synthetic, and natural. The latter category, natural, refers to the source of the API as being derived directly or extracted from natural sources. The category of semi-synthetic indicates that a starting "intermediate" for the preparation of the API was derived from natural sources. The "isolated" intermediate is then converted synthetically to the final API. Synthetic APIs are obtained directly by chemical conversion of intermediates. It is not uncommon to see the market introduction of an API pioneer compound as a natural product, which is subsequently produced by a semi-synthetic procedure. A recent example of the transitioning of an important API from "natural sourcing" initially to semi-synthetic sourcing is paclitaxel (3,4). In the arena of synthetic APIs, the transitioning that frequently occurs is that the initial drug product launch by the pioneer drug firm employed the API produced by a defined synthetic process. Subsequently, the pioneer product producer changes the API synthetic process. There is no requirement that the specific synthetic pathway be identified for the API as the product matures in the marketplace.

Recently, the USP has classified a category of drug substances as "complex actives" (5). This grouping of compounds includes biological and biotechnological drug substances, complex natural source drug substances. The traditional APIs are referred to as "Non-Complex Actives" (6).

This chapter will only focus on non-complex actives.

3. PATENT RESTRICTIONS AND EXCLUSIVITY GRANTED TO AN NDA SPONSOR

The filing of an NDA with the FDA for a drug product made with a NCE results in the listing of "relevant" patents and periods of "Exclusivity" for the approved drug product (frequently identified as the "listed drug") . This listing occurs in the FDA "Approved Drug Products with Therapeutic Equivalence Evaluations", and is referred to as the "Orange Book". The FDA now provides all of this information online at their website (fda.gov/cder). For an API supplier, the listed patents in the electronic Orange Book normally provides only those patents, which protect the NCE (compound and method of use) as well as formulation patents (presumably those relevant to the filed drug product) . Current issues concerning the listing of patents in the Orange Book are covered in Chapters 1 and 14 of this book. What is not a required listing in the Orange Book are process patents for the manufacture of the API or critical intermediates for the API, beyond the original patent(s) governing the NCE itself. This point is covered by a section of the Food Drug and Cosmetic Act, which authorizes an API supplier or an authorized party/agent for the API supplier to write to an NDA sponsor and request a listing of all relevant process patents which cover the filed NCE (7). This is a fee for service request, with a maximum allowed charge of $500 for the service. The relevant USC information concerning patent infringements and penalties for infringement cited in Ref. (7) can be found on the internet website for the USC.

With this list of process patents, the API supplier must now review all patents cited, as well as to conduct independent patent searches for all patents relevant to the NCE, which issued or were applied for in and outside the United States. This search should include not just the NDA sponsor but also any issued patent concerning the drug substance or any pivotal intermediate involved in the synthesis of the final drug substance. Specific aspects of the NCE that may be covered by process patents, and other non-listed patents in the Orange Book include particle size/surface area, morphic forms (polymorphs, hydrates, solvates), and impurity/purity characteristics. The objective of the patent search is to determine what synthetic route to exploit for the manufacture of the target API, which will be non-infringing, cost effective, and will yield finished API of appropriate quality and physical attributes suitable for formulation of the material into the targeted drug product for filing an Abbreviated New Drug Application (ANDA).

Finally, with respect to "Exclusivity" for the filing of an NDA, incorporating an NCE, the current regulations allow for a 5-year period of exclusivity before an ANDA can be filed incorporating the same API as the NCE. A different period of exclusivity is provided for the filing of formal supplements to NDAs, which is based on providing clinical data as part of the supplement. These points are covered in detail in Chapters 1 and 14.

4. COMPARISON WITH INNOVATOR API

The challenge that the API supplier/manufacturer faces in entering the market place is to assure the user of the material that the API will be comparable to the innovator or pioneer drug substance, which is employed in an approved NDA drug product. Current FDA requirements regarding the filing of an ANDA for a single component listed drug product is that the API must be the same chemical entity, which is contained, in the listed drug. The critical aspects of sameness or comparability for the "generic" API vs. the innovator API include three critical realms:

4.1. Chemical Structure

Same chemical entity including;

> salt or free base/acid form,
> isomeric composition,
> hydrate, solvate, or polymorphic form (see section below on Physical
>   Form for more details about the allowed latitude for variances).

4.2. Impurity Profile

Establish the total impurity profile for replicate batches of the final process material.

> identified as well as unidentified impurities,
> determine if there are impurities in the generic API, which are not present in the innovator API, and the relative level of such impurities.

The FDA Guidance, "ANDAs: Impurities in Drug Substances": Issued November 1999 (8), is the current benchmark for categorizing, quantifying, specifying, qualifying, and reporting on impurities in generic APIs. There is a very detailed "Impurities Decision Tree" in the guidance, which needs to be reviewed in depth when an issue arises about unknown impurities, or impurities whose safety profile cannot be gleaned from the literature and, more importantly, that impurity does not appear to be present in the innovator drug substance. Based on the Guidance above, the critical aspect of dealing with "impurities", which includes Organic Impurities (Process and Drug Related), Inorganic Impurities, and Residual Solvents, appears to focus on the issue of relating the levels found in the API to established pharmacopoeial standards or known safety data. A critical cut-off point for the organic impurities appears to be a level of 0.1 %. The API manufacturer is encouraged to try and reduce the level of detected, individual impurities to levels of less than 0.1 %. As far as impurity specifications are concerned, the issue is to have in place validated assay procedures than can assure a level of detection and a level of quantitation for all impurities. Maintaining individual impurities below 0.1 % and assuring that the total of all specified and unspecified, identified and unidentified impurities at a level of 1 % is likely to satisfy FDA concerns about the impurity profile for an API. On an individual basis, levels can be specified for individual impurities based on the process chemistry and stability history for the drug substance. The specification level has to meet benchmark issues of safety for use in the finished dosage form. The "ANDAs: Impurities in Drug Substances" guidance noted above goes into great detail about qualifying impurities and developing specifications for the impurities in APIs. Finally, the FDA advises in the Guidance (see Section L3b) that one should compare the impurity profile of the generic drug substance with the process impurity profiles found in the innovator's marketed drug product (looking at three or more different lots of the innovator's product). A final comment about this point is that today's innovator product may be made with the drug substance synthesized by a different process than the originally launched innovator product. The generic API may be synthesized with an expired patented process of the innovator resulting in an impurity profile which may be different from that found in today's innovator drug product. There is no benchmark "fingerprint" of the original innovator drug substance to make any comparisons of the original impurity profile with the current impurity profile of the innovator. An interesting issue is that if there was a USP monograph for the "innovator drug in place, prior to the point in time of submitting an ANDA for the drug product, a public standard would be available to establish "objective" boundaries for critical quality attributes for the drug substance". Subsequent changes in the pioneer impurity profile might require update of the USP monograph. However, the initial impurity profile testing requirements were presumably part of the original USP monograph testing requirements, and as such would still be available for comparative testing. Today's newer analytical technologies such as Near IR will permit more incisive analysis of the innovator drug product so that even in the absence of a USP monograph, the ability to carry out a fingerprint of the innovator product (search for the impurity profile of the drug substance therein) is within technical boundaries for getting reliable information.

4.3. Physical Form

Another critical aspect of the API comparability to the innovator API is the physical form. This generally falls in the domain of the "morphic form" including particle size distribution. The term "morphic form" includes variances in crystal form (amorphous vs. crystalline), polymorphism, solvates, and hydrates. Current precedents indicate that variants of the morphic form of the pioneer NCE can be incorporated into ANDAs, if the ultimate test for demonstration of the bioequivalence of the ANDA drug product to the pioneer listed drug product is successful.

Related aspects of the physical form of the API, such as particle size distribution, are important with respect to the in vitro dissolution performance of the finished dosage form. As noted above, the final dosage form developed by the ANDA sponsor must meet the FDA Office of Generic Drugs benchmark of "bioequivalence", which frequently is related to the in vitro dissolution performance of the dosage form. Thus, the physical form characteristics of the API discussed need to be controlled such that once bioequivalence is demonstrated vs. the innovator product, subsequent batches of the API will provide the same performance characteristics to the final dosage form.

Developing final specifications for the API is based on establishing the desired chemical and physical profile of the API. The API suppliers frequently develop particle size "grades" for individual customers of the same API. It is very important to have similar, preferably identical, test methods at the API source and the API user laboratory to avoid any confusing test results over time. An interesting practice that can serve the purpose of confirming the consistency of the physical form of the API is to employ optical microscopy as a routine inspectional test for individual batches of the API. The key in such a test is to assure that representative samples of the API batch must be examined in using the test to confirm the comparability of the product, batch after batch.

5. SPECIFICATIONS

The specifications developed for a new generic API must meet all USP monograph requirements, if an USP monograph exists for the API, as well as to satisfy all the current FDA/ICH guidance's concerning impurities, residual solvents, and other specified attributes. The scope of specifications for an API will typically include:

Identity testing

> active moiety (IR preferred as well as specific chromatographic procedures),
> identification of specific counter ions if API is a salt.

Impurity testing (includes degradants formed post-manufacture of the material)

> specified identified and specified but unidentified,
> individual and total,
> residual solvents (including USP organic volatile impurities),
> heavy metals and/or other specific elements.

Other specified tests

> morphic form including particle size,
> others (such as water, pH, assay)

The USP has recently posted on its website a guideline for describing the content of a typical USP monograph. The terminology in the guideline is consistent with all current ICH practices and descriptors (9).

All test procedures should be validated in accordance with standard practices. It is important to note that in the absence of any waiver, all specifications must be met through the designated shelf life or expiry dating or re-test date for the material. Part of the development of final specifications are the conduct of stability studies for the material in the final container closure system in which the material is sold to the API consumer. An important part of the API process is to establish user friendly "Certificates of Analysis". To the extent possible, all test results should be reported with actual findings and not left to the end point of "Complies". The test method employed should be easily identified if compendial methods are used, that is, specify the exact test method used. A critical factor in developing specifications is to have available well-defined reference standards for all tests that require a standard. In the absence of a USP monograph (or any other major compendia, such as the EP, BP, JP), which typically defines which tests need a reference standard, the API supplier needs to follow established practices to develop and provide to the drug product developer/manufacturer appropriate reference standards for the conduct of those tests requiring such standards.

6. DRUG MASTER FILE (DMF)

"A Drug Master File (DMF) " is a submission to the FDA that may be used to provide confidential detailed information about facilities, processes, or articles used in the manufacturing, processing, packaging, and storage of one or more human drugs. See the FDA website, http://www.fda.gov/cder/guidance/dmf.htm for full details. Upon submission of a complete DMF, the FDA assigns a number to the DMF. The number entry becomes part of the DMF database.

One can search the DMF database and obtain information such as the name of the article included in the DMF, the name and address of the sponsor or holder of the DMF and date of original submission. The filed DMF is typically used in the generic drug environment to support the filing of an ANDA. A DMF holder provides letters of authorization to the FDA and the ANDA sponsor indicating that the FDA can refer to information in the DMF to support the filed ANDA, which utilizes the API for the drug product, which is the subject of the filed ANDA. There are five types of DMF's. The Type II DMF is limited to the Drug Substance or Drug Substance Intermediate and the materials used in their preparation. A drug product can also be the subject of a Type II DMF. The FDA does not approve DMFs, but can question the content and hold up a filed ANDA, which employs the particular API, which is the subject of the DMF, until satisfactory responses are received. The DMF sponsor is required to update the filed DMF annually with information concerning any changes that were made in the manufacturing or controls employed for the production of the API, including specifications and test methods. As part of the procedure and practice of making any changes to a filed DMF for an API, the DMF holder is requested to notify all "customers" who purchase that API, and who have referenced the particular DMF in their ANDA, of such changes. The ANDA holder then is obligated to incorporate the information into its filed ANDA. Such incorporation may range from including the information in the Annual Report for the ANDA, file a Supplementary Changes Being Effected Supplement to the filed ANDA (CBE), or file a Prior Approval Supplement (PAS) with the FDA for the filed ANDA.

An important aspect of developing APIs is to have a complete understanding of the chemical class of the drug substance being produced and identifying at an early stage what special handling issues may be needed for the particular API at issue. These include APIs in the category of controlled substances (follow mandates and dictates of the Drug Enforcement Agency (DEA) for control and containment). Additional categories requiring special considerations are certain types of hormonal products and cytotoxic compounds. These handling precautions normally would get entered into batch manufacturing records, Material Safety Data Sheets (MSDSs), and on Analytical Test Methods. The required handling precautions should follow the trail of movement of the API all the way to the final user. There are a number of websites, including the USP where MSDSs can be reviewed for the terminology and handling precautions cited for compounds in all risk categories. An interesting approach is to "browse" the USP where a large number of monographs, both for the API and dosage forms, contain cautionary statements. The need for cautionary statements really falls into three sectors at the dosage form development site:

laboratory and quality assurance personnel who handle the compound for "testing";

drug product development personnel;

finished dosage form manufacturing, quality control, stability testing personnel.

Finally, there are consulting services that can provide counsel on environmental handling issues for the API and the drug product incorporating the API related to OSHA, EPA, and cleaning validation.

7. REGULATORY OVERSIGHT OF API MANUFACTURERS

For a new manufacturer or a new API manufactured at an established site previously registered in filed DMFs, the FDA normally requires that a successful pre-approval inspection occurs before the agency would grant approval to the filed ANDA, which incorporated the particular API. Typically, such inspections tend to be vigorous and cover both cGMP as well as scientific, technological, and related matters such as environmental, OSHA, compliance with DOT, and the like. A very detailed FDA guidance has been issued regarding "Good Manufacturing Practice Guidance for Active Pharmaceutical Ingredients (Q7A, August 2001)". This guidance covers every aspect of the API manufacturing operation, from start to finish, including documentation at all stages as well as distribution and recalls.

8. BACPAC (BULK ACTIVE CHEMICAL, POST APPROVAL CHANGES)

BACPAC I: Intermediates in Drug Substance Synthesis Formal Guidance, current update is February 2001

BACPAC II: Final Intermediate to Drug Substance PQRI final draft, representing consensual industry input will be provided to FDA for crafting a "Draft Guidance".

The BACPAC guidances concern post-approval changes to the API or bulk active ingredient, divided into the two sectors noted above. The information pools in the guidances cover all aspects of the API process ranging from manufacturing, ingredient sourcing, site changes, specifications, and test methods. In reviewing the guidance content, the two focal points that emerge are what impact does the change or changes have on the impurity profile and physical properties of the material as it relates to the end use of the API final intermediate or the final API. As far as the API manufacturer is concerned, any change will become incorporated into the Annual DMF report. With respect to the user of the API, the issue is how to report certain types of changes (Annual Report, Supplement Changes Being Effected, or a Prior Approval Supplement). As previously noted, the DMF holder has a legal obligation to notify an ANDA sponsor of changes that have been implemented in the "manufacture, processing, or controls of the API".

The critical point in the BACPAC guidance is that the API manufacturer is expected to obtain comparison data of the material, which underwent the change with the prior process material. Typically, a comparison of the pre- and post-material at the level of multiple batches is requested (10). Both the API-DMF holder and the ANDA holders need to have clear consensual views of what changes have been made and how to deal with the changes in a very consistent manner. The BACPAC concept came at the heels of the SUPAC concept for the finished dosage form. The simple fact is that some changes can be made, and based on the comparison data, may fall into the category of Annual Report in today's climate. This is a saving of time, energy, and resources for all parties concerned; DMF Holder, Approved ANDA holder, and the FDA.

9. TECHNICAL PARTNERSHIP BETWEEN THE API MANUFACTURER AND THE DRUG PRODUCT MANUFACTURER

A strong interactive working relationship between the API source and the API consumer is important to assure that there is harmony and consensus in the filing of ANDA specifications for the drug substance with the filed DMF of the API supplier. This relates in particular to specifications and test methods. The auditing of the API source by the API consumer should be based on mutual respect and understanding of differences. Such a relationship will lead to timely resolution of technical issues. Further with the implementation of BACPAC I and BACPAC II, it is even more critical that each side understand the issues and practices of the other side. An initial site audit of an API supplier is common practice when working with a new source of an API. This audit should be followed up on some periodic basis, particularly if some issues were discovered during the initial audit. As the FDA inspectional history for an API supplier evolves, some determination can be made about the need and frequency for follow-up audits.

10. IDENTIFYING AND QUALIFYING API SOURCES

The DMF track record and FDA inspectional history are typically a starting point for establishing the qualifications for an API source. As previously noted one can go online to the FDA web site for a listing of all DMFs for a particular API. The FDA inspectional history can be obtained under Freedom of Information from various search engine services for any given API manufacturer. One needs to know the particular site of manufacture for the API supplier for the particular API of interest, if the API manufacturer has multiple sites. The FDA inspectional history includes FDA "483s" and "EIRs". The FDA "483" is the inspection report listing "observations" issued to a firm immediately following a site inspection. The FDA "EIR" (Establishment Inspection Report) is the FDA's internal report about the inspection findings. For both types of documents, the FDA dockets management branch issues "purged" documents which excludes certain "confidential information".

A number of search engine services can provide detailed information about current manufacturers/marketers of specific APIs. The input requirements to get the search started are the CAS number, and any recognized/official names for the API. By pooling the information from the DMF database, FDA inspectional history, listings of identified suppliers (which often includes some marketing statistics for the firm and API), one can very quickly identify the pool of suppliers for just about any API. Following the identification of a primary source for an API, it is often common practice to establish alternate sources in case of an unexpected event, which might block the primary source from serving the needs of the ANDA drug product developer.

A critical factor in moving ahead with an alternate source of the raw material (frequently referred to as "ASRM") is to have established and well-defined specifications for all critical quality control attributes to minimize any adverse effect on the ANDA drug product formulation and manufacturing process. These specifications are provided to the potential ASRM and based on the response information provided, as well as the evaluation of samples of the API can provide the basis for determining whether the ASRM material will fit the "boundaries for the filed ANDA". Here the issue of comparability, previously discussed in the context of the primary source of the API vs. the "innovator" now becomes the comparability of the primary API source vs. the ASRM (10). The timing to complete the qualification of an ASRM typically can vary from 6 months to 12 months, if the testing includes manufacture and accelerated stability studies of test batches of the drug product. The completion of qualification would then be followed by filing an amendment to the filed ANDA.

A frequent issue for identifying an API source for an NCE is that at the early stages of the NCE history, there may not be any listed source for the API. Further, there may not be any solicitation for the compound. Here, the best approach is to understand the chemistry of the NCE and identify API sources that have been involved with that chemistry before. Alternatively, look for API sources that typically stay on the forefront of NCEs. A strategy that may be worth pursuing is to start the API sourcing process immediately after an NCE enters the marketplace, and when it is clear that the NCE will achieve an attractive market share.

11. CONCLUSION

The successful development of a generic drug product starts with the API. It is critical to understand the basic science underlying the targeted listed drug API as well as the intellectual property which "limits" the horizons for the synthesis and specifications for the generic API. Further, companion challenges that confront both the API supplier, and the generic drug product developer, are the evolving milieu of regulatory and compendial forces that provide acceptance boundaries for the purity, safety, efficacy for the API. Additionally, the regulatory milieu covering cGMP, including manual and electronic documentation, must be respected and enforced at both the site of production of the API and at the site of manufacture of the final dosage form targeted for marketing. On a going forward basis, the API supplier will be held accountable for the consistency of the chemical and physical properties of the material being produced on a routine basis. Good science and mutual respect for the technical issues must prevail in the relationship between the API manufacturer and generic drug product developer to assure the continued production of generic drug product which stays within the performance boundaries of the originally filed exhibit batch(s) in the filed ANDA.

REFERENCES

1. "Official and Official Articles", USP 26-NF 21, United States Pharmacopeial Convention Inc., Rockville, MD, 2003: 3.
2. Sheinin E, Williams R. Chemistry, manufacturing, and controls information in NDAs and ANDAs supplements, annual reports, and other regulatory filings. Pharm Res 2002; 19(3):217–226.
3. Montvale NJ, ed. "Taxol"[R], Physicians' Desk Reference. 48th ed. 1994: p.670.
4. Montvale NJ, ed. "Taxol"[R], Physicians' Desk Reference. 56th ed. 2002: p.1130.
5. USP 26-NF 21. 2003: p. xiv.
6. USP 26-NF 21. 2003: p. xvii.
7. US Code of Federal Regulations, Title 35, Part III, Chapter 28, Section 271(g); US Code of Federal Regulations, Title 35, Part III, Chapter 29, Section 287(b)(3)(6).
8. FDA CDER Guidance's for Industry can be found on the FDA CDER website. Key FDA Guidances include: ANDAs: Impurities in Drug Substances, November 1999, Q3C Impurities: Residual Solvents, December 1997, NDAs: Impurities in Drug Substances, February 2000, BACPAC I: Intermediates

in Drug Substance Synthesis/Bulk Actives, Post Approval Changes, CMC, February 2001, BACPAC II: Drug Substance Synthesis/Bulk Actives, Post Approval, Changes, CMC, PQRI Draft For Submission to FDA, November 2003, Q7A Good Manufacturing Practice Guidance for Active Pharmaceutical Ingredients, August 2001.

9. USP Guideline For Submitting Requests for Revision to the USP-NF (www.usp.org).

10. FDA Draft Guidance. Comparability Protocols—Chemistry, Manufacturing, and Controls Information. February 2003.

3

Analytical Methods Development and Methods Validation for Solid Oral Dosage Forms

Quanyin Gao and Dilip R. Sanvordeker
Watson Laboratories, Inc., Corona, California, U.S.A.

Robert Vita
Gram Laboratories, Inc., Costa Mesa, California, U.S.A.

1. INTRODUCTION

Development of oral pharmaceutical drug products presents many technical and regulatory challenges. Specifically, these include proper characterization of active pharmaceutical ingredient (API), assurance of compatibility of inactive ingredients with the active components over the shelf life of the product, processing and manufacturing and quality controls and compliance with current federal regulations and draft Federal Regulations under the CFR provisions for comments and approval process at the Food and Drug Administration.

Current Federal Regulations mandate that any generic drug product intended for human use must be approved by the Agency for marketing a generic drug product and its multi-strengths in the United States. These current Federal Regulations provide assurances to the consumer that these generic drug products are safe, therapeutically equivalent and effective in the same manner as the innovator or branded drug products approved previously as

New Drug Applications (NDAs) by the Food and Drug Administration. Additionally, the quality control information presented by a generic product manufacturer or sponsor in the Abbreviated New Drug Applications (ANDAs) documents the evidence that the API used in the dosage form— may it be a parenteral, oral solid dosage, topical, implant, or a specialized delivery system form—is rigorously tested to comply with the regulatory mandates of acceptable limits of compendial or regulatory specifications mutually agreed upon by the sponsor and the Office of Generic Drugs Division of the Food and Drug Administration. The reader is referred to numerous Current Federal Regulations and Guidance issues on this topic (1–8).

1.2. Method Development and its Importance

Development of a generic drug product begins with full analytical testing and reproducible characterization of the API for which there is a Drug Master File (DMF) registered with the Agency. The DMF provided by the API manufacturer contains details of the synthetic process, assurance of cGMP compliance, and information on the drug substance form and purity, along with identity of impurities listed in the API specifications.

Analytical method development and its validation play a very vital role in this process of API selection for generic dosage form development.

Typically, the analytical chemist utilizes numerous literature sources such as Summary of Basis of Approval (SBA) for the innovator drug product NDA and technical literature in numerous medicinal chemistry and analytical chemistry journals, as well as Internet web sites dedicated to publication of original articles on pharmaceutical entities and pharmaceutical drug product development. Frequently, the API supplier provides a starting point for a review of Material Safety Data Sheet (MSDS), a current analytical method used by the API manufacturer, such as an HPLC method to identify and quantify the active drug and presence of known and unknown impurities. This helps the method development chemist to get a head start in completion of preliminary method development work and establish preliminary API specifications for release of the API and support the formulation pharmacist in developing the dosage form for an ANDA filing.

Once the API method is developed, the analytical chemist can begin the method development for the dosage form. Typically, placebos of dosage forms such as tablets or capsules are utilized to assure that the inactive ingredients do not interfere in the process of a specific method in development for the drug. Establishment of method specificity, sensitivity, linearity, reproducibility, precision, and accuracy for quantification of the drug in a dosage form is pursued to assure that the method can be used for evaluation of dosage form stability and in vitro performance by such methods as dissolution profiles in physiological pH media. More frequently, specific methods for detection and quantification of trace amounts of impurities are developed to assure that the product complies with compendial (USP, BP, EP, etc.) or non-compendial specifications for organic and inorganic impurities to assure proper identity, purity, and safety of the drug product during the product shelf life, typically a minimum of two years from the date of its manufacture.

While scale-up of the new generic oral dosage form in one or more strengths is ongoing to prepare clinical supplies for pilot bioequivalence studies, in-process testing and methods for such testing are developed to assure proper control of the process and the quality of the drug product. Generally, test methods for finished dosage forms are stability indicating and the information generated from accelerated stability test results of the drug product in the final packaging intended for commercialization are used by the product development team of scientists and regulatory staff to determine the drug product specifications not specified by the compendia. The prime objective of the analytical chemist is to assure that the generic drug product in a final commercial packaging is in compliance with compendial standards of identity, potency, content uniformity, dissolution, and acceptable limits on impurities and related substances.

In this chapter, we have placed a strong emphasis on the importance of robust method development, in-process control methods, and validation approaches taken to finalize such methodologies for development. Also emphasized is the importance of documentation of dissolution and finished drug product specifications for the API and the drug product for submission in the Chemistry, Manufacturing, and Controls (CMC) sections of the ANDA. The reader is referred to several literature sources and CDER Guidances available on this topic (2–8).

2. METHOD DEVELOPMENT

Analytical test methods are used to generate data to establish the identity, potency, purity, and overall quality of the drug substance and drug product. A well-developed test method can control not only the quality of the product but also speed the development process by shortening the development time for raw material vendor selection, qualification and formulation screening. Further, a well-developed test method can enhance the efficiency for the down stream product launch and routine release tests. Analytical test methods are the stakeholders of product development by providing accurate and reliable data to support formulation, packaging, process development, characterization and process controls, stability and release, pharmacokinetics and bioequivalency, and regulatory filing.

The time and effort spent in developing a good test method are well worth it for the down stream method users such as laboratory technicians and chemists in the QC labs of the generic drug manufacturer. A test method with shorter run time and less use of solvents can save much labor and cost for the QC labs for years of future production.

The performance of a test method is determined primarily by the quality of the procedure itself. Timing is critical for method development since first to approve means substantially high profit vs. the latecomers.

Before developing a test method, one must a priori define the scope and requirements for the test method. The objectives for the test method will ultimately define the extent of the development and optimization. The requirements for the test method include the following issues to be addressed: (1) regulatory compliance; (2) technical requirements; (3) practical requirements; (4) validation requirements; (5) transfer requirements. Once these requirements have been addressed, the method development can start with a literature search and information gathering. A plan can be developed with clear objectives for the method, such as requirements for the separation of known compounds, chromatographic procedures, and a targeted timeline. Adequate resources should be allocated for method development prior to initiating the bench-work. Typical sample solution and standard solution can be used to evaluate different chromatographic conditions. It is suggested that one should fully utilize the ICH guidelines (9–11) regarding the reporting threshold, identification threshold, and qualification threshold. The ICH defined residual solvent classes and allowable limits can be used for method development and release specification. When the main objectives are met, the test method can be further optimized to make it more economical and user friendly. Once the optimization is completed, the method is challenged to see if it can be validated. For chromatographic procedures, the challenges are often method sensitivity and method selectivity. These method pre-validation evaluations can determine if the method is ready for validation.

The following are the commonly needed test methods in the development and manufacturing of generic pharmaceutical solid oral dosage forms.

2.1. API Test Methods

The objectives for the development of the API test methods are for raw material vendor selection and raw material release. Where multiple vendors of an API are available, test methods are needed to characterize each lot of API and evaluate the raw material quality. The quality and characteristics of the APIs can often influence the formulation development concerning the dissolution profile and stability of the final dosage form in development.

Typical test methods for the API release include identification, assay, chromatographic purity, organic volatile impurities, residual solvents, particle size measurement, and polymorph determination in addition to commonly required compendial tests such as water content (loss on drying or Karl Fisher test), residue on ignition, melting point and range, specific rotation, crystallinity, heavy metals, pH, sulfide, etc.

Very often, the assay and chromatographic purity tests are conducted using HPLC procedures. Most of these HPLC procedures are based on reversed phase chromatography. The knowledge, skill, and experience of the method developer in chromatography are critical for developing an accurate, precise, specific, rugged and robust test method with good linearity and range. The development of a chromatographic purity test method is often more challenging than the assay, since it is necessary to have the desired selectivity and sensitivity for separating all impurities at about 0.05% level. In particular, separating structurally similar isomers of the actives such as double bond shifts on a carbon ring structure or optical isomers (chiral molecules) poses challenges for the method developer. Figure 1 is a typical chromatogram for the chromatographic purity test of a pharmaceutical raw material.

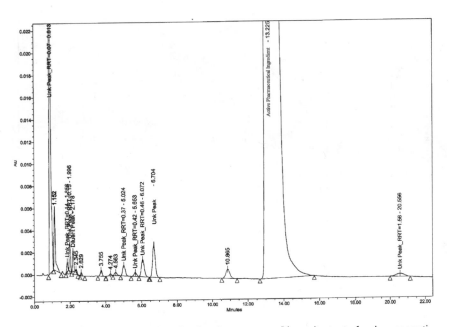

FIGURE 1   Typical chromatogram for the chromatographic purity test of a pharmaceutical raw material.

Sometimes, semi-quantitative TLC test methods are needed for testing of impurities in the API. The development of such test methods requires the selection of the appropriate TLC plate and optimization of the developing solvents. Due to the semi-quantitative nature of the TLC test method, an HPLC method is often used to quantitate the impurities.

The residual solvent test methods are often based on gas chromatography (12). Either headspace or direct injection mode can be used for the residual solvent test method. Since gas chromatography is a very mature field, separating residual solvents can often be resolved with limited development time due to the high selectivity of the modern capillary GC columns. Often, it is desirable to find a GC compatible solvent that can dissolve both the API and the target analytes of the residual solvents. Figure 2 is a typical headspace residual solvent test method where commonly used organic solvents are fully separated by gas chromatography.

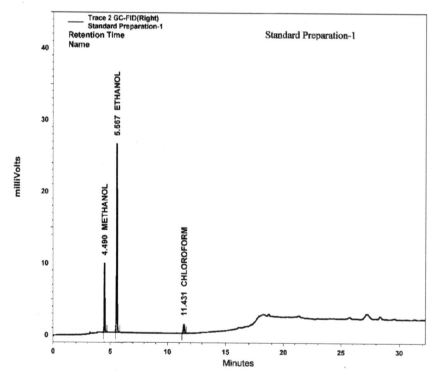

FIGURE 2   Typical headspace residual solvent test method chromatogram.

2.1.1. In-Process Test Methods

The objective of an in-process test method for oral solid dosage forms is to obtain information in order to control the pharmaceutical manufacturing process. Typical in-process test methods include loss on drying or use of Karl Fischer for water determination (to control the moisture content in the drying process), residual solvent (to control the residual solvent in the blend granules), and blend uniformity testing. The loss on drying (or Karl Fisher) test method is straightforward and usually does not require method development. The residual solvent test method and blend uniformity test method would require method development. Often, the blend uniformity (for granules), content uniformity (for finished dosage form), and assay (finished dosage form) share the same chromatographic conditions with separate sample preparation procedures. Therefore, method development is often conducted concurrently for these three tests (assay, content uniformity, and blend uniformity).

2.2. Finished Dosage Form Test Methods

The objectives for the development of the finished solid oral dosage form test methods include formulation identity, in vitro dissolution screening for acceptable performance within tolerance limits, and dosage form release. Very often, the dissolution test method is needed first for the in vitro characterization of the innovator's reference product vs. the in-house formulation. The screening dissolution test method is not necessarily the same as the dissolution test method for product release. The in vitro dissolution test method needs to be discriminative for different formulations and yet meet compendial requirements (13) for U.S.P./NF listed dosage forms. In particular, the selection of the dissolution medium and test conditions such as the type of apparatus and the rotational speed of either the paddle or the basket are critical for the success of the test method.

For a stable solid oral dosage form development, matching the in vitro dissolution profile with the innovator's or reference product is often the main concern for the formulator. Formulation support activity is then focused on the dissolution tests. When dosage form stability is also a concern for drug product development, assay and chromatographic purity test methods are often needed in addition to the dissolution test method. When possible, the use of the same chromatographic conditions for the assay and chromatographic purity tests can often save method development and method validation time.

Typical test methods for finished dosage forms include identification, assay, content uniformity, chromatographic purity, dissolution/

disintegration, and hardness/friability. Additional test methods needed to support the product development are cleaning test methods for the equipment release, confirmation methods for the absence of actives in the placebo tablets, etc.

Method development has the following deliverables:

1. Specificity, i.e., the method has to be able to separate the target analyte from other components and the method can quantitate this analyte without ambiguity.
2. Linearity, i.e., the method should operate in the linear response range of the detector. Although, linearity is usually obtainable, occasionally the linearity cannot be met due to the nature of the detector used. In such cases, a multiple-point calibration curve should be established and used for quantitation.
3. The method is optimized, i.e., the analyte can be fully extracted from the sample matrix, and the separation conditions are optimal.
4. Sensitivity, i.e., the test method can quantitate the target analyte at the required reporting threshold.
5. System suitability, i.e., all target analytes can be resolved, the requirements for the column performance is well-established, the instrument characteristics such as sensitivity and precision are established, and system reproducibility is established.

High performance liquid chromatography (HPLC) is commonly used for the assay and chromatographic purity determinations, since HPLC test methods can provide required accuracy, precision, linearity, sensitivity, ruggedness, and robustness. Many references have been published for HPLC method development and validation (14–18). The method development should consider the choice of columns for normal phase, reverse phase, or ion chromatography. The mobile phase selection and operational conditions should be optimized through the method development such as flow rate, column temperature, pH buffer, and use of ion-pairing agent. The detector used should have adequate sensitivity and dynamic response range. Where possible, an isocratic elution mode is preferred to a gradient elution mode.

The sample preparation, seemingly simple but very critical, is usually the first step of a test method. The solvent used for the extraction of target analytes should be studied to obtain the maximum performance. Without adequate extraction, it does not matter how good a chromatographic procedure is, the method would not be able to deliver reliable results.

For chromatographic purity methods, obtaining the required sensitivity and selectivity of the method is usually a challenge. The quantitation limit should guarantee that the test method can quantify components at the required reporting threshold concentration level. When the product strength is low, the method sensitivity will become more critical and challenging for method development. Hormonal oral solid dosage forms, such as oral contraceptives, is one of the examples of a low strength drug product. The strength of these products can be as low as a few micrograms per tablet. The test method should also have adequate specificity, particularly for stability-indicating capability. Forced degradation studies under thermal, acid, base, oxidation, and photo-degradation conditions should be conducted to verify that the test method can reliably quantify degradation products. Typical experimental conditions for the forced degradation studies are: storing solutions in a UV chamber, adding equal volume of 1 M phosphoric acid or HCl aq., adding 0.5 M sodium hydroxide solution, adding 2% hydrogen peroxide, or water, and heating to about 100°C for about 15 h. The recommended level of degradation is about 10–30%. The conditions should be adjusted depending on the stability of the actives. Efforts should be made to correlate the amount of active degradation vs. the amount of degradation products formed, even though it may not be possible to account for 100% of degradation products by the observed loss in actives. The method specificity becomes more challenging when the product contains multiple actives and the strength of these actives differs in orders of magnitude.

In developing a dissolution method, one should consider that the medium used for the test should meet the sink condition for the in vitro test. For water-insoluble compounds, the dissolution medium may contain surfactants or organic solvents, although the latter should be avoided if possible. The assay for the drug release method can be a chromatographic procedure such as HPLC, a spectrophotometric procedure such as UV, or other suitable procedures. Shorter run times for chromatographic procedures are necessary due to the large number of samples to be analyzed for dissolution profiling studies.

3. METHOD VALIDATION

Method validation is the process of demonstrating that the analytical method is suitable for its intended use. The validation process establishes documented evidence that provides a high degree of assurance that the test method will consistently provide accurate test results that evaluate a product against its defined specification and quality attributes.

3.1. Objectives of Method Validation

Validation of analytical methodologies is considered as an important task, occurring after method development and before method utilization, and is required in support of product registration applications.

3.2. Method Validation Requirements

3.2.1. Compendial Analytical Procedures

The validation of a test method normally depends on whether the test method is a compendial method or a non-compendial method. The validation of compendial methods is described in USP ⟨1225⟩. Users of analytical methods described in the USP and the NF are not required to validate accuracy and reliability of these methods but to merely verify suitability under actual conditions of use. The methods provided in official monographs have been validated by the laboratory submitting the monograph and may have also been verified by other laboratories designated by the USP. For chromatographic purity methods, method sensitivity and selectivity under the actual conditions of use should also be demonstrated.

For active ingredient (API) test methods, the compendial methods can be readily adopted for use with limited suitability verification. For finished dosage form product test methods, the suitability of the test methods to the specific formulation needs to be demonstrated through a validation procedure. Validation of compendial test methods for the finished product may include, where applicable, specificity, linearity, accuracy, precision, and solution stability. However, it should be noted that the compendial methods are not necessarily stability-indicating. When the compendial method is used for such purpose, forced degradation studies are needed to demonstrate method specificity.

One should keep in mind that USP monograph procedures are regulatory procedures. *A regulatory analytical procedure* is the analytical procedure used to evaluate a defined characteristic of the drug substance or drug product. The analytical procedures in the *US Pharmacopoeia/National Formulary* (USP/NF) are those legally recognized under section 501(b) of the Food, Drug, and Cosmetic Act (the Act) as the regulatory analytical procedures for compendial items. For purposes of determining compliance with the Act, the regulatory analytical procedure is used.

3.2.2. Non-compendial Methods

For the validation of non-compendial test methods, one should follow USP, FDA, and ICH guidelines. Four categories of analytical methods are classified in the USP ⟨1225⟩.

Category I: Analytical methods for quantitation of major components of bulk drug substances or active ingredients (including preservatives) in finished pharmaceutical products fall under category I.

Category II: Analytical methods for determination of impurities in bulk drug substances or degradation compounds in finished pharmaceutical products are in category II. These methods include quantitative assays and limit tests.

Category III: Analytical methods for determination of performance characteristics (dissolution, drug release) are considered category III.

Category IV: Analytical test method for identification purpose.

In addition, there are tests classified as specific tests such as particle size analysis, droplet distribution, spray pattern, dissolution (excludes measurement), optical rotation, and methodologies such as DSC, XRD, and Raman spectroscopy.

The elements recommended for validation for each category of the test methods are shown in Table 1.

Since the validation of a test method is a matter of establishing documented evidence that provides a high degree of assurance of the suitability of the test method for its intended use, the documentation process usually includes a validation protocol, test data, and a validation report.

One should keep in mind that even though a non-compendial procedure has been validated, when a compendial procedure exists, an equivalency study is needed for the regulatory submission in order to demonstrate that the non-compendial procedure is equivalent to the compendial procedure. The method equivalency study is discussed in Section 3.6. When a legal dispute occurs, the compendial procedure will be used to judge the product quality and compliance with the regulations.

3.3. Development of a Validation Protocol

The development of a method validation protocol should be based on the requirements of the product specification and regulatory guidelines. A protocol should include the target method to be validated, pre-approved validation elements, and acceptance criteria. It should also describe the requirements for protocol execution, experimental design, a plan or procedure when acceptance criteria are not met, and reporting items.

Typical validation characteristics are:

- accuracy,
- precision (repeatability and intermediate precision),
- specificity,
- detection limit,
- quantitation limit,

TABLE 1 Recommended Validation Characteristics of the Various Types of Tests

Type of tests/characteristics	Identification	Testing for impurities		Assay dissolution (measurement only), content/potency	Specific tests
		Quantitative	Limit		
Accuracy	−	+	−	+	+[a]
Precision-repeatability	−	+	−	+	+[a]
Precision-intermediate	−	+[c]	−	+[c]	+[a]
Precision[b]					
Specificity	+[d]	+	+	+[e]	+[a]
Detection limit	−	−[f]	+	−	−
Quantitation limit	−	+	−	−	−
Linearity	−	+	−	+	−
Range	−	+	−[f]	+	−
Robustness	−	+	−	+	+[a]

Note: see draft guidance for analytical procedures and methods validation of FDA (August 2000).

− Signifies that this characteristic is not normally evaluated.

+ Signifies that this characteristic is normally evaluated.

[a] May not be needed in some cases.

[b] Ruggedness is considered as intermediate precision.

[c] In cases where reproducibility has been performed, intermediate precision is not needed.

[d] Lack of specificity for an analytical procedure may be compensated for by the addition of a second analytical procedure.

[e] Lack of specificity for an assay for release may be compensated for by impurities testing.

[f] May be needed in some cases.

- linearity,
- range,
- robustness,
- solution stability,
- filter interference (where applicable).

System suitability evaluated during the method validation should be summarized in the method validation report and the finalized parameters for system suitability should be put in the test method. For example, the validation data indicate that the %RSD of six injections of the analyte in the working standard is close to but not more than 2.0, the resolution between two closely eluting standards is close to but not more than 2.0, the tailing factor for the analyte in the working standard is not more than 1.2, and the theoretical plate number of the analyte in the working standard is about 10,000. Then, the above mentioned parameters can be set as the system suitability requirements since the validation results have indicated that these parameters can provide assurance of the separation quality and repeatability of the test method.

Establishment of the acceptance criteria is based on the category of the test method. The typical validation elements and acceptance criteria for Category I methods of finished dosage forms are given in Table 2.

Typical validation elements and acceptance criteria for Category II method (chromatographic purity) are listed in Table 3:

Typical validation elements and acceptance criteria for the Category III test methods are listed in Table 4.

The Category IV validation element is specificity and the identification test procedure can be infrared spectrometry, TLC, wet chemistry, UV/VIS spectrophotometry, etc.

The protocol can also define the procedure for handling situations where one or more validation elements fail to meet the acceptance criteria during the method validation. When such a situation occurs, the study director with the assistance of the chemist executing the protocol can assess the situation and determine with management approval:

- Whether the results can still be accepted with justification.
- Whether a limitation to the method application can be set so that the failure of the method can be excluded outside of the method application range.
- Whether the failing results need to be confirmed and an investigation may be needed.
- Whether the method has a defect and needs to be modified and then re-validated.

TABLE 2 Validation Elements and Acceptance Criteria: Category I

Validation element	Acceptance criteria
Precision	The RSD of six determinations (injections) of each analyte must be NMT 2.0%
Accuracy	The average recovery for each analyte must be NLT 98.0% and NMT 102.0% for triplicate determinations at analyte concentrations of 80%, 100%, and 120% of the target concentration
Specificity	1. No peak interference in the diluent and placebo injections at the retention time of the target analyte 2. The target analyte peak is resolved from adjacent peaks 3. The target analyte peak is pure by PDA analysis for forced degradation conditions
Method linearity	These acceptance criteria must be met for a five point concentration range of at least 80% to 120% of the target concentration 1. The correlation coefficient (r) is NLT 0.995 2. The percent bias of y-intercept is NLT -5.0% and NMT 5.0%
Range	The precision, accuracy, and linearity criteria must be met from at least 80% to about 120% of the sample concentration. If the range is larger, report the largest range over which the acceptance criteria are met
Ruggedness (intermediate precision)	1. The RSD of the spiked sample preparations from a second analyst, on a 2nd instrument, and on a different day using a different column must be NMT 2.0% 2. The RSD of the spiked sample preparations from both analyst one and analyst two must be NMT 5.0%
Filter interference	The assay of a filtered sample must be NLT 98.0% and NMT 102.0% relative to the same sample prepared by centrifugation
Solution stability (ambient or refrigerated temperature)	1. The assay of the sample preparation must not change by more than 2.0% in a specified time period 2. The assay of the working standard must not change by more than 2.0% in a specified time period
Robustness	System suitability criteria are met for the following method variations: variation of organic component in the mobile phase $\pm 5\%$ (relative) variation of ion-paring concentration of $\pm 10\%$, when applicable variation of Mobile Phase pH of ± 0.1 pH units, when applicable variation of flow rate about $\pm 10\%$ variation of wavelength ± 2 nm variation of column temperature about $\pm 5°C$ (where applicable)

TABLE 3   Validation Elements and Acceptance Criteria: Category II

Validation elements	Acceptance criteria
Precision	RSD is NMT 10.0%
Accuracy	Recovery for target analyte is between 90% and 110% for spiked placebo samples for the method range
Linearity	1. The correlation coefficient (r) is NLT 0.99 for the method range 2. The 95% confidence interval of the intercept includes the origin. If not, the intercept is NMT 100 ± 10% of the response of the standard concentration (at the specification level)
Range	The concentration at which the precision, accuracy, and linearity criteria are met. This range should be from the LOQ to 150% of the specification level
Quantitation limit	The concentration at which the S/N ratio is about 10. The quantitation limit should be NMT the reporting threshold defined in ICH Q3B
Detection limit	The concentration at which the S/N ratio is about 3. The detection limit should be NMT half of the reporting threshold defined in ICH Q3B
Specificity	1. No peak interference in the placebo injection at the retention time of target analyte(s) 2. The known impurity peak(s) are resolved from each other and from the active substance peak(s) 3. The target analyte peak(s) are pure by PDA analysis under forced degradation conditions
Ruggedness	1. The precision and accuracy acceptance criteria for a second analyst must be met for a standard spiked placebo solution on a separate instrument using a different column with sample solution prepared on a different day at the specification limit concentration level 2. The combined RSD(s) of the analyte(s) for both analysts must be NMT 15.0%
Filter interference (where applicable)	The peak area of each known impurity peak must be within 100 ± 10% of the centrifuged solution
Robustness	System suitability criteria are met for the following method variations: variation of organic component in the mobile phase ±5% (relative) variation of ion-paring concentration of ±10%, when applicable variation of mobile phase pH of ±0.1 pH units, when applicable variation of flow rate about ±10% variation of wavelength ±2 nm variation of column temperature about ±5°C (where applicable)
Solution stability	The assay of the standard and sample solutions at room temperature (or refrigerated temperature) must not change by more than 5% in a specified time period at least as long as the time required to perform a typical analysis run (maximum analysis time from sample preparation should be defined in the test method)

TABLE 4 Validation Elements and Acceptance Criteria: Category III

Validation elements	Acceptance criteria
Precision	RSD is NMT 2.0%
Accuracy	Recovery for target analyte is between 98% and 102% for spiked placebo samples at the release tolerances (Q) level
Method linearity	These acceptance criteria must be met for the method range: 1. The correlation coefficient (r) is NLT 0.995 2. The percent intercept is NLT −5.0% and NMT 5.0%
Range	The concentration at which the precision, accuracy, and linearity criteria are met. This range should cover from the low concentration end of the stage 3 dissolution test to 120% of the drug release level
Quantitation limit	The concentration at which the S/N ratio is about 10. The quantitation limit should be NMT the reporting threshold defined in ICH Q3B
Specificity	1. No peak interference in the placebo injection at the retention time of target analyte 2. The target analyte peak is resolved from the neighboring peaks 3. The target analyte peak is pure by PDA analysis
Ruggedness (intermediate precision)	1. The RSD of single determinations (injections) of six preparations under dissolution conditions (second analyst, second dissolution system) must be NMT 3.0% 2. The RSD for the combined determinations (analyst 1 and 2) must be NMT 5.0%
Interference from the automated dissolution sampling system	The percent recovery for the sample collected by the auto-collector must be between 98.0% and 102.0% of the sample collected manually
Solution stability	The assay of the sample and standard preparations must not change by more than 2.0% in a specified time period at least as long as the time required to perform a typical analysis run (maximum analysis time from sample preparation should be defined in the test method)

All deviations to the validation protocol must be documented and authorized by laboratory management and reviewed and approved by the quality assurance (QA) department. These deviations are summarized in the validation report.

3.4. Validation Planning and Protocol Execution

Instrumentation Selection: The method validation is considered as a current good manufacturing procedure (cGMP) activity, requiring that the instruments used for the validation activity be fully qualified according to installation (IQ), operational (OQ) and performance qualification (PQ) protocols.

Standards Qualification and Handling: The standard used for the method validation must be qualified. A vendor's certificate of analysis with the purity factor is needed for establishing quantitative relationships such as relative response factors (RRFs). It is preferable to use compendial standards if available for method validation.

Optimization of the Experimental Sequence for Efficiency: Validation experiments should be designed that are efficient and optimized for resource utilization.

Resources and Timelines: The number of personnel needed for the validation should be well planned. The person involved in the method validation must be trained on cGMP compliance and method validation standard operating procedures (SOPs). The timeline for the method validation should be reasonable for full documentation, data and notebook review and signature and for quality review and approval process. Method validations must be completed before the methods' application for API testing in pilot-bio batch or exhibit batch release.

3.5. Validation Report

The validation report is a summary of the results obtained during execution of the validation protocol. The results are compared with the acceptance criteria. The validation report must discuss whether the results pass or fail the acceptance criteria.

The validation report must also discuss and document any deviation from the protocol, justify the deviation, and analyze the impact of the deviation.

During the method validation, some parameters of the test method may be required to be modified (such as system suitability parameters) or finalized (such as relative retention time and relative response factors, etc.). These suggestions should be documented in the method validation report along with the justification for the method change.

3.6. Method Equivalency Study

When an in-house method and a compendial method exist for the same test, a comparison to the compendial monograph test method must be established to demonstrate that the in-house method is equivalent or better than the compendial method. The assessment of method equivalency can be based on statistical principles such as F-tests and t-tests or approved acceptable criteria. One lot of the finished product can be chosen to compare both the in-house test method and the compendial test method. The sample with multiple preparations is assayed and the results from both methods are compared. If the results pass the pre-approved acceptance criteria or the statistical analysis, the two test methods are considered equivalent.

4. METHOD TRANSFER

After ANDA approval, the test methods will be applied to the validation batches and routine product testing conducted by quality control laboratories. Hence, the test methods must be transferred to the quality control laboratories. There could potentially be a difference in the geographic location of the R&D lab and the QC lab. The experience of the instrument operator and experience with the application of the test methods could vary from lab to lab. Therefore, the knowledge and experience must be passed to the new laboratories. The receiving laboratory must demonstrate its ability to perform the test method. A method transfer SOP or protocol must establish the requirements for satisfactory method transfer.

4.1. Objective of the Method Transfer

The method transfer is part of the technology transfer process. The method transfer can improve the understanding of the analytical methodology for both the originating and receiving laboratories. The receiving laboratory personnel performing the test method should be trained on the test method. The receiving laboratories must be cGMP compliant. When the receiving laboratory is a contract lab, appropriate auditing of the lab by quality assurance personnel is necessary. When a method transfer (crossover) study is performed, the results from both labs can serve as "intermediate precision" data.

4.2. Documentation of Method Transfer

4.2.1. Method Transfer Protocol

In order to confirm that the receiving laboratory has the full grasp of the test methods, the transfer process must be documented. If the transfer process is driven by a method transfer protocol, this protocol should define the manner of method transfer, the role and responsibility of the laboratories involved, the acceptance criteria for a successful transfer and reporting items.

One way of method transfer is by a crossover study involving both the originating laboratory and receiving laboratory. In executing the method transfer protocol, both labs can test the same lot of product and the results are compared for closeness. The second way of method transfer is for the receiving lab to perform a mini-method validation (for example, to reproduce the method accuracy, precision, and linearity) which demonstrates that the lab can fully reproduce the performance characteristics of the test method.

4.2.2.   Method Transfer Report

Upon the completion of the method transfer protocol, the test results are summarized and compared to the pre-approved acceptance criteria to determine whether the receiving laboratory is qualified to perform the test method. The transfer report should indicate whether the transfer is successful. All transfer data must be recorded and reviewed. Any deviation from the protocol must be documented and discussed. The report must include the justification for the deviation to the protocol and impact on the test method.

5.   ADDITIONAL VALIDATION AND RE-VALIDATION OF THE TEST METHOD

Additional method validation and re-validation of the test method may be needed when there are regulatory changes and when the expectation for the method performance characteristics is higher. Sometimes, an alternative raw material supplier is chosen and a different impurity profile is expected due to a different synthetic manufacturing route for the API. When an old analysis technique is replaced by new techniques, method validation will be required again. The last possibility is that the validated procedure requires modification due to a discovered defect and the modified method must be re-validated.

6.   SUMMARY AND CONCLUSIONS

Development of accurate and reliable analytical methods is an important element of pharmaceutical development. Good analytical methods support correct decisions being made from data for formulation development and stability studies. All analytical methods must be validated before they are used to generate data which will support a regulatory decision.

Analytical development can proceed efficiently if a thorough literature search is made of the available information on the API and drug product, including related compounds. A good source of information is the portion of the DMF that the API manufacturer is willing to share with its customers.

It is a good idea to work closely with the lab personnel from the API manufacturer in developing methods for the API and in identifying unknown impurities in the API.

Analytical development and validation must follow a timeline keyed to the other activities in developing a drug product. Analytical methods will usually be needed to support other plant activities such as cleaning validation or packaging development. The analytical method should be evaluated for robustness and reliability prior to committing the time and effort to validate a method.

A validated method can still be updated for special situations encountered during the method application. Such update may or may not involve an addendum or supplement to the method validation. This is usually part of the life cycle of the test method application.

The validation report is necessary for documenting the capability of the test method. All data that support the validation must be clearly identified and audited. These data will be scrutinized by the regulatory agency granting a drug product approval in a pre-approval inspection.

REFERENCES

1. US Food and Drug Administration, Title 21 CFR 314.94, Office of Federal Register, National Archives and Records Administration, 2003.
2. US Food and Drug Administration, Center for Drug Evaluation and Research. Guidance for Industry: Dissolution testing of Immediate Release Solid Oral Dosage Forms, Office of Training and Communications, Division of Communications and Management, Drug Information Branch, HFD 210, 5600 Fishers Lane, Rockville, Maryland 20857, August, 1997.
3. US Food and Drug Administration, Center for Drug Evaluation and Research. Guidance for Industry: Extended Release Oral Dosage Forms: Development, Evaluation and Application of In Vitro–In Vivo Correlations, Office of Training and Communications, Division of Communications and Management, Drug Information Branch, HFD 210, 5600 Fishers Lane, Rockville, Maryland 20857, September, 1997.
4. US Food and Drug Administration, Center for Drug Evaluation and Research. Guidance for Industry: SUPAC-MR: Modified Release Solid Oral Dosage Forms, Office of Training and Communications, Division of Communications and Management, Drug Information Branch, HFD 210, 5600 Fishers Lane, Rockville, Maryland 20857, September, 1997.
5. US Food and Drug Administration, Center for Drug Evaluation and Research. Guidance for Industry: Analytical Procedures and Methods Validation, Chemistry, Manufacturing and Controls Documentation, Office of Training and Communications, Division of Communications and Management, Drug Information Branch, HFD 210, 5600 Fishers Lane, Rockville, Maryland 20857, August, 2000.

6. US Food and Drug Administration, Center for Drug Evaluation and Research. Reviewer Guidance: Validation of Chromatographic Methods, Division of Communications and Management, Drug Information Branch, HFD 210, 5600 Fishers Lane, Rockville, Maryland 20857, November, 1994.

7. US Food and Drug Administration, Center for Drug Evaluation and Research. Draft Guidance: Stability Testing of Drug Substances and Drug Products, Division of Communications and Management, Drug Information Branch, HFD 210, 5600 Fishers Lane, Rockville, Maryland 20857, June, 1998.

8. The International Conference on Harmonization. The Common Technical Document (M4). (Internet).

9. The International Conference on Harmonization of Technical Requirements for Registration of Pharmaceuticals for Human Use. Q3B (R), Impurities in New Drug Products, October 1999.

10. The International Conference on Harmonization of Technical Requirements for Registration of Pharmaceuticals for Human Use. Q3C, Impurities in New Drug Products, July 1997.

11. The International Conference on Harmonization of Technical Requirements for Registration of Pharmaceuticals for Human Use. Q3A (R) Impurities in New Drug Substances, October 1999.

12. Miller JM, Crowther JB, eds. Analytical Chemistry in a GMP Environment. New York: Wiley, 2000.

13. USP 26/NF 21, ⟨724⟩ Drug Release and ⟨711⟩ Dissolution.

14. Snyder LR, Kirkland JJ, Glajch JL. Practical HPLC Method Development. 2nd ed. New York: Wiley, 1997.

15. Jenke DR. J Liq Chromatogr Relat Tech 1996; 19(5):719–736.

16. Jenke DR. J Liq Chromatogr Relat Tech Mar 1996; 19(5):737–757.

17. Jenke DR. Instrum Sci Technol 1998-01; 26(1):19–35.

18. Krull I, Swartz M. LC-GC North America 2000-06; 18(6):620, 622–625.

4

Experimental Formulation Development

Izzy Kanfer and Roderick B. Walker
Faculty of Pharmacy, Rhodes University, Grahamstown, South Africa

Peter Persicaner
Arrow Pharmaceuticals, Croydon, Victoria, Australia

The formulation scientist in the generic industry has a demanding role when developing generic oral solid dosage forms which not only need to match innovator products within tight acceptance criteria but should also circumvent restrictive formulation patents which makes it extremely challenging to achieve the desired generic product.

As the innovator companies come under increasing pressure from generic competition, it becomes important that valuable aspects of intellectual property acquired during the development of a specific drug product be sufficiently detailed in order to file a formulation patent. Their primary goal is to prevent, as far as possible, generic drug products from entering the market until after the benefits of basic patent coverage and subsequent formulation patent protection have been suitably exploited. Innovator companies may also file additional patents related to the synthetic process employed to produce the active pharmaceutical ingredient (API) (1), the specific crystal form (polymorph) (2), the formulation (3) and the combination of the drug with other active(s) which might provide synergistic benefits over the specific drug administered alone (4), specific "use" patents (5), and, of late, "paediatric exclusivity" (6).

Despite the fact that the literature abounds with numerous drug-product formulations, both qualitative and quantitative, it is rather surprising that formulation scientists struggle in their quest to match the innovator product from a bioequivalence point of view, resulting in failed biostudies. Possible reasons for not being able to match the innovator may well lie in the nature of the API material used (7,8), the composition of the formulation with respect to the excipients used (9,10) and the manufacturing process employed, amongst others (11). Table 1 lists the effects of excipients on the pharmacokinetic parameters of oral drug products clearly indicating the effect that excipients may have on bioavailability and bioequivalence (12).

It is very important to characterize the active ingredient to be used with respect to polymorph, particle size and also from a morphological point of view. The role of particle size cannot be overemphasized, especially in APIs of decreasing solubility and permeability (13). Failed bioequivalence studies are often due to issues of particle size and comparatively small differences of 5 μm (or even less in some cases) in mass median diameter (MMD) can spell the difference between success and failure (14). The fact that patents concerning particle size have been filed by drug companies testifies to the importance of that parameter in formulating effective drug products (15).

Different crystal forms of the same chemical entity (polymorphs), for example ibuprofen (16), can have varying solubilities, which could have significant implications with respect to bioequivalence if the incorrect form is used. Patent strategies pertinent to polymorph(s), provided that they are well thought-out and as far-reaching as possible, will continue to provide generic API manufacturers and formulation scientists considerable challenges. Drug manufacturers and formulation scientists have been able to counter most of the innovator polymorph strategies with considerable success, a fact which has prompted innovator drug companies to devise more elaborate patent strategies to protect their intellectual property.

TABLE 1 The Potential Effects of Excipients on Pharmacokinetic Parameters Following Oral Administration. Adapted From Ref. 12

Excipients	Example	k_a	t_{max}	AUC
Diluents	Microcrystalline cellulose	↑	↓	↑/—
Disintegrants	Sodium starch glycolate	↑	↓	↑/—
Enteric coat	Cellulose acetate pthalate	↓	↑	↓/—
Glidant	Talc	—	—	—
Lubricants	Magnesium stearate	↓/↑	↑	↓/—
Sustained-release agents	Methylcellulose, ethylcellulose	↓	↑	↓/—

In all cases, these effects may be concentration or drug dependent. The symbols represent: ↑ = increase, ↓ = decrease, — = no effect. ka = absorption rate, tmax = time to peak concentration, AUC = area under the plasma drug concentration time curve.

The morphology of APIs is of considerable importance especially in direct-compression (dry-blending) formulations of drug products where the active content is less than 20% of the formula. Regulatory authorities the world over (especially the FDA) have become increasingly aware of variations in active content in "blend samples" drawn to confirm homogeneity of active distribution after blending. In a recent report (17), lack of adequate potency and/or content uniformity was cited as the primary reason for the recall of solid dosage forms which, from a regulatory perspective, raises the issue of whether adequate process controls (including blend homogeneity testing) and release tests are in place. Due to the fact that the active ingredient and excipients rarely demonstrate comparable particle sizes/shapes, the compositional ingredients will flow into the "collection port(s)" of a sample thief at differing rates determined by their morphology. This will often give rise to the phenomenon of blends demonstrating considerable active ingredient variation (18), whereas the resultant tablets (compressed on modern tablet presses equipped with flow optimization attributes such as force feeders) will exhibit highly satisfactory content uniformities (usually within $\pm 5\%$ of label claim, with a concomitantly low relative standard deviation) which easily comply with the relevant compendial requirements. Consequently pharmaceutical manufacturers are required by law to provide evidence of the adequacy of their blending operations (19). Regulatory authorities require that a meaningful correlation between blend uniformity and tablet/capsule content uniformity exists, despite data from several reports where blend uniformity test failures were determined to be a result of sample size, sampling errors (position and depth in blender and hopper), sample thief design, and technique of sample collection (20–22). The formulation scientist is thus encouraged to seek creative sampling techniques to overcome sampling bias/disparity attributed to variances in morphology between active and excipient(s).

As a result of industry comment on a draft FDA guidance document (23), which has since been withdrawn, the Product Quality Research Institute (PQRI) Blend Uniformity Working Group (BUWG) published a recommendation to address the limitations with current sampling techniques. This proposal recommends the use of stratified sampling of blend and dosage units to demonstrate adequacy of mixing for powder blends (24). Stratified sampling involves the deliberate selection of units from various locations within a lot or batch or from various phases or periods of a process to obtain a sample. Such sampling specifically targets locations either in the blender or throughout the compression/filling operation where there is a high risk of failing content uniformity specifications.

Generally, differences observed between blend uniformity and drug-product content uniformity are less pronounced in wet granulation and compaction-type formulations compared to direct-compression formulations.

FORMULATION DEVELOPMENT STRATEGIES

1. Patent Search(es)

In the early days of the generic industry, once the basic patent had expired, generic pharmaceutical companies were free to launch their version(s) of the drug product(s) into the market. However, over the last 20 or so years, the innovator drug companies have sought to extend their product(s) life, focusing initially on "Process Patents" (the route of synthesis whereby the API is produced, including any unique crystal forms which may have resulted). The synthetic pathway has been explored to the full, and the widest possible claims registered. The leading generic bulk API manufacturers continue their quest to synthesize APIs that do not infringe process patents. Although generic bulk drug manufacturers were, at one time, content merely to produce non-patent infringing active(s), many have now taken it upon themselves to file patents of their own, a ploy which considerably increases the difficulty that other raw material manufacturers will face when attempting to synthesize the same active raw material.

1.1 Formulation Patents

In certain instances, innovator drug companies have valid reasons for filing formulation patents, particularly where a specific excipient (or blend of excipients) lends a particular uniqueness in terms of release or stability (25). However, some drug companies file patents which claim every excipient known, and such patents are clearly open to challenge.

It is more difficult to file formulation patents in the arena of immediate release dosage forms than in the case of modified/controlled release formulations, where creative solutions have been applied to modify the in vitro and in vivo release characteristics of active(s) so as to provide a dosage regimen which offers significant therapeutic advantages and improved patient compliance.

1.2 Combination Patents

Combination Patents are those which pertain to more than one active ingredient combined together in a single drug product, the resultant product ideally displaying a synergistic pharmacological response compared with each active ingredient administered on their own. One of the earliest examples of such a combination was co-trimoxazole, where sulfamethoxazole was combined with trimethoprim. More recent examples have focussed on decongestants in combination with antihistamines, for example loratidine and pseudoephedrine, antibiotic combinations such as amoxycillin and clavulanic acid, ACE-inhibitors in combination with diuretics such as enalapril and hydrochlorthiazide or perindopril and indapamide, and antihypertensives in combination with diuretics, such as atenolol and chlorthalidone.

1.3. Use Patents

In certain instances, a drug substance has been found to be of benefit in treating disorders other than those first known and recognized, as for example with omeprazole with its relatively new indication for use in Gastro-Esophageal Reflux Disease (GERD) and the amino-ketone antidepressant, bupropion with the additional claim for use in smoking cessation. New clinical studies are undertaken to provide the additional "use" which permits the innovator company to claim that particular new indication on both label and package insert. Use Patents prevent generic companies from making the additional claim(s), but do not prevent the generic product from being prescribed to treat conditions originally claimed in the basic patent. Consequently "Use Patents" do not carry the same impact as process and formulation patents, but nevertheless cannot be ignored.

2. Literature Search

A comprehensive literature search should be performed that focuses on the API material in question and the proposed formulation. The formulation patent(s) filed and information on the innovator's New Drug Application (NDA) can be obtained by requesting the Summary Basis of Approval (SBA) from the FDA at http://www.fda.gov/cder/foi/anda/index and provides an excellent source of background information. It is essential that such a literature search be embarked upon as early in the development process as possible.

3. Regulatory Strategy

Once all of the patents have been comprehensively analyzed, a regulatory strategy must be formulated to establish when the "earliest date of sale" of the generic drug product can legally be made. In this respect, the Approved Drug Products (Orange) Book (26) provides useful information relating to the expiration date of appropriate patents of drug products that are the subject of approved applications but excludes process patents. The reader is referred to Chapter 14 for a more comprehensive account. Such strategies need to embrace "first to file", "exclusivity", and a whole host of "legal implications" which need to be encompassed within the project plan, which will ultimately lead to a "first to market" strategy (27). This scenario has evolved over the past fifteen years, and gained prominence for the first time when ranitidine (Form 1) ANDAs were reviewed by the FDA in the mid 1990s (28).

Once patent hurdles have been fully investigated, and regulatory strategies put in place, it is up to the formulation scientist to ensure that a non-patent infringing raw material can be incorporated into a non-patent infringing formulation which will be at least as stable as the innovator drug product and also bioequivalent.

4. Sourcing of the Active Raw Material(s)

Purchasing an API raw material can be quite demanding and is not as straightforward as one might perceive. Data bases are consulted as to which manufacturers have the required material available and once the potential vendors are identified, each is requested to furnish the following information:

1. The detailed synthetic pathway whereby the API is produced, including all solvents, catalysts, materials, etc. utilized at every step.
2. A statement indicating that the process pathway does not infringe any patent(s) that may be in force and must be verified by the generic company's patent lawyers.
3. A statement indicating the possible polymorphic nature of the active drug in question, where relevant.
4. The batch size(s) of API which have been manufactured to-date.
5. Any validation data which may be available to provide some degree of assurance that the synthetic process has been evaluated/controlled.
6. Fifty to one hundred gram samples from three discrete batches of material manufactured according to the synthetic pathway provided. In each case, the batch-size should be made available.
7. A complete list of synthetic impurities and potential degradation products which may be used to fingerprint the API, together with full chemical characterization of each as well as 50–100 mg samples of each synthetic impurity/degradation product alluded to. Appropriate methodologies such as mass spectroscopy, high performance liquid chromatography (HPLC), X-ray diffraction (where polymorphs may be present), nuclear magnetic resonance (NMR), electron spin resonance (ESR), amongst others are generally used for the characterization. In some instances, one of the recognized international compendia such as the United States Pharmacopoeia (USP) (29) and/or Pharmacopoeial Forum (30), the British

Pharmacopoeia (BP) (31) and the European Pharmacopoeia (EP) (32) may list potential impurities and/or degradation products for the API in question. Depending on the route of synthesis followed, there may be no possibility for a listed impurity to be present in the API. Should such a situation present itself, the onus is on the API manufacturer to provide a statement as to why there is no possibility for the stated impurity to be present. *Note*: Such a statement would have to be supported by actually demonstrating the absence of said impurity by HPLC analysis, and in order that this be done, it is essential that the impurity be synthesized (and chemically characterized), either by the API manufacturer or by a contract laboratory.

8. A complete list of solvents used in the synthetic process (which should relate to those claimed in the detailed synthetic pathway) together with those which should be monitored in the API. Where appropriate, a statement must be made by the API manufacturer claiming that none of the organic volatile impurities (OVIs) listed in the USP are present.

9. Specifications pertinent to raw material particle size, which may become better defined as the drug-product manufacturer closes in on a final formulation.

10. A Technical Package, which embraces the information requested, plus stability data to confirm suitability of the raw material in question and validated analytical methods pertinent to assay, related substances/degradation products and residual solvents.

11. A commitment by the API manufacturer to undertake the necessary validation of the synthetic process, and the batch-size envisaged for future commercial production.

The vast amount of data required (not to mention the sensitivity of the information requested) will necessitate the signing of Confidentiality/Secrecy Agreements between the API manufacturer(s) and the generic pharmaceutical company. Once the information has been received and reviewed, the choice can be made as to which raw material supplier to select.

The reader is referred to the Drug Information Association (DIA) Fourth Symposium on APIs held in Baltimore during November, 1998 and the subsequent publication of several relevant articles in the Drug Information Journal (33–39) as well as Chapter 2 of this book.

Although the strength of the Drug Master File (DMF) or Technical Package supplied by the vendor may be the most important criterion on which to base the selection, past experiences with the bulk drug manufacturer (promptness of supply, quality, working relationships, ability to respond to competitive pricing) should enter into the decision-making process as well.

The relationship between API manufacturer and generic drug company is far closer today than it ever was in the past; this is due to the considerable amount of intellectual property and strategies that need to be shared between the companies. In this respect, it is important to maintain a close liaison with the API manufacturer to ensure that any change in API manufacture is promptly communicated.

One of the most important difficulties facing both companies is the phenomenon of scale-up from R&D laboratory samples through pilot-batch manufacture to full commercial production, since it is widely known and accepted that increasing the batch-size can sufficiently stress the process thereby resulting in higher levels of impurities, residual solvents, and altered particle-size characteristics (39).

Once the exhibit-batches (whose documentation is part of the sub-mission dossier) have been produced, the API manufacturer will be in a position to file a relevant DMF with the appropriate government agency. A DMF may be used to provide confidential detailed information about facilities, processes, or articles used in the manufacturing, processing, packaging, and storing of the API (40). The information contained in the DMF may be used to support an Abbreviated New Drug Application (ANDA). Any updates/amendments to the DMF must only be made after consultation with the drug-product manufacturer since such changes may jeopardize approval of the finished product. Frequently, API manufacturers will supply drug-product manufacturers with the "open part" of a DMF, since the information therein may be necessary and useful in formulating a drug-product. An open part of the DMF would typically include the following:

A.   Drug Substance,

    1.   description of API,
    2.   manufacture of drug substance (synthetic pathway only) which includes:

       flow chart,
       impurity profile,
       demonstration of chemical structure, and
       physical characteristics of the product (spectroscopic analysis),

    3.   Purity of the reference material, and
    4.   packaging and labeling,

B. Laboratory Controls,

1. specifications and test methods used for the API,
2. scheme of the stability evaluation protocol, and
3. batch size,

C. Complaints File, and
D. Environmental Impact Analysis.

4.1 Alternate Vendor Sourcing

It is useful to secure approval of an alternate API manufacturer. However, different API manufacturers may have applied different strategies to overcome process patents. In such cases, there is a high probability that the impurity and residual solvent profiles will vary significantly, necessitating full analytical methods re-validation.

Where polymorphism is an issue, it is essential that both suppliers provide the identical form. From a regulatory perspective, the preferred situation would be if both manufacturer's materials were synthesized utilizing the same (very difficult to achieve if patent(s) have been filed) or a similar synthetic approach, which is likely to result in similar impurity and residual solvent profiles and polymorphic form.

The need to change sources of raw material during formulation development is unfortunately not a rare occurrence. Such situations may arise when there may initially only be a single source of supply of R&D quantities of API. Formulation development thus commences with relatively costly raw material and often, in time, additional bulk API suppliers emerge to provide raw material at more favorable prices. If the formulation scientist is required to change the raw material source for scale-up or exhibit-batch manufacture, the formulation may need to be re-developed, since the physico-chemical characteristics of the new supplier's raw material may bear scant resemblance to that used initially and as a consequence, this may slow the project down considerably.

Even if another supplier's raw material is similar, if not identical to that employed initially, a simple substitution of the latter by the former may not result in an identical product being produced even when the raw material specifications appear identical. When faced with such a situation, it is always in the formulation scientist's best interests to undertake a series of trials, preferably at pilot-batch scale, to confirm acceptability of the alternate API from both production and analytical points of view. Hence, when adding an additional source or contemplating the replacement of one source of active raw material with another, all necessary precautions must be taken to ensure interchangeability and this holds true for key excipients as well.

5. Formulation Development

Formulation development should only commence once the following issues have been suitably addressed:

1. relevant patents have been accessed and investigated,
2. the appropriate literature search has been undertaken,
3. regulatory and formulation strategies have been established, and
4. the desired API(s) have been ordered and received.

A beneficial approach to formulation development is to critically evaluate and, where possible, to characterize the innovator product with respect to composition, type of granulation (wet granulation or direct compression) and any other qualitative and/or quantitative analyses which may be practical or feasible. Additional useful information relating to the innovator product may be gleaned by measuring in vitro drug release over a range of pHs and rotational speeds used in dissolution testing as well as inspection of brand labeling for stability information. Conventional microscopy and visual observation may well provide useful information regarding the granulation method used although caution should be exercised since the results may prove inconclusive and possibly erroneous.

A simple and very useful approach is to determine the pH of the innovator drug product dispersed in a small volume of pH adjusted Purified Water, and then to compare the result with that yielded by a similar dispersion of the trial formulation. This approach is based on the premise that if the two dispersions provide comparable pHs, the excipient compositions of both innovator and generic formulations are probably similar. Once again circumspection is necessary since this simple test may sometimes not be sufficiently discriminatory.

Initial trials should be undertaken employing the identical excipients referenced in texts such as the Physicians' Desk Reference (41), Compendium of Pharmaceuticals and Specialities (Canada) (42), Dictionnaire Vidal (43), and the Repertorio Farmaceutico Italiano (44).

Selection of appropriate quantities of key excipients such as binders, disintegrants/dissolution enhancers, compressibility aids, glidants, lubricants, anti-adherents, and surface-active agents is an important consideration for the formulation scientist. In this regard, a valuable reference that should be consulted is *The Handbook of Pharmaceutical Excipients* (45).

It would be reasonable to presume that provided the same excipients, as outlined in referenced texts, are used, possible instability/incompatibility issues may be circumvented. However, should it be deemed necessary to use an excipient(s) not present in the innovator product, it will be prudent to evaluate such an excipient(s) for compatibility with the active ingredient using techniques such as a stability indicating HPLC assay, TLC and/or Differential Scanning Calorimetry (DSC) (46,47).

It is recommended that all compression trials be undertaken with trade dress requirements in mind, using the same punches and dies envisaged for future commercial production. This approach circumvents future compression problems such as sticking, picking, and poor friability upon subsequent exhibit-batch/commercial-batch production. In addition, it may be difficult to predict hardness/compression force settings if tooling of different dimension(s) and shape were used at development level, which in turn may affect dissolution profiles to a considerable degree (48–50).

The need to optimize tablet punch design and even consider the nature of the stainless steel used is often overlooked at the formulation stage. The fifth edition of the *Tablet Specification Manual* provides comprehensive information on specifications and quality control programs for tablet tooling (51). In order to achieve acceptable tablet compression characteristics, optimization of binder(s), lubricant(s), glidant(s), and anti-adherents in the formula(e) are also important considerations. Relatively small changes in the amount of such key excipients can dramatically alter the appearance and physical attributes of tablets, whereas the impact of such changes on drug product stability and dissolution profiles can be significant (46,52,53).

Finally, all formulation trials should be compressed on a high-speed, rotary tablet-press that is preferably instrumented (54) to provide the scientist valuable information relating to pre-compression, main compression, ejection, and take-off forces. In many instances, the active pharmaceutical ingredient may be very expensive or in short supply. In such cases, valuable information regarding compressibility of the granule blend under high-speed conditions may be obtained by use of a tablet-press tooled with as few as four sets of punches and dies or by use of commercially available tablet-presses with a small number of tooling stations.

The formulation of a capsule follows the same guidelines advocated for tablets. As was the case with the development of tablets, powder(s) intended for encapsulation can be produced by dry blending/compaction or wet granulation. Dry-blending formulations are, as the name implies, merely a blend of the active with excipients which may be included as disintegrants/ dissolution enhancers, glidants, lubricants, anti-adherents, surface-active agents, and diluents, where necessary. Should the powder blend need to be compacted, due care must be given to the incorporation of dry binder as well as well as anti-frictional agents and other necessary excipients since these could have significant implications with respect to their effects both intra- and inter-granularly. Where a wet granulation approach needs to be adopted in order to densify the powder, the same degree of attention regarding formulation and processing as for tablets must be adopted.

The development of a capsule formulation is not only dependent on capsule shell size and shape, but attention must be given to the degree of capsule fill, the quantity of lubricant to be included as well as the type and quantity of surface active agent used to impart improved dissolution profile characteristics (55).

The polymerization (56) of gelatin involving cross-linking and hydrogen bonding has been previously identified as a significant factor affecting dissolution rate of active principles from solid oral dosage forms containing gelatin or encapsulated, either in hard or soft gelatin capsules. The reduction in dissolution rate may be attributed to pellicle formation due to an insoluble cross-linked portion of the gelatin, which remains intact and can be seen by observation of the capsules in the dissolution medium. Various factors influence the dissolution rate of soft gelatin capsule shells, such as temperature, plasticizer, and various other additives (57). This has significant bioavailability implications (58,59). Stability and dissolution testing of gelatin based formulations thus require special attention during product development and subsequently (60,61a,61b).

Where possible, the capsule contents should fill the body of the shell as much as possible, since if too much head space is present, the stability of the active(s) in the formulation may be compromised and susceptible to degradation reactions such as oxidation.

During the initial formulation process, it is extremely important to validate/characterize each key process, such as:

1. screen-sizes and milling rates (pre-granulation),
2. dry blend mixing times (pre-granulation),
3. the quantity and rate of addition of the granulating vehicle,
4. the specific granulating time(s),
5. the temperature and air flows employed during the drying process,
6. loss on drying of the granules,
7. screen-sizes and milling rates (post-granulation), as well as granulometry assessment (pre-blending),
8. times and speeds used during all blending operations where the active granule is blended with the inter-granular/extra-granular phase(s), and
9. all coating parameters and conditions.

When the formulation scientist is satisfied with the compressibility characteristics of the formulation, aesthetic appearance and disintegration profile of the tablets/capsules produced, samples should be submitted to the laboratory for dissolution profile testing.

The use of dissolution profile testing at the formulation development stage is extremely important, and consequently it is essential that time and effort be devoted to developing discriminatory dissolution methods, which are sufficiently sensitive to highlight differences between innovator and test products. Caution must be exercised since it is possible to develop an over-discriminatory dissolution test whereby dissolution rate differences between innovator and test products may not be clinically significant, suggesting bio-inequivalence in cases where bioequivalence does indeed exist (62–70).

There are various approaches which can be taken to develop a discriminatory dissolution method and conditions. One process would be to determine the dissolution profiles of a drug product in a minimum of three different media, whereas another would be to devise dissolution conditions such that the active will be released gradually over a 30–45-min period. Matching dissolution profiles between generic and innovator products usually augurs well for future in vivo performance of the generic product. This is particularly probable for drug products containing highly soluble and highly permeable active ingredients and if the product is rapidly dissolving, in vivo bioequivalence testing may be waived (71).

The effect of hardness on dissolution profile must be considered for each viable tablet core formulation, and the formulation which demonstrates the least variation in release rate and extent over the widest possible hardness range (while still retaining the desired appearance and disintegration characteristics) will invariably become the "final formulation". It is this formulation and associated manufacturing process which must be scaled-up in the course of further development.

6. Equipment Selection for Formulation Development

During the early era of generic drug-product manufacture, formulation development was often commenced using different equipment to that used for pilot production, exhibit batch and/or in the commercial scale manufacturing facility. The process of scale-up is more often than not a daunting task even when employing equipment of the same type and operating principle during the initial stages of formulation development (small-scale) through pilot-batch (exhibit-batch) production to final full-scale (commercial) batch manufacture. As far as possible, the type of tablet compression equipment and tooling or encapsulator machinery should be identical in principle to those used for scale-up manufacture of the exhibit batch/commercial batches resulting in technology transfer from pilot scale to production batch occuring with few difficulties for the formulation scientist. Hence the use of different types of equipment between the different phases of development is not recommended. A comprehensive account of scale-up and technology transfer is portrayed in Chapter 5 of this book.

Of all the processes that need to be controlled, the most critical is wet granulation since it is particularly vulnerable with respect to consistency using different types of equipment. Careful monitoring of (a) mixer and chopper speeds, (b) rate of addition of the granulating vehicle, (c) the quantity of granulating vehicle, and (d) the processing time necessary to yield an evenly textured granulate in order to result in satisfactory granules after subsequent drying (72–76). It is, however, possible to vary the type of mill used, and yet achieve the desired granulometry by adroit use of screen dimension and milling-rate (77).

Drying of wet granulate can be undertaken effectively using either a fluid-bed dryer or a circulating air oven, the most noticeable difference between the two techniques manifesting itself in the granulometry of the dried granule, since the fluid-bed technique tends to provide a "finer" (less dense) granule than an oven (78,79).

Wet-granulation formulations tend to suffer less from non-homogeneity of (active) distribution than do direct-compression formulations, since the active/excipients are far more intimately mixed prior to granulation than can be effected by traditional dry blending. Each granule yielded by wet granulation should thus comprise a homogenous blend of active and excipients, whereas in the case of direct-compression formulations, the blending is far less vigorous and the materials being blended are usually not of the same size and morphology, these two differences being the main contributing factors to dry-blends demonstrating greater (active) variation than those produced by wet granulation (80).

The type of blender used can also affect the compressibility and, to a lesser extent, the encapsulation characteristics of a granule/powder blend. Blenders which offer too intimate a mix between granule and inter-granular excipients (as in the case of wet granulation formulations) can result in granules for compression which provide tablet cores demonstrating:

- prolonged disintegration times (due to excessive hydrophobic layer build-up because of "overblending" with hydrophobic lubricants such as magnesium stearate) (81), and
- low hardness, which again is a symptom of too intimate a contact between granule, lubricant(s), and some inter-granular disintegrants.

The selection of blender and blending times can also impact the final granule with respect to active/excipient homogeneity and compressibility (17). In the case of direct-compression formulations, over-blending can result in de-mixing of active (82), in addition to prolonged disintegration times and soft tablets (83). Similarly, under-blending can give rise to homogeneity and compressibility/encapsulation problems. Consequently, the formulation scientist must optimize the blending conditions during formulation development, with the realization that these may well vary from product to product.

Many pharmaceutical companies employ a perforated pan (for example Accela-Cota) coating system to film coat tablets. Sugar-coating has almost entirely been eclipsed by film-coating. Once again, it would be in the company's best interests to ensure that the formulation scientist is provided with a smaller version (12 or 24 in. pan(s)) of the same equipment used in the production facility. In addition, environmental, safety, and cost concerns have necessitated the change to aqueous based film-coating dispersions or water soluble polymers from organic solvent based coating solutions. However, the use of organic solvents may in certain cases be unavoidable.

7. Assessment of the Final Formulation and Exhibit-Batch Production

The most promising formulation, selected on the basis of consistent/ satisfactory *in vitro* drug release over a broad hardness range, is then scaled-up from an initial development batch-size of 5000 units to about 20,000 units. Samples of the drug product (which may be in the form of uncoated/coated tablets or capsules) are then packaged in all possible configurations intended for future commercialization, and placed on "informal stability" (investigative stability assessment) together with the appropriate packaging(s) of innovator product, both of which have been analyzed for potency, degradation products, and dissolution profile. By so doing, it is possible to evaluate the comparative stability of the generic product against the product of original research.

"Informal stability" is carried out under "accelerated" conditions of elevated temperature/humidity (normally 40°C/75% RH) and light (where applicable) for a period of 2–3 months. It is also useful to place the Reference Listed Drug (RLD or Brand) on accelerated stability. The generic product is analyzed at monthly intervals for active content/potency, related substances/degradation products and dissolution profiles are generated. Should stability problems manifest with the generic product stored under a specific storage condition then testing of the RLD stored under the same conditions can be extremely informative.

It is preferable to analyze the samples using validated analytical procedures since those would be the analytical methodologies employed during full stability evaluation of samples derived from the exhibit-batch manufacturing program.

Should the generic product prove to be stable over a 2–3 month period of exposure to accelerated conditions, there would be a high degree of probability that the formulation scientist has succeeded in formulating a stable drug product.

It is also vitally important to ensure that all desirable characteristics observed during the manufacture of the final formula at development-level are maintained as closely as possible when the formulation is scaled-up. The dissolution and disintegration profiles at the pre-determined hardness levels (where applicable) should be consistent. The bulk and tapped densities of the powder/granule, prior to compression/encapsulation, as well as the pertinent granulometries should be similar and the "loss on drying" values of the granule/powder prior to compression/encapsulation should be consistent with previous data.

Once the generic drug product has demonstrated a minimum of two months satisfactory stability, attention must be focused on the following:

1. Development of specifications for both raw material (API) and the dosage form.
2. Ordering of the API and excipients for exhibit-batch manufacture.
3. Ordering of all relevant tooling, change parts, and capsule shells (if required).
4. Completion of a Development Report.

It is essential that the raw material specifications are set in conjunction with the API manufacturer, in order to avoid setting specifications which may be considered too restrictive by the latter. The debate invariably involves limits with respect to related substances/impurities/degradation products, residual solvents, particle size and, in certain instances, microbial limits, especially where the active raw material(s) is produced by fermentation at some stage during the synthetic pathway. Only once both parties are in full agreement, should the requisite specification(s) be confirmed and signed by the responsible persons.

8. The Development Report

A Development Report is a summary of the complete development process and will be the subject of keen regulatory agency scrutiny during a Pre-approval Inspection (PAI) (FDA) or any other similar audit.

This report must make detailed reference to the following:

a. An overview of the actions and uses of the particular active, as well as any information pertinent to the relevant pharmacokinetics.
b. A brief description of the innovator product and the pack-sizes commercially available and appropriate to all markets where the product is destined to be sold.

c. A detailed summary of the innovator product's physical characteristics (such as appearance, size, shape, and weight). The inclusion of a photograph, as visual confirmation, is desirable.

d. A comprehensive account of the APIs used during the formulation development process including sources of supply. All information pertinent to the polymorphic form used in development as compared to that used by the innovator (which is usually easier to determine in drug products containing more than 25% of active) as well as particle sizes of the APIs, bulk/tapped densities information and the mechanism whereby the appropriate specifications were established. Generally three lots of API from an approved supplier should be analyzed and on the basis of the resultant data, specifications need to be set. Compendial monograph(s) may be too lenient as far as impurity limits are concerned and often data relating to residual solvent presence, particle size, polymorph, and polymorph ratio are either absent or scant.

e. A section dealing with the development of a discriminatory dissolution method including profiles of the generic and RLD product(s) using this method and conditions. The dissolution methodology outlined in the USP, BP, or EP may not be sufficiently discriminatory to serve formulation development needs. Because the particular compendial method serves as a "batch release" specification for the commercial product, it is essential that both the innovator and generic drug products meet applicable compendial specifications.

f. A detailed account of all experimentation undertaken to arrive at the "final formulation". Reference should be made (ideally in the form of an "Appendix") to each formula employed, details of granulometries, bulk and tapped densities, loss on drying and ranges of tablet core hardness together with associated disintegration times and dissolution profiles.

g. A detailed account of all experimentation undertaken to prove:

- "ruggedness" of process [investigating such effects as "under" and "over" granulation; "over" and "under" blending; the impact of varying the screen-size(s) and milling rates during the comminuting process(es), etc.], and
- "ruggedness" of formulation (by varying the percentages of all "key" ingredients as permitted by the SUPAC (84) "level 1" change) and a comparison of all "trial" formulations to a "control" (the derived "final formulation") with all batch-sizes identical to those produced at the formulation development stage.

Instead of varying excipient ranges at the level advocated by SUPAC "level 1" change, many formulation scientists prefer to investigate the effect(s) of raising and lowering the percentages of all key excipients by 20% of their level in the final formulation since this is thought to provide more meaningful data reflecting the robustness of the formulation.

Only where the coating confers some functionality to the formulation (controlled or delayed-release), need the coating levels be varied as detailed above.

For each trial formulation, only the pertinent physicochemical attributes need be assessed, such as content uniformity and dissolution profile, the latter employing a discriminatory dissolution method.

> h. An account of the formulation(s) to be progressed to exhibit-batch level, as well as a brief outline of the desired manufacturing pathway.

9. Master Manufacturing Document

This document must be drawn up by a team comprising the formulation scientist and his/her counterpart in the exhibit-batch manufacturing section. Once agreement has been reached, a draft of the "Master" document is forwarded to Plant Operations for comment and acceptance.

A copy of the signed Master Manufacturing Document is then provided to the Process Validation Department for generation of the Process and Cleaning Qualification protocols. In general, the validation process requires at least three batches of each strength of drug product to be assessed whereas the qualification process relates to a single batch of each strength of drug product only.

The Process Qualification Protocols must monitor and control all key processes in the manufacturing pathway such as:

- volume and rate of addition of granulating vehicle,
- exact drying conditions,
- milling rates, screen-sizes, etc.,
- blender rotation speeds and mixing times,
- blend uniformity after blending,
- blend uniformity after discharge of the granule into "holding bins" (to evaluate if active segregation has resulted on discharge), and
- granulometry assessments, bulk and tapped density determinations and loss on drying measurements before and after granule discharge from the blender.

Prior to compressing the batch of granules into tablets at the optimum hardness and speed, the following parameters need to be established:

a. "low" and "high" hardness levels at which the tablets can be compressed meeting all pre-determined acceptance criteria, with specific reference to dissolution profiles,
b. the highest speed at which the particular press can be operated to provide tablets meeting pre-determined acceptance criteria, with specific reference to content uniformity, and
c. humidity and temperature (these are controlled in plant operations by SOPs whereas specific conditions are imposed by product-specific demands during formulation development).

Samples must be drawn at pre-determined intervals during the compression cycle, and then grouped into sets reflecting the beginning, middle, and end of the run. Samples from each stage must be tested for assay, content uniformity, and dissolution profile, in addition to full physical characterization (hardness, disintegration, friability, average weight, individual weights, etc.).

A Qualification Report embracing all the results must be completed once the batch(es) have been manufactured and the analyses completed.

Once the specifications have been set, the API and excipients ordered, received and tested, the necessary tooling received and verified, the Development Report written, the Master Manufacturing Document approved and signed-off, the Process and Cleaning Qualification protocols written and the third month's satisfactory informal stability results (which indicate drug product stability) generated, the exhibit-batch manufacture can be progressed.

10. Exhibit-batch Production

Manufacture of the exhibit batch is the responsibility of the formulation scientist/technician(s) associated with the development of the final formulation together with the scale-up or "technical transfer" team. The formulation and process should be tested by manufacturing a sub-batch using similar equipment as the scale-up equipment and using the same raw materials intended for exhibit-batch manufacture. For example, using a 15 kg capacity granulator, consider the need to manufacture $150, 000 \times 500$ mg tablets (i.e., 75 kg batch-size). In this case, five granulation sub-lots would be required ($75/15=5$) to complete the batch manufacture. Hence one sub-lot or more can be used to optimize the granulation parameters and once this has been done, these parameters are applied to the actual exhibit batch. In so doing, the granulation, drying, milling, and blending operations can be optimized in advance thereby obviating the possibility of problems occurring during subsequent batch production.

This preliminary sub-batch must be progressed to completion and samples submitted to the laboratory to confirm both physical and chemical attributes of the dosage form. Only once the testing has revealed an acceptable comparison to the development batches produced to the same formula and process, should the actual exhibit-batch manufacture be undertaken.

Clearly all exhibit-batch manufacture is required to be carried out under cGMP conditions (85).

Samples from the exhibit batch must be submitted to the laboratory, and only when the pre-determined acceptance criteria have been met (imposed at both "Batch Release" and "Process Qualification" levels), can the generic product be randomized and subsequently packaged.

Randomization is required so that any bias in the manufacturing process is removed. This involves blending a batch of drug product in a blender of sufficient size, for example a "drum roller" blender, following validation of the process. Validation involves the addition and mixing of an equal mass of tablets/capsules of the same size but different colors (red and blue for example) and their distribution evaluated after rotating the blender for a set number of revolutions. The process may be deemed to be validated, if, after three consecutive tests, the different color drug products are uniformly distributed with approximately $\pm 20\%$ variation in the samples drawn (usually 100 units). For example, draw ten 100 tablet samples of the blended lot of red and blue tablets to characterize the blending process. Determine the number of red and blue units in each sample. Acceptable randomization would thus be 30:70 (red:blue) or 70:30 (red:blue). In the case of coated tablets, the rotation of the coating-pan automatically confers acceptable randomization on the coated tablets.

Prior to packaging of the batch(es), the necessary Packaging Documentation needs to be prepared. This describes the actual packaging disposition of each batch. It is customary to package each batch (in its entirety) into equal quantities (taking the actual batch "yield" into account) of each packaging configuration to be utilized after initially removing sufficient quantity for "large pack" evaluation under controlled warehouse conditions. For example, if 50,000 tablets/capsules are removed for "large pack" evaluation, the balance can be packed into various sizes such as 50s, 100s, 250s, 500s, and 1000s. Each of the container closure systems must be of identical material/chemical composition as the large storage container for the 50,000 batch. The packaging operation must be carried out under cGMP conditions, using large-plant equipment.

Once the product has been packaged, samples of each pack size are incorporated into formal stability programmes (usually 40°C/75% RH;

30°C/65% RH and 25°C/60% RH) (86,87) according to a Stability Protocol, which outlines the pack sizes and types to be evaluated, the manufacturer(s) of the packaging components and actual composition thereof, the pre-determined times at which samples must be drawn, the necessary testing that needs to be undertaken and the pre-determined acceptance criteria that are required to be met. Refer to Chapter 6 for further details on stability testing.

Drug product(s) containing APIs sensitive to light should be tested in appropriate photostability chambers according to an approved protocol. Samples of innovator product(s) should be included as controls for each accelerated condition specified.

Details on stability protocols and testing can be found in Chapter 6 of this book.

It is generally considered that the formulation of tablets is somewhat more complex than capsules, hence the manufacturing processes required to produce tablets are necessarily more rigorous than those required to manufacture capsules. The foregoing processes have thus focused on the development of tablet dosage forms whilst at times occasional references were made to capsules. Nevertheless, similar considerations apply to the development of a capsule dosage form.

An appendix is provided herewith to outline the processes and sequences involved in the development of a generic tablet dosage form.

REFERENCES

1. Stowell GW, Whittle RR. Form A of fluoxetine hydrochloride. The present invention provides novel processes for the preparation of Form A of fluoxetine hydrochloride. United States Patent 6,313,350, November 6, 2001.
2. Stowell GW, Whittle RR. Form A of fluoxetine hydrochloride. The present invention relates to novel polymorphic Form A of fluoxetine hydrochloride. United States Patent 6,316,672, November 13, 2001.
3. Lovgren KI, Pilbrant AG, Yasumura M, Morigaki S, Oda M, Ohishi N. Pharmaceutical formulations of acid-labile substances for oral use. United States Patent 4,853,230, filed April 20, 1987.
4. Carlson EJ, Rupniak NM. Treatment of depression and anxiety with fluoxetine and an NK-1 receptor antagonist. United States Patent 6,319,953, filed December 8, 1999.
5. Archer S, Glick SD. Method for treating nicotine addiction. United States Patent 5,965,567, filed July 15, 1997.
6. The Pediatric Exclusivity Provision: January 2001 Status Report to Congress—01. US Food and Drug Administration. Washington, DC: FDA, 2001. http://www.fda.gov/cder/pediatric/reportcong01.pdf
7. Ansbacher R. Bioequivalence of conjugated estrogen products. Clin Pharmacokinet 1993; 24(4):271–274.

8. Meyer MC, Straughn AB, Jarvi EJ, Wood GC, Pelsor FR, Shah VP. The bio-equivalence of carbamazepine tablets with a history of clinical failures. Pharm Res 1992; 9(12):1612–1615.

9. Varley AB. The generic inequivalence of drugs. J Am Med Soc 1968; 206:1745–1748.

10. Lund L. Clinical significance of generic inequivalence of three different pharmaceutical preparations of phenytoin. Eur J Clin Pharmacol 1974; 7:119–124.

11. Welling PG, Patel RB, Patel UR, Gillepsie WR, Craig WA, Albert KS. Bio-availability of tolazomide from tablet: comparison of in vitro and in vivo results. J Pharm Sci 1982; 71(11):1259–1263.

12. Shargel L, Yu Y, eds. Biopharmaceutic Considerations in drug product design. Applied Biopharmaceutics and Pharmacokinetics. 4th ed. New York: McGraw-Hill, Chapter 6, 1999:137.

13. Posti J, Katila K, Kostianen T. Dissolution rate limited bioavailability of flutamide, and in vitro–in vivo correlation. Eur J Pharm Biopharm 2000; 49(1):35–39.

14. Jounela AJ, Pentakinen PJ, Sothmann A. Effect of particle size on the bio-availability of digoxin. Eur J Clin Pharmacol 1975; 8:365–370.

15. Stamm A, Seth P. Fenofibrate pharmaceutical composition having high bio-availability and method for preparing it. United States Patent 6,277,405, filed May 18, 2000.

16. Burger A, Koller KT, Schiermeier WM. RS-Ibuprofen and S-Ibuprofen (dexibuprofen)—binary system and unusual solubility behaviour. Eur J Pharm Biopharm 1996; 42(2):142–147.

17. Prescott JK, Garcia TP. A solid dosage and blend content uniformity troubleshooting diagram. Pharm Technol 2001; 25(3):68–88.

18. J Berman and Blanchard JA. Blend uniformity and unit dose sampling. Drug Dev Ind Pharm 1995; 21(11):1257–1283.

19. Code of Federal Regulations Title 21 Food and Drugs, 21CFR § 211.110 (a). http://www.access.gpo.gov/nara/cfr.index.html.

20. Berman J, Schoeneman A, Shelton JT. Unit does sampling: a tale of two thieves. Drug Dev Ind Pharm 1996; 22(11):1121–1132.

21. Mohan S, Rankell A, Rehm C, Bhalani V, Kulkarni A. Unit-dose sampling and blend content uniformity testing. Pharm Technol 1997; 21(4):116–125.

22. Berman J. The compliance and science of blend uniformity analysis. PDA J Pharm Sci Tech 2001; 55(4):209–222.

23. Guidance for Industry. ANDAs: Blend Uniformity Analysis. US Department of Health and Human Services, Food and Drug Administration, Center for Drug Evaluation Research (CDER), August, 1999. (Withdrawn)

24. Product Quality Research Institute (PQRI) Blend Uniformity Working Group (BUWG). The use of stratified sampling of blend and dosage units to demonstrate adequacy of mix for powder blends. PQRI 2002. www.pqri.org

25. Kulkarni PK, Shah BB, Maitra A, De Vito JM. Pharmaceutical composition containing bupropion hydrochloride and a stabilizer. United States Patent 6,242,496, filed September 28, 1999.

26. Approved Drug Products with Therapeutics Equivalence Evaluations. 21st Ed. Department of Health and Human Services, Public Health Service, Food and Drug Administration, Center for Drug Evaluation and Research, Office of Information Technology, Division of Data Management and Services. Washington, DC, USA: 2001. http://www.fda.gov/cder/ob/default.htm.

27. Abbreviated New Drug Application Regulations: Patent and Exclusivity Provisions. Federal Register, 59, October 3, 1994, 50338–50369.

28. Minsk AG. . To Grant or Not to Grant (180 Days of Market Exclusivity) : That is FDA's Question. Regulatory Affairs Focus, December, 1997:25–27.

29. The United States Pharmacopeia, 26 (2003) Incorporating the National Formulary 21, 12601 Twinbrook Parkway, Rockville, MD 20852: United States Pharmacopeial Convention, Inc.

30. Pharmacopeial Forum. The Journal of Standards Development and Official Compendia Revision, 12601 Twinbrook Parkway, Rockville, MD 20852: United States Pharmacopeial Convention, Inc.

31. The British Pharmacopeia 1 and 2 (2002). Incorporating the 4th edition of the European Pharmacopoeia (2002). London: The Stationery Office.

32. European Pharmacopoeia. Wallingford: Council of Europe, Pharmaceutical Press, 2001.

33. Fabian AC. Guest Editors Note: 4th Symposium on Active Pharmaceutical Ingredients: "Issues at the Development, Production, Regulatory Interface". Drug Inf J 1999; 33(3):737–738.

34. Angelucci LA III. Current good manufacturing practice design trends in active pharmaceutical ingredients facilities. Drug Inf J 1999; 33(3):739–746.

35. Fabian AC. Principles for effective regulatory active pharmaceutical ingredients policy. Drug Inf J 1999; 33(3):747–753.

36. Möller H, Oldenhof C. The active pharmaceutical ingredients starting material (APISM) and other materials in API manufacture: scientifically-based principles for the common technical dossier. Drug Inf J 1999; 33(3):755–761.

37. Oldenhof C. Bulk actives post approval changes (BACPAC): a European perspective. Drug Inf J 1999; 33(3):763–768.

38. DeTora DJ. GMP compliance during development. Drug Inf J 1999; 33(3):769–776.

39. Gold DH, Byrn S. Product quality research initiative and bulk actives post approval change. Drug Inf J 1999; 33(3):777–784.

40. Guideline for Drug Masterfiles. Center for Drug Evaluation Research, Food and Drug Administration, Department of Health and Human Services. Washington, DC, USA: September, 1989. http://www.fda.gov/cder/guidance/dmf.htm

41. Physician's Derk Reference (PDR). Litton Industries Inc. Oradell, NJ, United States of America: Medical Economics Company, A Litton Division, 2003.

42. Compendium of Pharmaceuticals and Specialties (CPS). Ottawa, Canada: Canadian Pharmaceutical Association, 2003.

43. Le Dictionnaire VIDAL®. Paris, France: OVP-Editions du Vidal®, 2001.

44. Repertorio Farmaceutico Italiano. Milan, Italy: Farmindustria, Associazione Nazionale dell'Industria Farmaceutica, CEDOF EDITORE.

45. Rowe RC, Sheskey PJ, Weller PJ, eds. Handbook of Pharmaceutical Excipients. 4th ed. The American Pharmaceutical Association and the Pharmaceutical Press, 2003, Washington, DC, USA and London, UK.

46. Wells JI. Excipient compatibility and resumé. Pharmaceutical preformulation: The physicochemical properties of drug substances. In: Rubenstein MH, ed. Ellis Horwood Series in Pharmaceutical Technology. Chapter 8, 1988:219–219, Ellis Horwood Ltd, Chichester, UK.

47. Brown ME, Antunes EM, Glass BD, Lebete M, Walker RB. DSC screening of potential prochlorperazine–excipient interactions in preformulation studies. J Thermal Anal Calorimetry 1999; 56:1317–1322.

48. Mechtersheimer B, Sucker H. Effects of punch face geometry and different magnesium stearate/talc combinations on tableting properties. Pharm Technol 1986; 10(2):38–50.

49. El-Din EE, El-Shaboury MH, El-Aleem HA. Effect of tablet shape on the in vitro and in vivo availability of directly compressed, non-disintegrating tablets. Pharm Ind 1989; 51(6):694–696.

50. Chowan ZT, Amaro AA, Ong JTH. Punch geometry and formulation considerations in reducing tablet friability and their effect on in vitro dissolution. J Pharm Sci 1992; 81(3):290–294.

51. Tableting Specification Manual. 5th ed. 2215 Constitution Avenue, NW, Washington, DC 20037-2985: Tableting Specification Steering Committee, American Pharmaceutical Association.

52. Carstensen JT. Compatibility testing. Pharmaceutical Preformulation. Lancaster Basel: Technomic Publishing Co. Inc. Chapter 14, 1998; 259–275.

53. Hartauer KJ, Arbuthnot GN, Baertschi SW, Johnson RA, Luke WD, Pearson NG, Rickard EC, Tingle CA, Tsang PKS, Wiens RE. Influence of peroxide impurities in povidone and crospovidone on the stability of raloxifene hydrochloride tablets: identification and control of an oxidative degradation product. Pharm Dev Technol 2000; 5(3):303–310.

54. Watt PR. Tablet Machine Instrumentation in Pharmaceutics: Principles and Practice. In: Rubenstein MH, ed. Ellis Horwood Series in Pharmaceutical Technology, Part 1, 1988: 19–23, Ellis Horwood Ltd, Chichester, UK. Chichester: 1988.

55. Murthy KS, Ghebre-Sellassie I. Current perspectives on the dissolution stability of solid oral dosage forms. J Pharm Sci 1993; 82(2):113–126.

56. Cooper JW, Ansell HC, Cadwallader DE. Liquid and solid interactions of primary certified colorants with pharmaceutical gelatins. J Pharm Sci 1973; 62(7):1156–1164.

57. Hom FS, Veresh SA, Miskel JJ. Soft gelatin capsules I: factors affecting capsule shell dissolution rate. J Pharm Sci 1973; 62(6):1001–1006.

58. Meyer MC, Straughn AB, Mahtre RM, Hussain A, Shah VP, Bottom CB, Cole ET, Lesko LL, Mallinowski H, Williams RL. The effect of gelatin cross-linking on the bioequivalence of hard and soft gelatin acetominophen capsules. Pharm Res 2000; 17(8):962–966.

59. Digenis GA, Gold TB, Shah VP. Cross-linking of gelatin capsules and its relevance to their in vitro–in vivo performance. J Pharm Sci 1994; 83(7):915–921.

60. Bottom CB, Clark M, Carstensen JT. Dissolution testing of soft shell capsules—acetominophen and nifedipine. J Pharm Sci 1997; 86(9):1057–1061.

61. (a) Singh S, Manikandan R, Singh S. Stability testing for gelatin-based formulations: rapidly evaluating the possibility of a reduction in dissolution rates. Pharm Technol 2000; 24(5):57–72; (b) Singh S, Rama KV, Rao, Venugopal K, Manikandan R. Alteration in dissolution characteristics of gelatin-containing formulations: A review of the problem, test methods and solutions. Pharm Technol 2002; 26(4):36–58.

62. Rekhi GS, Eddington ND, Fossler MJ, Schwartz P, Lesko LJ, Augsburger LL. Evaluation of in vitro release rate and in vivo absorption characteristics of four metoprolol tartrate immediate release tablet formulations. Pharm Dev Technol 1997; 2(1):11–24.

63. McGilveray IJ. Overview of workshop: in vitro dissolution of immediate release dosage forms: development of in vivo relevance and quality control issues. Drug Inf J 1996; 30(4):1029–1037.

64. Story DE. The role of dissolution testing in the design of immediate release dosage forms. Drug Inf J 1996; 30(4):1039–1044.

65. Shiu GK. Dissolution methodology: apparatus and conditions. Drug Inf J 1996; 30(4):1045–1054.

66. Qureshi SA. Calibration—The USP dissolution apparatus suitability test. Drug Inf J 1996; 30(4):1055–1061.

67. Grady LT. Third generation dissolution testing: dissolution as a batch phenomenon. Drug Inf J 1996; 30(4):1063–1070.

68. Shah VP. Concept of mapping. Drug Inf J 1996; 30(4):1085–1089.

69. Lucas G. Critical manufacturing parameters influencing dissolution. Drug Inf J 1996; 30(4):1091–1104.

70. Polli JE, Rekhi GS, Shah VP. Methods to compare dissolution profiles. Drug Inf J 1996; 30(4):1113–1120.

71. Guidance for Industry. Waiver of In Vivo Bioavailability and Bioequivalence Studies for Immediate-Release Solid Oral Dosage Forms Based on a Biopharmaceutics Classification System. US Department of Health and Human Services, Food and Drug Administration, Center for Drug Evaluation Research (CDER), August, 2000. http://www.fda.gov/cder/guidance/3618fnl.pdf

72. Rangaiah KV, Chattaraj SC, Das SK. Effects of process variables and excipients on tablet parameters of norfloxacin tablets. Drug Dev Ind Pharm 1994; 20(13):2175–2182.

73. Faure A, Grimsey IM, Rowe RC, York P, Cliff MJ. Methodology for the optimization of wet granulation in a model planetary mixer. Pharm Dev Technol 1998; 3(3):413–422.

74. Faure A, Grimsey IM, Rowe RC, York P, Cliff MJ. Importance of wet mass consistency in the control of wet granulation by mechanical agitation: a demonstration. J Pharm Pharmacol 1998; 50(12):1431–1432.

75. Johansen A, Schaefer T. Effects of interactions between powder particle size and binder viscosity on agglomerate growth mechanisms in a high shear mixer. Eur J Pharm Sci 2001; 12(3):297–309.

76. Klenebudde P. ed. Granulation Theme issue. Eur J Pharm and Biopharm 2001; 52(3):267–394.

77. Badawy SI, Menning MM, Gorko MA, Gilbert DL. Effect of process parameters on compressibility of granulation manufactured in a high shear mixer. Int J Pharm 2000; 198(1):51–61.

78. Emory H, Yoshizawa T, Nishihata T, Mayumi T. Prospective validation of high shear wet granulation process by wet granule sieving method. Part 1. Selection and characterization of sieving parameters for wet granules. Drug Dev Ind Pharm 1997; 23(2):193–202.

79. Emory H, Sakuraba Y, Nishihata T, Mayumi T. Prospective validation of high shear wet granulation process by wet granule sieving method. Part 2. Utility of wet granule sieving method. Drug Dev Ind Pharm 1997; 23(2):203–215.

80. Gayot A, Blouet E, Leterme P, Traisnel N. Study of content and uniformity of content of tablets prepared with a low concentration of active ingredient. Boll Chim Farm 1988; 127:218–220.

81. Steffens KJ, Koglin J. The magnesium stearate problem. Manufacturing Chemist, 1993; 64(12):16–19.

82. Kornchankul W, Parikh NH, Sakr A. Effect of process variables on the content uniformity of a low dose drug in a high shear mixer. Pharm Ind 2000; 62(4):305–311.

83. Shah AC, Mlodozeniec AR. Mechanism of surface lubrication: influence of duration of lubricant–excipient mixing on processing characteristics of powders and properties of compressed tablets. J Pharm Sci 1977; 66(Oct):1377–1382.

84. Guidance for Industry: Immediate Release Solid Oral Dosage Forms. Scale-Up and Post-Approval Changes: Chemistry, Manufacturing and Controls, In Vitro Dissolution Testing, and In Vivo Bioequivalence Documentation. US Department of Health and Human Services, Food and Drug Administration, Center for Drug Evaluation and research (CDER), November, 1995. http://www.fda.gov/cder/guidance/cmc5.pdf.

85. Code of Federal Regulations, Food and Drug Administration, Current Good Manufacturing Practice for the Manufacture, Processing, Packing and Holding of Drugs, 21 CFR—parts 210 and 211. March, 1979, revised April, 1997.

86. Guidance for Industry: Q1A Stability Testing of New Drug Substances and Drug Products. United States Department of Health and Human Services, Food and Drug Administration, Center for Drug Evaluation and Research (CDER), Center for Biologics Evaluation and Research (CBER), ICH, August, 2001. http://www.fda.gov/cder/guidance/4282fnl.pdf

87. ICH Harmonised Tripartite Guideline: Stability Testing of New Drug Substances and Products (Revised). International Conference on Harmonsation of Technical Requirements for Registration of Pharmaceuticals for Human Use, November, 2000. http://www.ich.org/pdfICH/q1arstep4.pdf

88. Moore JW, Flanner HH. Mathematical comparison of dissolution profiles. Pharm Technol 1996; 20(6):64–74.

89. Guidance for Industry: Dissolution Testing of Immediate Release Solid Oral Dosage Forms. US Department of Health and Human Services, Food and Drug Administration, Center for Drug Evaluation and Research (CDER), August, 1997. http://www.fda.gov/cder/guidance/1713bp1.pdf.

APPENDIX 1:

PRODUCT DEVELOPMENT FLOW CHART

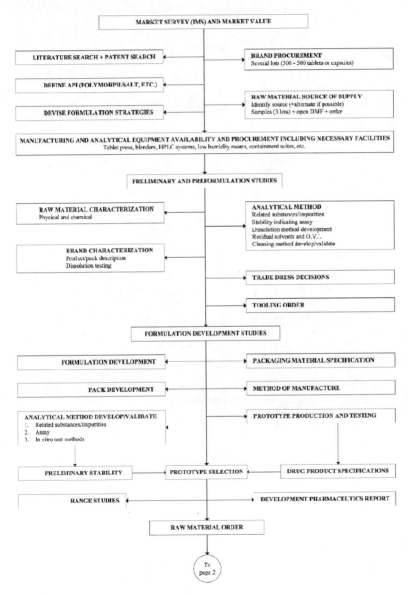

To
page 2

(Continued)

APPENDIX 1: (Continued)

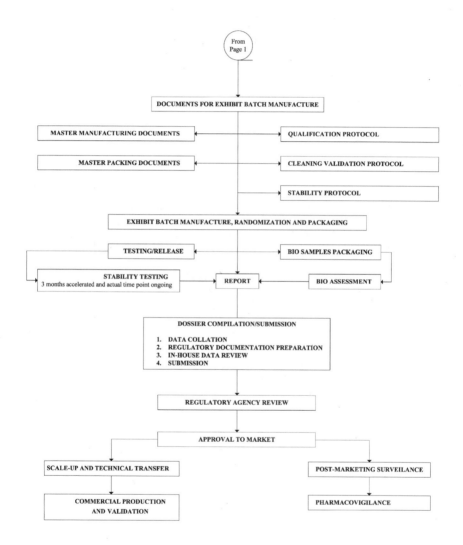

APPENDIX 2:

DESCRIPTION OF THE FORMULATION-DEVELOPMENT AND SUBSEQUENT EXHIBIT-BATCH MANUFACTURE OF A GENERIC SOLID ORAL DOSAGE FORM (TABLET)

A. Acquisition of API and Technical Package Following Comprehensive Literature and Patent Reviews

A full set of all specified impurities, together with a characterized working reference standard and a list of residual solvents must be included with the Technical Package (which is also known as the Open DMF).

B. Preformulation studies on the API

    a. Appearance and color, e.g., a white crystalline powder.
    b. Polymorphism—Differential Scanning Calorimetry (DSC)/ Differential Thermal Analysis (DTA); Infra-red and X-Ray Diffraction; tests to confirm identity and in some cases, the ratio of the desired polymorph-mix.
    c. Solubility in various solvents including water.
    d. Particle-size determination.

It is advisable to set an in-house particle-size specification which is then submitted to the supplier describing the method used. A relevant specification can then be set in collaboration with the supplier. A three-tier specification such as those initially adopted by the Canadian TPD and subsequently by various European Regulatory Agencies, FDA and more recently the Australian Therapeutic Goods Administration is recommended.

A typical specification is described hereunder:

$$d(0.9) \leq 60\,\mu m; \quad 10\,\mu m \leq d(4.3) \leq 25\,\mu m; \quad d(0.1) \geq 2\,\mu m$$

which indicates that 90% of the particles are less than/equal to $60\,\mu m$; the "volume mean" lies between 10 and $25\,\mu m$, while 10% of the particles are greater than/equal to $2\,\mu m$. By setting a three-tier specification as outlined , the normal "bell-shaped" distribution curve is implied.

C. Innovator Product Characterization

    a. Qualitative composition—refer to all available sources of information; e.g., Physicians Desk Reference (PDR), Canadian Compendium of Pharmaceuticals and Specialties (CPS) from which relevant information can usually be obtained.

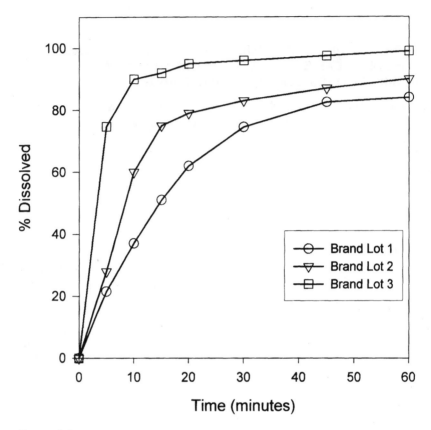

Figure A.1

b. Comparative dissolution rate studies should be conducted on several different lots of commercially available product using an appropriate method (Figure A.1). Dissolution test methods should be adequately discriminatory to identify true differences in dissolution rate and extent, if and where they do exist. Compendial methods (if shown to be discriminatory) are preferable.

D. Formulation Development

Formulation development is undertaken on comparatively small batches between 2000 and 5000 units. Physical data are captured from all batches (LOD, bulk/tapped density, sieve analysis [granule] and hardness, friability, disintegration, compressibility characteristics [tablets]).

Once a satisfactory formulation from a physical characterization point-of-view has been arrived at, samples are submitted to the laboratory for chemical testing (dissolution profile, assay, content uniformity, etc) as deemed appropriate.

It is recommended that dissolution-profile testing be undertaken on samples compressed at several hardnesses, so that the effect of varying the hardness on dissolution profile can be established.

The development process is continued until one of the trial-formulations demonstrates a close correlation to the Brandleader drug product as regards both physical and chemical results.

An example of such a formulation follows.

	Active/Excipients	mg/tablet	Comment
(i)	API	250.0	Required
(ii)	MCC	87.2	Diluent/compressibility enhancer/disintegrant/ dissolution aid
(iii)	Povidone	10.0	Binder (2.5%)
(iv)	Starch	20.0	Disintegrant (5%)
(v)	Citric acid	8.0	Stabilizer
(vi)	Starch (as paste)	20.0	Binder (5%)
(vii)	Stearic acid	4.0	Lubricant (1%)
(viii)	Magnesium stearate	0.8	Lubricant (0.2%)
(ix)	Purified water	q.s.	Granulation liquid

The Handbook of Pharmaceutical Excipients (45) should be consulted to confirm the quantities of the excipients selected.

This formulation is then scaled-up in size to 10,000–20,000 units to provide sufficient samples for stability assessment. The physical/chemical testing is repeated to confirm that the larger batch provides comparable data to that yielded by the smaller trial.

D.1.   Manufacturing Method

Items (i)–(iv), screened through an appropriate mesh (e.g., 20 mesh), are added to a suitably sized granulator/mixer bowl and mixed for 5 min under conditions of high-speed mix and shear. The citric acid (item (v)) is dissolved in a portion of purified water (ix) in a suitable stainless steel container. The starch (item (vi)) is added to form a slurry and then additional boiling purified water is added and vigorously stirred until a paste is formed. The paste is allowed to cool to ambient temperature and then added to the previously mixed powders and granulated for 5 min under controlled conditions using approximately 10–30% by weight of granulating vehicle. The granules are dried in a fluidized bed drier (50–60°C) to a moisture level not exceeding 2% loss on drying. The dried granules are milled and transferred to a suitable tumble-blender. Stearic acid (item (vii)) is screened through a 40 mesh and blended with the granule for 10 min, prior to the addition of Magnesium stearate (also pre-screened through a 40 mesh) with final blending effected for 5 min.

Granules should be analyzed for LOD, bulk and tapped density, and sieve analysis. The resultant granules are compressed to a target weight of 400 mg.

Tablets should be compressed at three hardness ranges [low (2–8 kP), target (6–10 kP), and high (11–17 kP)] and friability, hardness, thickness, disintegration, and dissolution profiles determined.

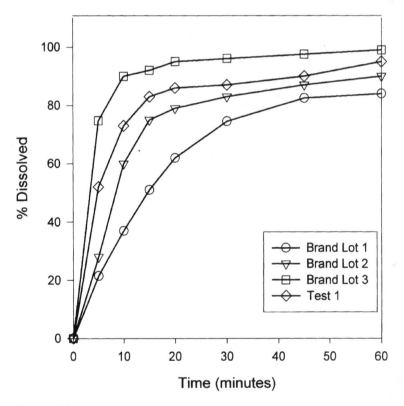

Figure A.2

It is important that tablets meet all physical and chemical acceptance criteria at both the lower and higher end of the hardness range.

Results revealed that the target hardness generic formulation (Test 1) has a dissolution profile similar to Brand Lot 2 which is slower than Brand Lot 3 (faster releasing Brand Lot) and faster than Brand Lot 1 (slowest releasing Brand Lot) (Figure A.2).

E. Range Studies—Investigation of Formulation and Process Variables

Should the formulation prove stable under "accelerated" conditions of high temperature/humidity, "range studies" should be progressed in order to verify and assess the robustness of the formulation and process of manufacture.

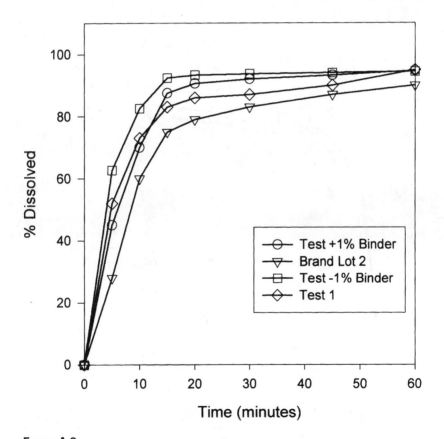

FIGURE A.3

The batch-size should be the same as was employed for formulation-development (2000–5000 units), and the campaign must contain a "control" batch, so that differences in excipient-level and process of manufacture can be correctly interpreted.

E.1.   Formulation Variables

Effect of Binder Level.   Consider the effect of increasing/decreasing the binder level, e.g., by 1% of the total weight of this formulation. Provision for varying the binder level must be accommodated by reducing/ increasing the amount of diluent to maintain a consistent tablet weight. Bulk and tapped density as well as sieve analysis of the final blend should be determined. In addition, granule flow and compressibility must be carefully monitored. Friability, disintegration, and dissolution rate testing must be performed in each case.

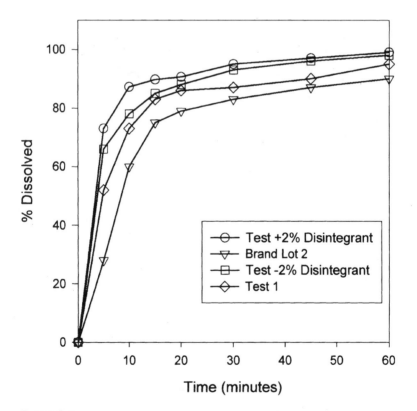

FIGURE A.4

Figure A.3 depicts the dissolution results which show that the effects of binder level variation by 1% were not significant.

However, non-uniform flow was observed in the tablets containing a lower binder concentration. This, together with the fact that the in vitro release rate did not decrease with increased binder concentration, demonstrates that an adequate amount of binder has been used.

Effect of Disintegrant Level. Similar experiments to those described above but increasing and decreasing instead, the level of disintegrant (starch) by a specified amount (for example, by 2%) are depicted. In both trials, compressibility was found satisfactory while dissolution profiles (shown in Figure A.4) were comparable.

This demonstrates that a satisfactory level of disintegrant has been used.

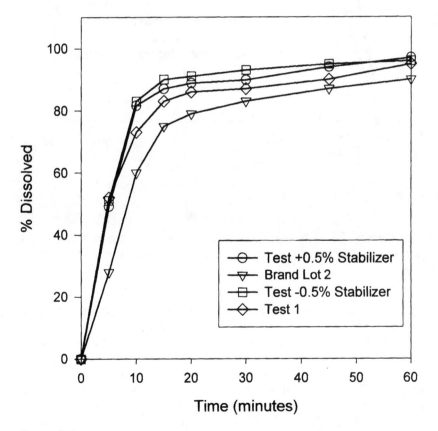

FIGURE A.5

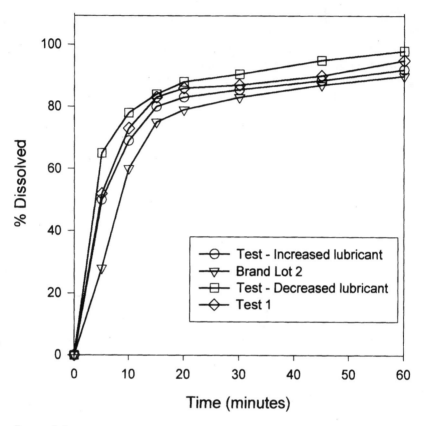

It must be borne in mind that since microcrystalline cellulose itself possesses disintegrant properties, these may well over-ride the effect(s) of starch.

Effect of Other Formulation Components. Further experiments describe the evaluation of a change in stabilizer concentration (increase/ decrease by 0.5%); lubricant (increase stearic acid and magnesium stearate by 1.0% and 0.25%, respectively/decrease stearic acid and magnesium stearate by 0.5% and 0.1%, respectively) and granulation liquid (±10.0%).

Increasing or decreasing the level of stabilizer did not impact the dissolution profiles, but the full impact of change in stabilizer concentration requires assessment by comparing impurity profiles following accelerated stability testing. Changes in the lubricant levels affected the in vitro release profiles and the trial employing lower levels of both lubricants demonstrated

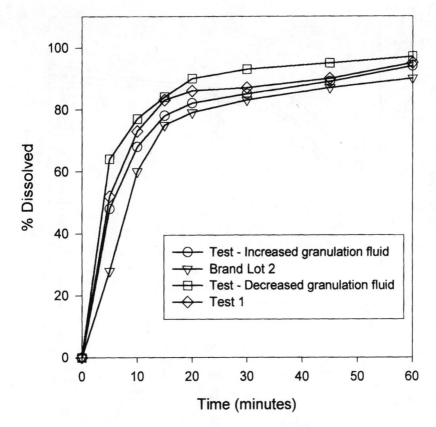

sticking problems. The increase in magnesium stearate had a negative effect on tablet hardness and resulted in a slower dissolution rate.

Changes in the quantity of granulation vehicle had a slight effect on the dissolution profiles, but compression related difficulties such as poor granule flow (due to under-granulation) were apparent.

In general, too little granulating vehicle can result in too fine a granule with associated poor flow, whereas too much granulating vehicle usually results in comparatively coarser granules providing tablets having a slower dissolution profile.

Dissolution profiles for each of these experiments are depicted in Figure. A.5–A.7.

Further increases in lubricant level from 1% to 2.5% of stearic acid and from 0.2% to 0.5% of magnesium stearate to reduce sticking were evaluated and the resultant dissolution profiles can be seen in Figure A.8.

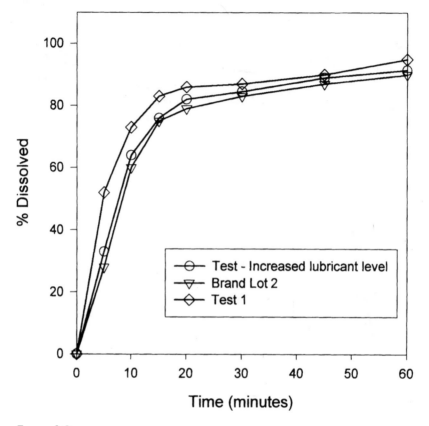

E.2.   Process Variables

Typical variables that should be assessed include amongst others, the granulation process (rate and quantity of granulation liquid addition, mixer and chopper conditions, over/under granulation, and the effects of over/under blending), dry-powder mixing time/speed, and the mesh size used for screening.

Samples from the resultant tablet batches should then be tested for compliance to specifications for hardness, disintegration, friability, and dissolution profile.

Effect of Increasing Lubricant Mixing Time. Doubling the mixing time should be evaluated to establish robustness. In this instance, no adverse effect on in vitro release profiles was seen (Figure A.9).

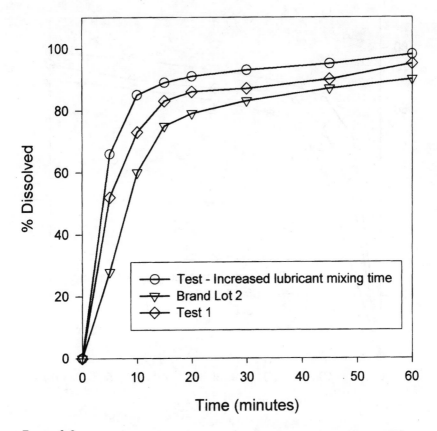

Effect of Increasing Granulation Time.   Similarly, doubling the granulation time was evaluated for robustness and the in vitro release profile is
depicted in Figure A.10.

Once again, no marked changes to the dissolution-profile were
observed. In spite of satisfactory dissolution rates exhibited by the test
formulations (Figures A.9 and A.10) the longer manufacturing times miti-
gate against using these process parameters for full-scale production.

Since the above series of trials challenging both the ranges of excipients
and process variables provided results which confirmed that the formulation
and process were sufficiently robust, and since data were available to
demonstrate that the formulation was stable, exhibit-batch manufacture
(comprising a minimum of 100,000 units or 10% of the envisaged commercial batch size, whichever is the greater) can now be embarked upon.

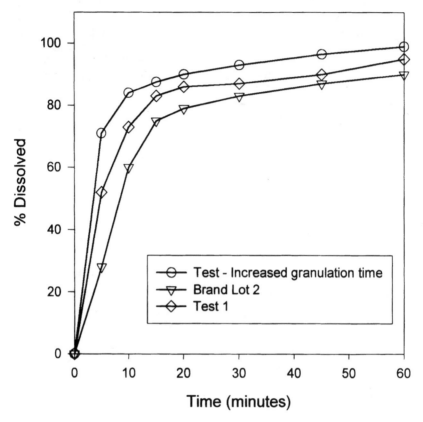

FIGURE A.10

SIMILARITY AND DIFFERENCE FACTORS

As confirmation of acceptance of each formulation of the test product, difference (f_1) and similarity (f_2) factors (88) should be determined by performing the requisite dissolution rate testing on 12 units of each according to the FDA's Guidance on Dissolution Testing of Immediate Release Solid Oral Dosage Forms (89).

The difference factor (f_1) is a measurement of the relative error between the two curves, whereas the similarity factor is a measurement of the similarity in the percent (%) dissolution between the two curves. If the f_1 values range between 0 and 15 and f_2 values range between 50 and 100 the dissolution curves being compared are considered similar or equivalent. The closer f_1 and f_2 are to 0 and 100, respectively, the better the comparability of the curves.

These factors can be determined using the following formulae:

$$f_1 = \left\{ \frac{[\sum |R_t - T_t|]}{[\sum R_t]} 100 \right\}$$

$$f_2 = 50 \log \left\{ \left[1 + \frac{1}{n} \sum w_t (R_t - T_t)^2 \right]^{-0.5} 100 \right\}$$

where: f = fit factor; R_t = reference assay at time t (percent dissolved); T_t = test assay at time t (percent dissolved); n = number of sample points; w_t = weighting at time t (optional); $\sum$ = summation from $t = 1$ to $t = n$.

In the example above, it was noted that the dissolution profile depicted in Figure A.8 for a formula with increased lubricant levels represented the formulation of choice. Calculated f_1 and f_2 values for this formulation relative to Brand Lots 1, 2, and 3 indicate that the test product is equivalent, in vitro, to only Brand Lot 2. The table below is a summary of all the calculated f_1 and f_2 values.

	Brand Lot 1 vs. Test[a]	Brand Lot 2 vs. Test[a]	Brand Lot 3 vs. Test[a]
f_1	39.8	4.6	14.4
f_2	30.5	72.8	42.2

[a]Test formulation—increased lubricant, depicted in Figure A.8 (target hardness 6–10 kp)

5

Scale-Up, Process Validation, and Technology Transfer

Salah U. Ahmed and Venkatesh Naini
Barr Laboratories, Inc., Pomona, New York, U.S.A.

Dilip Wadgaonkar
Interpharm, Inc., Hauppauge, New York, U.S.A.

1. INTRODUCTION

Generic product development aims at the formulation of a product bio-equivalent and/or pharmaceutically equivalent to a specific reference product. The product should be manufacturable and the manufacturing process must be validatable. The formulation and manufacturing process developed by scientists at a pilot scale must be capable of manufacturing large scale production batches. Scale-up and technology transfer are crucial steps in pharmaceutical product development process. During this stage, process validation activities establish the robustness and limitation of the manufacturing process and assure that the product consistently meets predetermined quality attributes. Critical process steps and product properties are thoroughly examined as per a validation protocol. The process is scaled up to a batch size close to the bio-batch or production batch after the initial development work. Experimental design may be employed to study and optimize critical parameters. Depending on the complexity of manufacturing processes involved, such as dry blending, wet granulation, roller compacting, tableting, encapsulation, coating, etc., appropriate process parameters are carefully monitored and viable ranges established. The process may be further validated at the extremes of these ranges to set up controls for the manufacturing process.

The manufacturing process is transferred to the manufacturing floor typically prior to product approval and launch. This may involve further scaling up of the batch size, change in manufacturing equipment and site, and other changes in the manufacturing process. These changes may be considered minor or major in a regulatory review and may require additional work, as per the scale-up and post-approval changes (SUPAC) guidelines.

This chapter will focus on several issues related to these essential processes in generic drug development. All topics related to process validation, optimization, equipment qualification, personnel training and documentation, cleaning validation, and analytical and regulatory issues are discussed.

2. PRODUCT DEVELOPMENT

Scale-up, process validation, and technology transfer take place at the terminal phase of the development cycle of generic products. However, the performance of these phases is somehow affected by formulation composition, manufacturing process, and in process and finished product specifications. Since many of these are established at early stages of product development, it is imperative to address formulation and process development issues that have pronounced effect on the manufacturing process, scale-up, and process validation. Once a product is identified for generic development, various activities are initiated and a stepwise approach is taken in the development work, to include the following:

1. Preformulation studies
2. Formulation development and process optimization
3. Scale-up of manufacturing process
4. Process validation
5. Process demonstration and technology transfer
6. Documentation
7. Post-approval changes—SUPAC

2.1. Preformulation Studies

The manufacturing process utilized is affected by the physical properties of the drug and the excipients (1). If the drug component comprises the predominant portion of the dosage form, its physico-chemical properties would influence mixing, granulation, flow, compression, and coating. Typically, the composition of the branded product is used as a guide in selecting excipients for the corresponding generic product. The formulation scientist needs to perform extensive work to identify the particular type or grade of excipient suitable for the product. The type of excipient not only influences dissolution and bioequivalence, it also affects the manufacturing performance of the product and quality attributes of the finished dosage form. Excipient selection must be made keeping in mind the final manufacturing process (2) that will be utilized for the product. This critical parameter is often ignored in the early stages of product development, and many a time, improper selection of excipients contributes to significant scale-up and process validation problems. Table 1 provides a list of common excipients and their effect on manufacturing process and scale-up.

The formulation scientist must carefully review various physico-chemical parameters of the excipients and dosage form in selecting excipients and the manufacturing process. Excipients not only help in achieving target quality attributes, but proper excipient selection also influences the manufacturing process, ability to scale-up, and successful process validation. In many instances, various excipient grades are available differing in particle shape, size, degree of crystallinity, moisture content, flowability, and compressibility. Careful evaluation of the excipient properties in light of manufacturing process to be utilized is important. For example, lactose is available in several grades including anhydrous direct tableting grade, a free flowing spray-dried form (Fast-Flo®), and several particle size grades of lactose monohydrate. While lactose monohydrate is useful both for dry mix and wet granulation, the anhydrous type should be avoided in aqueous granulation processes. The conversion of the anhydrous form to the monohydrate during aqueous granulation may contribute to about 5.3% weight gain, resulting in accountability problem. Drug and excipient properties critical to the manufacturing process and scale-up of solid dosage forms are identified here:

1. Particle shape, size, and surface area
2. Solubility in water or granulating fluid
3. Crystallinity and polymorphism
4. Moisture sensitivity and equilibrium moisture content (EMC)
5. Bulk and tapped densities of major components
6. Flow parameters
7. Granulation properties
8. Drying properties
9. Compaction behavior

TABLE 1 Properties of Some Commonly Used Diluents for Tablets and Capsule
Products

Component	Remarks
Dibasic calcium phosphate	Used in dry granulation (unmilled type) and wet granulation (milled type). Provides good hardness. High amounts in formulation may cause tablet hardness sensitive to compression force and may lead to lamination and capping.
Dibasic calcium phosphate dihydrate	Used in dry granulation (unmilled type) and wet granulation (milled type). Under certain conditions can lose the water of crystallization. Due to irreversible dehydration, accelerated stability of formula containing high amounts may lead to erroneous results.
Tribasic calcium phosphate	Used in dry granulation and wet granulation. Not a clearly defined chemical entity. High amounts in dry mix tablet formulation may cause capping and lamination.
Calcium sulfate	Used in dry granulation and wet granulation. Avoid anhydrous form that may convert into dihydrate during wet granulation or under accelerated stability conditions.
Microcrystalline cellulose, cellulose powder	Used in dry granulation and wet granulation. Improves tablet hardness if added dry. Improves granulation process and helps avoid batch failure due to overgranulation. High amounts in formulation increase tablet thickness.
Dextrose anhydrous (granular), dextrose monohydrate	Used in direct compression, primarily in chewable tablets. Both the anhydrous and monohydrate forms are hygroscopic in nature and require handling at relatively low %RH. Tablets are likely to harden on aging. Offers improved stability for drugs prone to oxidation. The anhydrous form may convert to monohydrate form on long term exposure to high humidity.
Lactose monohydrate	Used in dry granulation and wet granulation. Select appropriate particle size grade. Fine particle grade impalpable lactose improves mixing uniformity of potent micronized drugs. Excessive amount may cause compression problem.
Lactose anhydrous	Anhydrous form in wet granulation may convert into monohydrate and contribute to a 5.2% higher accountability. Spray-dried formulation is more susceptible to Maillard reaction and browning effect.
Maltodextrin	Various grades of particle size and bulk density exhibit difference in flow properties. Produces hard tablet. Formulations containing relatively high amount of maltodextrin should be processed at less than 50% RH. Tablet hardness may increase with aging.

(Continued)

Table (Continued)

Component	Remarks
Mannitol	Used for chewable and regular tablets. It has high bulk density and good flow property. Not hygroscopic in nature. Produces hard tablets. Can be used in direct compression and wet granulation.
Starch	Used in dry mixing or wet granulation. A wide variety of grades vary in particle size, rate of hydration, compaction properties, etc. Facilitates mixing of potent drug and colors if used as a diluent. High amounts in formulation may result in poor compression and lubricant sensitivity. Avoid high amounts of lubricant.

2.1.1. Particle Shape, Size, and Surface Area

Particle shape and size and the size distribution of drugs and excipients significantly affect their flow behavior. This is especially significant for products intended for manufacturing using the direct compression method. Spherical particles are ideal for dry mixing, whereas rod and needle shaped particles are difficult to process in dry mixing. Most pharmaceutical components (drug and excipients) are in between these two extremes. It is important to perform a thorough microscopic evaluation of the drug and other major components of the formulation. The shape, size, surface morphology, and relative amounts of these components should be considered in selecting the manufacturing process. It is also possible to modify particle characteristics of materials for ease in the manufacturing process. For example, Povidone K90 is available as flakes and powder. The powder form is suitable for dry mixing whereas flakes can be used as a binder dissolved in the granulating medium.

2.1.2. Solubility in Water and Granulating Fluid

If the manufacturing process utilizes the wet granulation method, the solubility of the drug and major excipients in the granulation fluid is critical. Water-soluble components solubilize during the granulation process with water and may form a doughlike mass, quickly resulting in overgranulation, making drying difficult. If all components are water insoluble, the resulting granules will be soft due to poor binding, and the advantage of wet granulation to improve flowability and content uniformity remains questionable. A powder mass containing a mixture of soluble and insoluble components in appropriate proportions provides excellent granules. For components that are susceptible to hydrolysis or require drying under milder temperatures, use of organic solvents such as ethanol or isopropanol may be the only alternative.

2.1.3. Crystallinity and Polymorphism

Many pharmaceutical materials exist in multiple crystal forms or polymorphs. Depending on the crystallization solvent and conditions, the drug substance may also form hydrates or solvates, usually referred to as pseudopolymorphs. A careful evaluation of the crystal form of a drug substance is important to avoid processing effects on crystalline transformations and amorphous to crystalline transitions, which may have implications for finished product stability, dissolution behavior, and bioavailability. Prior to formulation development, it is important to establish the crystal properties of drug substances and critical excipients using x-ray powder diffraction (XRPD) and thermal analysis. These techniques can also be used to monitor crystallinity changes during processing and in the finished product on storage.

2.1.4. Moisture Sensitivity and Equilibrium Moisture Content (EMC)

Since water is typically used as the granulating medium, the moisture binding property and EMC of the formulation play a significant role in the granulation and drying processes. Hygroscopic materials such as polyethylene glycol (PEG), if present in large amounts in a formulation, are difficult to dry. In some instances, the hygroscopic nature of the drug may necessitate the use of special manufacturing facilities with strict humidity control. The EMC of major components generally dictates the final moisture content of the dried granules. The drying rate (drying curve) of a formulation can be theoretically estimated from the drying rate of the individual components. If the drug component is moisture sensitive, water should be avoided as the granulating medium. In such cases, ethanol or isopropanol may be used; however, the drying equipment (tray or fluid bed dryers) needs to be explosion proof, since alcohols have low flash points. Furthermore, the rate and extent of alcohol emission to the environment must be considered, since EPA has strict guidelines on alcohol emission that may vary from state to state.

2.1.5. Bulk and Tapped Densities of Major Components

The bulk and tap densities of formulation components are easy to measure, yet provide valuable guidance for the flow property and in selecting the manufacturing equipment and processes. Low bulk and tap densities indicate poor flowability of a material and require additional processing such as roller compaction or wet granulation, to avoid production problems. Bulk densities of the major components affect the load size in the processing equipment, i.e., mixture, dryer, etc., and govern the batch size. Eq. (1) can be useful in estimating the batch size from the bulk densities of the individual components:

$$B = V/\{(a/D_a) + (b/D_b) + (c/D_c) + \cdots\} \qquad (1)$$

where B is the batch size (kg), V is the working volume of the mixer (L), a, b, c are the major components in the batch in kg, and D_a, D_b, D_c are the bulk densities of the components $a, b, c, \ldots$ in kg/l. Once the value of B is known, a batch size of 80–105% of the B value can be considered to be optimum depending on the type of equipment used.

2.1.6. Flow Parameters

The flow characteristics of individual components and the blend remarkably affect the manufacturing process. In addition to bulk and tapped densities, other flow characteristics such as angle of repose, angle of spatula, floodability, and flow through a hopper should be evaluated for the blend. Typically, a material with high angles of repose, low floodability, and low bulk density contributes to manufacturing problems if not processed using wet granulation, slugging, or roller compaction.

2.1.7. Granulation Properties

The granulation properties of the drug and excipients are important for products manufactured using wet granulation. The ability of formulation components to hold the granulating fluid (kg of fluid per kg of material) can be measured alone or in combination. This information can be utilized in estimating the granulating fluid requirements for a scale-up using Eq. (2):

$$W = (A_1B_1 + A_2B_2 + A_3B_3 + \cdots) \times f \qquad (2)$$

where, $A_1, A_2, A_3, \ldots$ are the amounts (kg) of components 1, 2, 3, $\ldots$ in the batch, B_1, B_2, B_3 are fluid holding capacities (kg of fluid per kg of material) of components 1, 2, 3, $\ldots$, and f is a scale-up factor typically between 0.7 and 1.

The amount of fluid required for the scale-up batch depends on other factors such as type of equipment, atomization, rate of addition, etc.

2.1.8. Drying Properties

The drying performance of a material is its ability to dry from a wet mass formed during the granulation process. Although various processing conditions such as drying temperature, relative humidity of the drying air,

air velocity, and exposed granule surface area affect drying, the material affinity for the solvent dictates the drying rate. Small to medium molecular weight materials with low to medium water solubility lose water quickly and dry rapidly, e.g., lactose, calcium sulfate, and dicalcium phosphate. Some materials such as high molecular weight povidone, hydroxypropylmethylcelluloses (HPMCs), starch, hydrophilic gums, and PEG are difficult to dry, especially if present in relatively high proportions in the formulation. However, an efficient drying technique such as use of the fluid bed dryer, is useful to overcome the drying problem for otherwise difficult to dry material.

2.1.9. Compaction Behavior

The compaction behavior of tablet components plays a key role in the tableting process. The compaction property of the final blend is dictated by the individual components. Manufacturing processes such as wet granulation, roller compaction, and slugging can significantly alter compaction characteristics. In early preformulation, compaction behavior can be conveniently studied using an instrumented single station press (Carver or Korsch).

2.2. Formulation Development and Process Optimization

Development of a pharmaceutical product is essentially a technique wherein the physico-chemical properties of the active ingredient, excipients, and the manufacturing process are manipulated to achieve desired quality in the finished dosage form. Certain goals such as product specifications, ease of manufacturing, cost, etc., are defined for a dosage form prior to initiating development work. The traditional trial and error approach may be less dependable and more time consuming, and often provides an apparently (or marginally) acceptable formulation and process rather than an optimum one. In today's competitive market, statistically designed experiments in product and process development are becoming increasingly necessary since they are quick and cost effective. Analysis of data from statistically designed experiments, also known as optimization, enables one to generate a mathematical model and contour plots that elucidate formulation and process parameters affecting the product properties. Various software packages (3–4) are available for designing experiments, developing polynomial equations, and generating contour plots. However, the success of statistical design depends on careful selection of factors, the ranges of these factors, and a specific experimental design to be utilized in the study. Optimization requires statistical skill in addition to an understanding of the physico-chemical properties of the materials involved and their effect on the process. Identification of independent (cause) and dependent (effect) variables, and an understanding of the expected relationship between cause and effect, is crucial to the success of this approach. A brief description of experimental design applicable in process optimization is given here. A list of process variables and their responses relevant in solid dosage forms is given in Table 2. For understanding the effect of multiple process variables on product quality, factorial design is widely chosen in process optimization. The independent variables in experimental design must be carefully selected, since increasing the number of variables results in a large increase in the potential number of experiments. However, the number of experiments can be minimized by carefully modifying the design and level of factor to be studied. Accordingly, one may choose to use full factorial, fractional factorial, orthogonal composite, nonorthogonal symmetrical composite, central composite, or noncentral composite design. The composite design is made by adding extra points (star points) to the two level factorial or fractional factorial design. If n is the number of factors to be studied, the additional points required for the composite design is $2n + 1$, one at the center and the remaining $2n$ in pairs along the coordinate axis. An example of a central composite design is given in Table 3. In this orthogonal composite design, the value of 1.215 (axial point) at the six composite points (experiments 9–14) depends on design specifics such as number of factors and experiments. Table 4 shows the total number of experiments and the values of axial points for several designs. It also shows the benefit of a composite design over a three level factorial design. The increase in number of experiments due to an increase in the number of factors is significantly higher in case of a three level factorial design compared to a fractional composite design.

Details of experimental design are available in various publications (6–9). It is recommended that some initial trials be performed for gaining an understanding into the effect of each variable. This adds tremendous value in developing a design with minimal number of experiments, yet capturing the optimum formulation and processing conditions.

2.3. Scale-Up of Manufacturing Process

High speed production of large scale batches using modern technology has become essential in minimizing manufacturing costs to improve the profit margin in today's competitive market. Increases in batch size or scale-up are accomplished by using larger, high speed equipment that may require adjustments to the process parameters established using small scale equipment. However, the in process and finished products must meet all predetermined specifications, and the products from scaled-up and pre-scaled-up batches must be physically and chemically equivalent.

TABLE 2 Parameters to be Considered in the Optimization of the Pharmaceutical Process for Oral Solid Dosage Forms

Pharmaceutical unit operation	Independent variables (process parameters)	Dependent variables (product attributes)
Dry mix	Mix time, impeller/chopper speed, lubricant mix time	Flow parameters,[a] mix uniformity, compression parameters,[b] dissolution.
Wet granulation	Mixer load, granulating fluid addition rate, total amount of granulating fluid, impeller/chopper speed, wet mix time	Granulation end point, torque, granule size distribution, drying rate, dissolution.
Drying (tray dryer)	Powder bed thickness, i.e., load/tray, total load in oven, temperature, %RH of drying air, duration in oven	Moisture content (LOD) as a function of time, drying time, end point (%LOD)
Fluid bed drying	Load, inlet temperature, bed temperature, airflow rate, %RH of drying air	Moisture content (LOD) as a function of time, drying time, end point
Milling/screening	Screen size, blade setting (hammers/knives), blade speed, feed rate	Particle size, bulk/tapped densities, flow parameters,[a] dissolution
Compression	Precompression force, compression force, machine speed, dwell time, force feeder setting	Tablet hardness, weight variation, dissolution
Encapsulation	Tamper setting, aspiration setting, encapsulation speed	Capsule weight variation, dissolution
Roller compaction	Roller type, clearance between rollers, compaction pressure and speed	Particle size, bulk/tapped densities of milled compacts, dissolution
Film coating	Spray rate, pan speed, airflow rate, pan load, inlet/exhaust temperatures Spray nozzles and guns assembly	Coating weight gain, weight variation, dissolution
Fluid bed coating	Inlet temperature, bed temperature, airflow rate, spray rate, rotor speed	Coating weight gain, assay to determine drug layering, bead bulk/tapped densities, dissolution

[a]Angle of repose, bulk/tap density, flow through hopper, etc.
[b]Compression force versus hardness, ejection force, maximum hardness achievable, capping, sticking, etc.

TABLE 3 Example of Central Composite Design Used in Optimization

Experiment	Factor A	Factor B	Factor C	$n = 3$
	Factors (independent variables)			
1	+1	+1	+1	Factorial design (2^n)
2	+1	+1	−1	
3	+1	−1	+1	
4	+1	−1	−1	
5	−1	+1	+1	
6	−1	+1	−1	
7	−1	−1	+1	
8	−1	−1	−1	
9	+1.215	0	0	Composite points ($2n$)
10	−1.215	0	0	
11	0	+1.215	0	
12	0	−1.215	0	
13	0	0	+1.215	
14	0	0	−1.215	
15	0	0	0	Center point

The first and foremost step in scaling up is the establishment of batch size requirements. Batch sizes in generic industries are often determined arbitrarily and may require further scale-up or scale-down, depending on future market demand. It is important to identify an optimal batch size, rather than the maximum size possible. Several factors that need to be considered in determining batch sizes are:

TABLE 4 Number of Experiments and Axial Points for Several Designs

Variables	Three level factorial	Composite design	
n	3^n	$2^n + (2n + 1)$	Axial point
2	9 (full factorial)	9 (full factorial)	1.000
3	27 (full factorial)	15 (full factorial)	1.215
4	81 (full factorial)	25 (full factorial)	1.414
5	243 (full factorial)	43 (full factorial)	1.596
5	81 (1/3 fractional)	27 (1/2 fractional)	2.041
6	729 (full factorial)	77 (full factorial)	1.761
6	243 (1/3 fractional)	45 (1/2 fractional)	1.724

1. Market demand
2. Available production capacity
3. Raw material cost
4. Stability of the finished product
5. Analytical testing issues

The manufacturing process and operating parameters utilized in smaller batch manufacturing are to be considered in the scale-up plan. The technology and equipment used in the development process often impose several constraints during scale-up work. Since pharmaceutical products are usually manufactured using several discrete batch processes, it would be appropriate to discuss the scale-up of each of these batch processes. The following are some of the most common pharmaceutical unit processes used in the manufacture of solid dosage forms:

1. Dry blending
2. Wet granulation
3. Roller compaction
4. Milling
5. Drying
6. Extrusion/spheronization
7. Compression
8. Encapsulation
9. Coating

2.3.1.   Dry Blending

Dry blending is often the most common unit operation in the pharmaceutical industry, due to its simplicity and use of less-complicated equipment. However, several factors are to be considered while scaling up a dry blending process. Equipment considerations such as blender type and design, blender load, mixing speed, use of auxiliary dispersion equipment such as intensifier bars, choppers, etc., and the dynamics of mixing action produced within the mixer need cautious evaluation. Formulation variables that influence a mixing operation are particle shape and size distribution and cohesiveness of major components, their bulk densities, and the order of addition of various components into the blend. Mixer selection should be based on the cohesive nature and the flowability of the ingredients to be mixed. Low shear tumble blenders, such as the V-blender (Patterson–Kelley) and double cone blender (Gemco) are well suited for mixing free flowing and slightly cohesive powders. V-blenders are widely used in handling potent drugs due to their ability to mix by geometric dilution. However, improper load (too high or too low), as well as wide difference in particle size and shape, may lead to segregation. Intermediate shear mixers such as the orbiting screw mixer (Nauta), ribbon blender, and shaking mixer (Turbula) are used for blending free flowing powders that are moderately cohesive. High shear mixers (Diosna, Collette-Gral) are recommended for powders that are highly cohesive and not free flowing, to break up lumps and improve mixing. The drug components are often sandwiched between other excipients, to improve dispersion and prevent loss of drug (especially low dose) due to their preferential adherence to the interior surface of the mixer. If the drug ingredient is highly cohesive, it may be beneficial to screen the premix prior to final blending. To avoid segregation of free flowing powders, particle size reduction of one or more components of the blend prior to mixing may be essential. This can be achieved by including a milling step in the compounding process. Geometric dilution is often employed to aid uniform mixing of low dose actives. In scaling up in tumble blenders of similar design, rotational speed may be reduced relative to the smaller mixer, to achieve dynamic similarity, i.e., similar Reynolds number. However, mixing times may be increased to provide a constant number of rotations (10). In some instances, increased mixing times may have an adverse effect on the manufacturability of the product, e.g., tablet capping due to overlubrication or increased segregation potential due to overmixing. Several manufacturers of tumble blenders provide scale-up factors for determining the mixing times in large mixers from experiments performed in small mixers. Table 5 summarizes the working capacities, blender load levels, and scale-up factors for twin-shell blenders without the agitator bar. These factors are useful in calculating mixing times during blending scale-up operations.

Usually such factors are not applicable when dry blending in high shear mixers. These are very efficient in mixing cohesive powders by increasing shear forces and thus improving deagglomeration efficiency. Mixing times are usually kept constant when scaling up in such mixers, providing constant impeller tip speeds. However, segregation potential increases in high shear blending, especially when components with large differences in particle shapes and sizes exist within the blend. Blend uniformity is usually recognized by following a well-established sampling plan based on the mixer type and geometry. The drug content assay of the sampled blend must meet pre-established criteria.

2.3.2. Wet Granulation

The wet granulation process offers several advantages over dry blending. Wet granulation provides effective distribution of low dose actives, increased densification of low bulk density materials, and improved flowability and compressibility of the final blend. Although several wet processes are

TABLE 5 Scale-up Factors for Selected Twin-Shell Blenders[a]

Working capacity (ft^3)	Total capacity (ft^3)	Shell diameter (in.)	Scale-up factor[b]
1	1.68	11.5	1.3
3	5.16	16.5	1.6
5	8.42	19.5	1.7
20	33.83	31.0	2.0
50	82.95	42.0	2.2
100	174.95	54.0	2.8

[a]Source: Patterson–Kelley Company, East Stroudsburg, PA.
[b]blending time in large blender $= \frac{\text{scale–up factor for larger blender}}{\text{scale–up factor for small blender}} \times$ blending time in small blender

feasible, granulation employing low/high shear mixers and a fluid bed are more often used in the pharmaceutical industry and will be discussed here.

Low shear granulation employs mechanical agitation at slow speed, such as in ribbon and paddle mixers, planetary mixers, orbiting screw mixers, and sigma blade mixers, or rotating granulators such as twin-shell blenders with an intensifier bar/spray head combination. These granulators usually produce fluffier granules with lower bulk density compared to high shear granulation, which may be the desired property for some products. Important factors to consider during scaling up in rotating blenders include liquid addition rate, spray droplet size, intensifier bar/spray head design, and shell and intensifier bar rotation speeds.

Successful scale-up in mechanically agitated low shear mixers depends on the ability to monitor the granulation process during liquid/binder addition and subsequent wet massing. Researchers have suggested several techniques, such as infrared moisture sensors, torque measurement, current monitoring, and power consumption, to detect granulation end point. Luenberger (11) identified five distinct phases during wet granulation in a planetary mixer using a power consumption meter, and stated that useful granules could be produced during the third phase. Landin et al. (12) and Faure et al.(13) used the concept of relating power consumption to several process and formulation variables in scaling up granulations in planetary mixers. The variables evaluated were impeller rotation speed and dimensions, wet mass density and consistency (measured using a mixer torque rheometer), and fill ratio (height of wet mass/bowl diameter). Using data obtained for mixers of different sizes, they came up with a relationship between the power number (Np) and Reynolds number (Re), Froude number (Fr), and the bowl fill ratio i.e. $Np = f(Re, Fr, \text{fill ratio})$. The Reynolds number represents the ratio of dynamic to viscous forces, whereas the Froude number represents the ratio of dynamic force in the mixer to the gravitational force. This relationship is useful in predicting consistent granulation end points during scale-up (12,13).

Lately, wet granulation in high shear mixer granulators is the method of choice due to shorter process time, superior granule properties, and process reproducibility. High shear granulation offers several advantages, including densification of low bulk density materials, lower binder requirement, control over porosity of granules, and easy cleaning. Several designs of bowls, impellers, and choppers are available from different manufacturers. The most common design has the impeller shaft rotating in the vertical plane. The impeller could be bottom driven inside a fixed bowl, such as in Diosna, Fielder and Powrex mixers. In a variation of this design, the impeller and chopper are top driven inside a detachable bowl, such as in Collette-Gral, GMX/Vector and Bohle mixers. Several of these granulators are available as single-bowl systems where the product can be granulated and vacuum/microwave dried inside the same bowl. Some of these mixer/granulators have been thoroughly characterized with respect to their processing parameters (14–16).

Several reports have been published dealing with the issue of scale-up in high shear granulators (17–22). Some important parameters and terminology used in the scale-up of high shear granulation are depicted in Figure 1. Table 6 lists critical scaling-up parameters for Collette-Gral high shear mixer/granulators. Rekhi et al.(23) studied the effect of scale-up in three geometrically similar Fielder high shear mixers. They concluded that three factors govern successful scale-up: (a) impeller speed adjustment to keep the tip speed constant, (b) linearly scaled-up amount of granulating fluid based on batch size, and (c) granulation time adjustment based on ratio of impeller speeds in different sized mixers (23). In one study, normalized impeller work was used for predictable end point control in high shear granulation containing high amounts of microcrystalline cellulose(21). Horsthuis et al. (19) studied lactose formulations in 10, 75, and 300 l Gral mixers and obtained different power curves for each of these mixers, since Gral mixers are not geometrically similar. However, they found good correlation between granulation end point and the Froude number (Fr), but not a predictable relation with tip speed or relative swept volume. Landin et al. (22) and Faure et al. (18) used relationships between dimensionless numbers (power, Reynolds and Froude numbers) and bowl fill ratio for scaling up in fixed bowl (Fielder) and removable bowl (Gral) mixers, respectively, with some success. In spite of such reports on scale-up in high shear mixers, this topic is not a well-developed science (17).

Fluid bed is the other commonly used approach for wet granulation and concurrent drying. Some important factors to consider during scaling

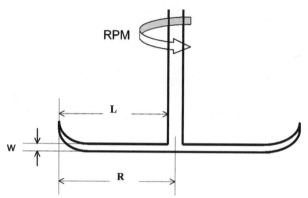

Angular velocity, $\omega = 2\pi/60 * RPM$

Tip Speed, $V_T = \omega * R$

Projected Impeller Blade Area, $A_b = N * w * L$

Swept Volume $= \omega * R * A_b$

Relative Swept Volume $(s^{-1}) = W/(\rho\omega R A_b)$

Bowl Fill Ratio $= \rho R_b^3/W$

Power Number, $Np = \Delta P/(\rho\omega^3 R^5)$

Reynold's Number, $Re = \rho\omega R^2/\mu$

Froude Number, $Fr = R\omega^2/g$

Where:

R is the Impeller radius

N is the number of blades on impeller

L is the effective length of blade

w is the width of blade

W is the amount of wet mass

ρ is the wet mass bulk density

Rb is the bowl radius

ΔP is the net power consumption of the mixer

μ is the wet mass consistency

(measured using torque rheometer)

g is the gravitational constant

FIGURE 1   Description of several scale-up terms and concepts used in wet granulation.

up in a fluid bed granulation are: fluidization velocity of process air, ratio of granulation spray rate to drying capacity of fluidization air, inlet air temperature, bed depth, and droplet size of the sprayed binder (24,25). It is recommended that one use the same inlet temperature, droplet size, and air velocity (airflow/area of screen size) and achieve the same fluidization level when transferring the process from smaller equipment to production scale. The spray rate for the larger unit may be calculated using Eqs. (3)(26):

$$R = (B/b) \cdot r \tag{3}$$

where R is the spray rate in the larger unit (g/min), B is the bowl screen area for the larger unit (ft^2), b is the bowl screen area for the smaller unit (ft^2), and r is the spray rate in the smaller unit (g/min).

TABLE 6 Upscaling Gral High Shear Mixer-Granulators[a]

GRAL (liters)	10	25	75	150	300	400	600	1200
Bowl content (l)	7.9	27.0	77.0	153.0	303.0	400.3	614.0	1166.0
Height in cm	18.0	26.0	38.0	45.0	60.0	60.0	70.0	70.0
Width in cm	24.6	37.5	52.5	69.2	84.2	96.2	109.2	149.2
Radius of mixing arm in cm	11.9	18.0	25.4	33.5	40.0	46.0	52.5	72.50
Width of mixing blade in cm	2.5	3.5	5.5	7.0	6.0	6.4	8.0	11.0
Thickness of mixing blade in mm	6.0	8.0	12.0	15.0	15.0	20.0	20.0	25.0
Surface of mixing blade in cm^2	23.8	48.0	110.0	198.0	197.0	242.0	348.0	610.0
Angle of inclination of mixing blade	55.0	55.0	55.0	55.0	55.0	55.0	55.0	155.0
Speed 1 (rpm)	430	283	206	145	120	103	95	79
Speed 2 (rpm)	650	423	300	218	185	155	135	119
Tip speed @ speed 1 in m/s	5.36	5.33	5.48	5.09	5.03	4.96	5.22	6.00
Tip speed @ speed 2 in m/s	8.10	7.97	7.98	7.65	7.75	7.47	7.42	9.03
Froude number @ speed 1	2243	1470	1099	718	587	497	483	461
Froude number @ speed 2	5125	3283	2330	1623	1396	1127	975	1047
Swept volume in dm^3	0.764	2.356	7.536	18.234	20.998	30.129	45.635	130.842
Relative swept volume@ Speed 1 (s^{-1})	0.6931	0.4116	0.3360	0.2880	0.1386	0.1292	0.1177	0.1477
Relative swept volume@ Speed 2 (s^{-1})	1.0477	0.6152	0.4894	0.4330	0.2137	0.1944	0.1672	0.2226

[a]Source: Collette-Gral Division, Niro Pharma Systems, Columbia, MD.

Small adjustments may need to be made to such theoretical calculations to account for differences in bed depth (26).

2.3.3. Roller Compaction

Roller compaction involves continuous compaction of drug–excipient blends into ribbonlike compacted material, which is subsequently milled, lubricated, and either compressed into tablets or encapsulated. Roller compaction as a pharmaceutical unit process has several advantages over other particle enlargement techniques such as wet granulation. For high dose water-soluble drugs, aqueous granulation is not the preferred method due to inadequate water distribution and formation of lumps. For drugs that are chemically unstable in the presence of water or the granulating solvent, roller compaction offers an effective alternative for granulation. Several equipment and process parameters have to be addressed when scaling up a roller compaction granulation:

1. Roll configuration or design—smooth, corrugated, or concavo-convex
2. Roll diameter, nip angle, and area
3. Screw feed rate
4. Roll speed
5. Compaction pressure
6. Feed screw orientation—vertical or horizontal
7. Vacuum deaeration of precompacted blend.

Nip angle is the angle made by the powder being compacted by the rolls in the compaction (nip) region (27). Highly compressible materials have large nip angles compared to incompressible materials. Corrugated rolls have a higher capacity to drag material between the rolls compared to smooth rolls and hence provide greater compaction forces. It is important to maintain these design similarities between compactors when scaling up from a laboratory or pilot unit to the production equipment. Sheskey et al. (28) studied the effect of several process parameters during scale-up of an HPMC containing controlled release matrix formulation of theophylline. They scaled up the roll speed by maintaining the same linear velocity as that obtained from the laboratory unit, thus providing similar dwell time for the material in the compaction zone. Keeping the parameter force/linear inch constant, the compaction force was scaled up to the production unit. Finally, the screw speed to roll speed ratio was kept constant for all units. Using these scale-up factors, reproducibly consistent granules and finished tablets were produced in the laboratory, pilot, and production scale equipment. However, dissolution similarity (f_2 factor) was only established for the laboratory and pilot scale formulations but not the production scale one. Based on the predicted in vivo performance of these formulations, the authors concluded that the production scale equipment produced a faster releasing formulation compared to smaller units (28). For successful scale-up, it is important to evaluate compaction rate (kg/min) and applied pressure as well as milling parameters, i.e., milling rate (kg/min/screen surface area) and mill speed. The particle size distribution of the processed material provides valuable information about the reproducibility of the process.

2.3.4. Drying

Drying is a commonly employed unit process in the manufacture of solid dosage forms. Drying in the pharmaceutical industry is accomplished using static bed dryers (tray or truck ovens), moving bed dryers (turbo-tray dryers), fluidized bed dryers, and spray dryers. More recently, single-pot systems incorporating high shear mixer-granulators with vacuum, microwave, or infrared drying are also becoming popular (29). Depending on the desired final product characteristics, any of these dryers may be employed. The commonly used dryers in solid dosage form manufacture, i.e. tray dryers and fluid bed dryers, are discussed here. Critical factors governing the drying process include the EMC of the formulation blend, the exposed surface for solvent transfer, and the vapor carrying capacity of the drying air. Psychrometric principles for calculating the vapor carrying capacity of air should be employed in scaling up a drying process. Some important factors while scaling up a tray-drying process are the number of trays, product load per tray (bed thickness), temperature, and humidity of the circulating air inside the oven. Maintaining the same bed thickness (kg/tray) and providing similar drying air capacity will facilitate successful scale-up from pilot scale to production scale dryers.

Fluid bed drying processes are more challenging to scale up (30,31). Several factors impacting the drying process include airflow, air temperature, bed depth, and product characteristics. The fluidization air volume should be adjusted to keep the same air velocity (ft/min) between different sized units. Inlet temperature and dew point and the product bed temperature in the scaled-up larger batch should be maintained as in the smaller unit. However, some adjustments to these parameters may be made, depending on relative differences in fluidized bed heights between different units.

2.3.5. Milling

Milling is commonly employed to reduce particle size of granulations, bulk drug substances, and excipients to facilitate uniformity of powder mixes.

This process is also used to manipulate the dissolution profile of the dosage form. Following wet granulation, wet milling is often employed to improve the granule surface area for more efficient drying. Sizing of granulation is typically accomplished using either low energy mills (oscillating granulators) or high energy mills (hammer, conical, and centrifugal impact mills). The hammer mill is the most common and versatile machine used in the manufacture of solid dosage forms. It consists of either a swinging or fixed rotor, which forces the material against a fixed screen. Various factors such as rotor shaft configuration (vertical/horizontal, fixed/swinging), granulation feed rate, blade type (hammer or knives), rotor speed, and screen size and type (mounting, screen thickness, rasping, or regular screens) are to be considered while scaling up a hammer mill process. The particle size of the milled material is smaller than the corresponding screen size since particles enter the screen holes tangentially (32). This effect is more pronounced at higher rotor speeds. Narrow particle size distributions are obtained at medium and high speeds compared to low speed. Several scale-up factors for Fitzpatrick hammer mills are summarized in Table 7.

A conical mill (Comill) consists of a conical screen inside a milling chamber along with a rotating impeller. Comills use less energy than hammer mills and are well suited for milling heat sensitive and difficult to mill materials. The impeller configuration (knife, round, or sawtooth edges), impeller speed, and screen size affect the properties of the milled product in a comill.

2.3.6. Extrusion/Spheronization

This technique is primarily used to produce approximately spherical granules in a narrow particle size range for controlled release products. The major advantage of this process is its ability to incorporate high drug loads in the granulation. The dry mixing, wet granulation, and drying aspects of this technique are similar to those of most pharmaceutical wet granulations.

During the extrusion process, a wet mass (granulation) is forced through dies and shaped into small cylinders (extrudates). As the mass comes out of the extruder, the extrudate particles usually break at even length due to their own weight. The granulating fluid usually serves as the binder to form the extrudate, which is usually a small strand or rod shaped like spaghetti. The wet extrudate is further processed in the spheronizer to form pellets. Extruders come in a variety of sizes and shapes, and are usually classified according to the feeding mechanism. These include screw, gravity, and pistons to feed the wet mass into the extruder. The wet mass is essentially a wet granulation of the drug with a binder and inert excipient, which is

TABLE 7 Scale-Up Parameters for Fitzpatrick Hammer Mills[a]

Model	Chamber			Rotor			Machine limits		Approximate dimensions[b]		
	Capacity factor[c]	Nominal width (in.)	Screen area (in.[d])	Diameter (in.)	Number of blades	Tip speed factor[d]	Maximum rpm[e]	Maximum horse power[f]	Length (in.)	Width (in.)	Height (in.)
L1A	0.07	1	8.5	5.4	8	1.42	9000	0.5	18.5	15.4	20
Homoloid	0.4	2.5	43	6.625	12	1.73	7200	10	38	30	52
M5A	0.7	4.5	76	8	16	2.09	4600	3	32	26	55
D6A	1	6	109	10.5	16	2.75	4600	5	35	31	63
DASO6	1	6	109	10.5	16	2.75	7200	15	42	30	66
DKASO12	2.36	12	257	10.5	32	2.75	6000	30	48	32	66
FASO8	1.83	8	199	14.375	16	3.7	6800	40	60	36	72
FASO12	2.83	12	309	14.375	24	3.7	6000	75	60	36	72
FASO20	4.85	20	529	14.375	48	3.7	3000	75	60	44	72
FHASO20	4.85	20	529	14.375	48	3.7	3600	75	60	44	72
HASO30	9.05	30	986	17.25	80	4.45	2400	150	68	60	75

[a]*Source*: Fitzpatrick Company, Elmhurst, IL.
[b]With typical throat and 36 in. (91.4 cm) between chamber discharge and floor.
[c]Throughput relative to Model D-6 at same tip speed.
[d]Tip speed = factor × operating speed.
[e]With type 125, 225, or 425 blades.
[f]With V-belt driven at maximum rpm.

typically a plastic deforming material like microcrystalline cellulose (Avicel). The extruder screen size directly controls the final particle size of the pellets, thus controlling drug dissolution and release.

The formulation components, amount of granulating fluid, and consistency of the wet mass can also affect the final particle size of the pellets. The extrusion speed and water content are also critical factors in achieving a desired pellet configuration. Hasznos et al. (33) have studied some factors influencing the characteristics of pellets made by an extrusion/spheroniza-spheronization process. They concluded that the extrusion variables are less important than granulating fluid level and spheronization parameters (33). Goodhart et al. (34) studied the effect of extruder design on the extrusion process. The effects of granulating fluid, end plate open area, number of mixing anvils, and screw speed were evaluated, and it was found that the granulation fluid type and end plate open area had a significant effect on granulation density. Extrusion can be a batch, semibatch, or continuous process. Most pharmaceutical extrusion processes are batch processes. The following extrusion parameters are usually monitored and are useful during scale-up:

1. Feed rate
2. Feed temperature
3. Extrudate temperature
4. Coolant
5. Inlet/outlet temperature
6. Die temperature
7. Compression pressure

The twin screw type extruder is available in different sizes for pilot scale to production size batches. The rate of extrusion can range from 30 to 2000 kg/hr. Scale-up factors depend on size of extruder wet granulation final consistency.

A spheronizer is a device made up of a vertical hollow cylinder with a horizontal rotating disk. The extrudate is charged onto the rotating disk and broken into small segments, which further spin on the disk, causing them to deform and form small spherical particles. The transformation of the wet mass into spherical particles is due to frictional forces between the particles and the equipment walls. Spheronization disks play an important role in the shape and size of the final spheres. Disks normally come in two types, cross-hatched and radial. Radial disks are relatively faster and are commonly used. Spheronization is a batch process, the spheronized material being further dried in either fluid bed or tray dryers. The residence time in the spheronizer depends on the feed rate from the extruder. Often, the extrusion operation is a continuous one and several spheronizers are used to speed up the process. The variables affecting the overall spheronization process include:

1. Spheronizer size
2. Feed rate (charge)
3. Disk type and speed
4. Residence time

In general, compared to the extrusion variables, the spheronization variables affect the end product more significantly. Higher disk speed and increased residence time increase the mean diameter of pellets. This combination also tends to produce more spherical particles. Higher charge reduces moisture loss during the process and produces more plastically deformed particles. Several investigators have studied the various factors affecting the extrusion/spheronization process using factorial design and response surface methodologies (35–37). The effect of disk speed and residence time was examined, and it was found that the friability of pellets increased with increased residence time. Increase in screen size reduces friability. Besides these variables, several formulation variables significantly control the final pellet attributes. Scale-up in the spheronization process is generally dependent on the size of the spheronizer. No systematic studies demonstrating scale-up factors in extrusion/spheronization have been reported in the literature. The effect of scale-up is reduced because the process is primarily considered as a batch process.

2.3.7. Compression

Tablet compression process parameters are independent of the batch size, and large scale batches are typically manufactured by performing compression for a longer period of time or using multiple tablet presses. Modern tablet presses are capable of self-adjustment to produce a consistent finished product during high speed production. However, scaling up a tableting operation is still largely empirical. Scale-up parameters have been suggested in the literature based on dwell times and total work of compaction. Superior powder flow is obviously very important for producing uniform tablets in a high speed production press. Levin (38) has identified the following critical factors that effect tablet properties due to increased compression speeds during production:

1. Decrease in tensile strength of tablets with viscoelastic materials like Avicel
2. Decreased tablet friability

3. Increased tendency for lamination and capping
4. Increase in tablet temperature, which may be important for formulations containing low melting point materials

In addition, several equipment parameters (differences in tablet press designs) require attention during tableting scale-up. These include capacity of the tablet press to compress to constant thickness (most commercial presses) or to constant compression force (Courtoy), method of die filling (gravity or force feeder), size of feeder chamber, and speed of the feeder motor. During formulation development, it is important to evaluate the compaction parameters of a particular formulation (40). These would include the effect of compaction force and speed and lubricant sensitivity of the formulation (level of lubricant and lubrication time). Formulations that are sensitive to overlubrication and also requiring a force feeder should be evaluated more thoroughly. In such instances, it is useful to estimate powder residence times inside the force feeder using Eq. (4) as described below:

$$T = 1000(Vd)/wrn \tag{4}$$

where T is the powder residence time in the force feeder (min), V is volume of the force feeder (ml), d is the bulk density of the blend (gm/ml), w is the tablet weight (mg), r is the tablet press speed (rpm), and n is the number of stations.

The residence time of such formulations should be minimized since additional mixing inside the feed frame will adversely affect tablet hardness and/or dissolution. These trials should be performed preferably on tablet presses similar to production machines. If the tablet crushing strength declines rapidly with increasing compaction force or higher speed of compaction, the tablet may face potential capping problems during production. The rate of decrease in crushing strength with small changes in lubricant levels provides insight into the lubricant sensitivity of the formulation, which may later cause problems during production. More recently, small scale sophisticated equipment such as compaction simulators or single station rotary press simulators (Presster™, MCC Corporation) are available for determining various compaction parameters during trial batches. The advantage of machines like the Presster™ is that they match compression forces and dwell times of any production size press and mimic its punch displacement profile. Using a Presster™ and the approach of dimensional analysis, Levin and Zlokarnik (39) successfully predicted parameters for scaling up from a Manesty Betapress (16 stations) to a 36 station Fette P2090 production press.

2.3.8. Encapsulation

Many issues important in the scale-up of the tableting operation are also important during encapsulation. Some of the problems encountered during encapsulation scale-up include powder flowability, content uniformity, plug formation and densification behavior, powder feed, and lubricant sensitivity of the blend. In addition, the type of encapsulation equipment used during development and large scale production often dictates the success of scale-up, due to differences in operating mechanisms (41). Most equipment use the piston tamp method for plug formation along with either a dosator (MG2, Zanasi and Matic) or a dosing disk (Hofliger-Karg). The equipment may also be differentiated based on its motion during encapsulation, such as intermittent motion machines (Zanasi E and F series and Hofliger-Karg) or continuous motion machines (MG2, Zanasi Z500 series, Farmatic). The type of production scale equipment usually dictates the powder blend properties that need to be built into a formulation. Ullah et al. (42) evaluated the scale-up of cefadroxil encapsulation from the Zanasi LZ-64 development scale to Hofliger-Karg GFK-1500 production machine. The blend containing 1% magnesium stearate as lubricant gave satisfactory dissolution in the small batch low speed encapsulated product but showed severe slowing down of dissolution in the high speed production batch. Further investigation revealed that the powder tamping process used in the high speed machine exposed the powder to additional shear forces, causing overlubrication and resulting in slower dissolution. It was concluded that reducing the amount of magnesium stearate to below 0.6% resulted in a powder blend less prone to shear effects in the large scale encapsulation process (42).

2.3.9. Coating

Coating is typically the last step in the production process. Coating performance significantly affects the appearance of the finished product and other quality attributes influencing the drug release and in vivo performance. Although sugar coating and microencapsulation approaches are available, film coating using pan and air suspension techniques is the most popular and will be the focus of this section. Coating serves many purposes, including taste masking, improving product appearance, light and moisture protection, and controlled release (enteric or sustained release). Several water-soluble and -insoluble polymers and ready to use coating systems are commercially available. In recent times, water based aqueous systems have gained in popularity due to environmental issues related to the use of organic solvents. However, for certain applications, organic coatings may be the only alternative.

Pan coating in the batch approach uses a perforated pan equipped with a special air handling system and coating guns. Campbell and Sackett (43) have identified several key parameters affecting the film coating process in a perforated pan:

1. Process airflow and evaporative rate
2. Inlet/exhaust temperature
3. Spray rate, number of guns, spray pattern, and achievable droplet size
4. Pan speed
5. Atomization air pressure
6. Product load and gun to bed distance

Pans may be partially perforated (Hi-Coater®—Vector/Freund and Driacoater®—Driam) or fully perforated (Procoater®—Glatt, Fastcoat®—O'Hara and Accela Cota®—Thomas Engineering). Many of these machines are available from small laboratory scale to production size equipment. Table 8 summarizes the dimensions and brim volumes for Vector Hi-Coater® pans available in production sizes. One of the important factors governing the scale-up of the film coating process is the evaporative capacity of process air. The following equation (Eq. (5)) is useful in estimating this evaporative capacity during scaling up (43):

$$R = \frac{\text{CFM} \times C_p \times d \times \min \times [(T_{in} - T_{out}) - H_L(T_{in} - T_{out})]}{\text{LHV}} \tag{5}$$

where R is the evaporative rate of water in lb/hr, CFM is the actual process airflow in ft^3/min, C_p is the specific heat capacity of air (0.241 Btu/lb m °F),

TABLE 8 Standard Hi-Coater® (Vector Corporation, Marion, IA) Production Coating Pan Specifications[a]

Model	Pan diameter (in.)	Brim volume (l)	Number of spray guns	Process air CFM range	Overall dimensions (in.) ($W \times D \times H$)
HC-100	39	90	2–3	530–880	$55 \times 63 \times 69$
HC-130	52	225	4	765–1275	$65 \times 68 \times 80$
HC-150	59	350	4	1016–1690	$70 \times 78 \times 89$
HC-170	67	550	4–6	1270–2120	$81 \times 88 \times 99$

[a]Source: Vector Corporation, Marion, IA.

TABLE 9 Scale-Up Considerations in Pan Coating[a]

Parameter	Scale-up equation
Batch size	Batch size $(L) = \dfrac{\text{Batch size (S)}}{\text{volume(S)}} \times$ volume (L)
Pan speed	Pan speed $(L) = \dfrac{\text{Pan diameter (S)}}{\text{Pan diameter (L)}} \times$ pan speed (S)
Spray rate/gun	Spray rate $(L) = \dfrac{\text{Gun spacing (L)}}{\text{Gun spacing (S)}} \times$ spray rate(S)/gun Assuming same gun to bed distance
Spray time	Spray time $(L) =$ Spray time $(S) \times \dfrac{\text{batch size (L)}}{\text{batch size (S)}} \times \dfrac{\text{spray zone (S)}}{\text{spray zone (L)}}$
Airflow	Airflow $= \dfrac{\text{total spray rate (L)}}{\text{total spray rate (S)}} \times$ airflow (S)

L = large coating pan; S = small coating pan.
[a]*Source*: G. Sackett, BASF/Vector Coating Seminar Notes, Vector Corporation (www.vector-corporation.com), Marion, IA.

d is the density of air (0.0634 lb m/ft^3), min is the number of minutes per hour, T_{in} is the process inlet temperature, T_{out} is the process outlet temperature, H_L is the percent heat loss of the system, and LHV is the latent heat of vaporization of water (1040 Btu/lb m).

Sackett (44) has discussed in detail the factors governing scale-up of a pan coating process, and these are summarized in Table 9. Usually scaling up involves increasing the spray rate with a corresponding increase in the pan speed. However, in such circumstances, tablet attrition and overwetting should be closely monitored.

Air suspension or fluid bed coating is a more complicated process and requires additional parameter optimization compared to pan coating. Air suspension coating can be broadly classified into three types of processes: (1) Top spray, (2) rotary fluid bed with tangential spray, and (3) Wurster/zbottom spray. Top spray is well suited for large particle coating, while rotor and Wurster processes are applicable for fine particle coating and drug layering onto nonpareil seeds. Operating parameters important in pan coating such as process airflow (fluidization), inlet/outlet temperatures, and spray rate are also important for air suspension coating. Besides factors such as rotor speed in rotary fluid bed, partition height and distribution plate inside the Wurster column play a critical role in scale-up (45,46). A summary of scale-up parameters and other considerations during air suspension coating are summarized in Table 10 (44).

TABLE 10 Scale-Up Considerations for Air Suspension Coating Processes[a]

Parameter	Scale-up equation
Batch size	Top spray and rotary processes:
	Batch size (L) $= \dfrac{\text{volume (L)}}{\text{volume (S)}} \times$ batch size (S)
	Wurster process:
	Batch size = product bulk density [column volume − (number of partitions × volume of partitions)]
Fluidization air volume	Air volume (L) = air velocity (S) × cross sectional area (L)
	Air velocity (S) = air volume (S)/cross sectional area (S)
Spray rate	Total spray rate (L) = spray rate (S)/gun $\times \dfrac{\text{number of guns (L)}}{\text{number of guns (S)}}$
Rotor speed	Rotor process:
	Rotor speed (L) = rotor speed (S) $\times \dfrac{\text{rotor diameter (S)}}{\text{rotor diameter (L)}}$

L = Large fluid bed system; S = small fluid bed system.
[a]*Source*: G. Sackett, BASF/Vector Coating Seminar Notes, Vector Corporation (www.vector-corporation.com), Marion, IA.

2.4. Process Validation

Process validation for solid oral dosage forms in the generic industry is required by the Current Good Manufacturing Practices (cGMP) for finished pharmaceuticals (47). According to the FDA's guideline (48), process validation is defined as follows:

> Process validation is establishing documented evidence which provides a high degree of assurance that a specific process will consistently produce a product meeting its pre-determined specifications and quality characteristics.

Process validation establishes the flexibility and constraints in the manufacturing process controls in the attainment of desirable attributes in the drug product while preventing undesirable properties. It involves systematic work and documentation of performance so that the crucial parameters in the pharmaceutical manufacturing process will consistently produce a quality product. Although process validation features in the final stages of product and process development, several validation concepts are incorporated in the laboratory/pilot scale development, scale-up and process optimization stages. Typically, for generic solid dosage forms, the formulation development team is closely involved with the validation personnel at the early stages of product development. Depending on the complexity of the manufacturing process, several equipment, process, and product parameters are optimized at a smaller scale compared to the production size batch. Once the formulation composition and manufacturing process are optimized at the smaller scale, the next stage involves optimizing the process at a larger scale, usually using production equipment. At this stage, the experience and input of the production personnel are vital for the success of the project. The production batches may be of the same size or greater than the bio-batch, which has a minimum requirement of 100,000 units as per the FDA (49). During this process, the product and process are challenged to the extremes of the proposed specifications and necessary adjustments made if required. Depending on the pharmaceutical unit operations (dry blending, wet granulation, milling, roller compaction, compression, encapsulation, coating, etc.), several critical process parameters are varied while the product properties are measured and evaluated thoroughly.

The formal validation process may begin during the manufacture of the bio-batch if the intended production batch size is the same. As per the regulatory requirement, three consecutive production size batches are required for the completion of process validation (50). The objective is to qualify and optimize the process using full scale production equipment. The validation is performed as per a written and approved validation protocol defined by the FDA guideline (48) as follows:

A written plan stating how validation will be conducted, including test parameters, product characteristics, production equipment, and decision points on what constitutes acceptable test results.

This protocol driven, three batch validation usually forms part of what is termed as prospective process validation. Here, the validation is conducted before the distribution and sale of a new generic product or an existing product made using a revised manufacturing process, which can affect the product or quality attributes of the finished product. Many companies validate their manufacturing process well ahead of approval, if the risk is considered minimal and if it is expected that the FDA review letter will not challenge the process or product specifications. In some instances, a retrospective process validation is performed on existing products to establish that the manufacturing process is under control satisfactorily. A third option of concurrent process validation is used during the production stage to develop further acceptance criteria for subsequent in process control. The last and fourth option of process validation is revalidation and is used when changes in process equipment or manufacturing site occur. Usually these changes are deemed major or minor as per the SUPAC guidelines (51) and a decision is made as to the requirement for revalidation. The SUPAC guidelines are discussed in greater detail in later sections of this chapter and elsewhere in this book.

A well-written validation protocol forms the backbone of the validation master plan and should include the following items:

1. Purpose of the study
2. Personnel responsibilities
3. Critical process steps
4. Critical process and product parameters
5. Sampling plan
6. Testing plan
7. Acceptance criteria

The writing of the validation protocol is the primary responsibility of the validation department. However, critical process and product attributes and their specifications are included after careful consultation with the product development team and engineering and production personnel. In the manufacture of solid dosage forms, depending on the complexity of the manufacturing process, several process and parameters may be specified for testing. A general guideline for process and product parameter inclusion in the process validation protocol is summarized in Table 11. The amount of samples collected and tested will depend on the type of manufacturing process used, e.g., blend content uniformity to validate a blending operation or dissolution profile to validate tablet hardness range. Mixing of powder components is probably the most common manufacturing step in pharmaceutical industries. The mix uniformity of the blend is evaluated from samples, which itself may contribute to the outcome of the result due to variation in the sampling procedure, device, amount of sample, etc. The problem in blending validation due to sampling error has been investigated and various recommendations made (52–59). As per the Barr decision, the recommended sample size in blending validation is three times the weight of an individual dose. If difficulties arise, larger samples may be taken, but the petitioner should provide adequate justification for doing so and the FDA reviews such applications on a case-by-case basis. In many instances, when validating low drug content noncohesive powders blends, it was found that although failing blend content uniformity, the compressed tablet or capsule product satisfactorily met finished product content uniformity. This

TABLE 11 Process and Product Parameters Considered During Generic Solid Dosage Form Manufacture

Pharmaceutical unit operation	Process parameters	Product attributes
Wet granulation	Granulator loading capacity Binder or liquid addition rate Impeller/chopper speed (high shear mixer) Wet massing time	Granule size distribution
Tray drying	Number of trays loaded (tray dryer)	Moisture content (LOD) Solvent residue such as alcohol used in granulation
Fluid bed drying	Loading capacity (fluid bed dryer) Inlet temperature Bed temperature Airflow rate	
Milling/screening	Screen size Milling throughput Use of hammers/knives Mill speed	Particle size of milled granules Bulk/tapped densities of the milled granules
Blending	Blender capacity Mixing time Speed of mixing	Blend content uniformity in mixer Blend content uniformity in drums (after discharge) Particle size and bulk/tapped densities of final blend
Compression	Tablet press speed (speed study) Compression force (hardness study) Weight and compression force (thickness study) Powder feed rate into dies (hopper study)	Tablet weight, thickness, hardness and friability Content uniformity Dissolution/disintegration Assay or potency
Encapsulation	Fill volume Tamper setting Encapsulation speed Aspiration setting	Capsule weight Content uniformity Dissolution Assay or potency

(Continued)

Table 11 (Continued)

Pharmaceutical unit operation	Process parameters	Product attributes
Roller compaction	Roller type	Granule size of milled compacts
	Clearance between rollers	Bulk/tapped densities of milled compacts
	Compaction speed and pressure	
Film Coating	Spray rate	Coating weight gain
	Pan speed	Weight variation analysis (Mocon)
	Airflow rate	Assay or potency
	Pan loading	Dissolution/disintegration
	Inlet/exhaust temperatures	Mottling or speckling
	Spray guns assembly and nozzles	
Fluid bed coating	Inlet temperature	Coating weight gain
	Bed temperature	Assay to determine drug layering
	Airflow rate	Content uniformity
	Spray rate and type (top, Wurster/bottom or tangential)	Bead bulk/tapped densities, porosity etc.
	Rotor speed	Dissolution
Liquid filling hard gelatin capsule	Product temperature during filling	Capsule weight
	Product congealing rate	Content uniformity
	Viscosity of fill	Dissolution
	Fill volume	Assay or potency
	Encapsulation speed	

has led to the belief that several inadequacies and sampling biases exist with the present techniques. The thief employed for blending validation may itself cause segregation and perturbation of the blend when sampling in static powder beds. Although several alternative sampling devices have been suggested in the literature (57), the sampling thief is still the most commonly used sampling device during blending validation. FDA's recently issued draft guidance to the industry for blend uniformity analysis for ANDAs is based on amount of active component present in the dosage unit and suggests the use of tighter limits for blend uniformity (90–110% of label claim with RSD $\leq$ 5%). This will provide added assurance that such a blend will meet the USP criteria for finished dosage units of 85–115% label claim with RSD $\leq$ 6% (58). Recently, Prescott and Garcia (59) proposed a troubleshooting diagram for blend content uniformity in solid dosage forms. They attribute poor blend and/or content uniformity to possible causes such as nonoptimum blending, thief sampling error, segregation after discharge, analytical error, and insufficient particle distribution and suggest solutions to these problems. However, the presence of a validation engineer trained in the proper technique for sampling powders in blenders and drums is important. A well-laid-out validation protocol for solid dosage forms should include details of the sampling plan for the specific equipment being employed. The number of samples (blender and/or drum), sampling locations, and sampling thief to be used are specified in the protocol. The collected samples are tested using validated analytical methods and the results analyzed using appropriate statistical tests.

During the manufacturing process, several samples are collected and tested to validate the process and product parameters identified in Table 11. The samples are subjected to appropriate testing using approved analytical methods. These validation studies are thoroughly documented and summarized in a process validation report. The validation report should include the following items:

1. Aim of the validation study
2. List of raw materials used in the manufacturing process
3. List of manufacturing equipment
4. Critical process steps studied
5. Data collected and their analysis
6. Product and process acceptance criteria evaluation
7. Statistical analysis of results
8. Recommendations by the validation department
9. Attachments of copies of the executed batch records

The manufacturing process is released for regular production after careful evaluation of the validation documentation.

2.4.1. Equipment Qualification

Equipment qualification is an important part of the overall validation program. Qualification for new equipment or a new facility incorporates extensive testing, verification, and documentation to establish that a particular piece of equipment meets the design specifications, and its installation is appropriate to execute the functions required (60). The procedures involved not only assure the current state of the equipment, but also help maintain them in peak working condition and calibration status. Equipment qualification usually involves the following aspects:

1. Installation qualification (IQ)
2. Operation qualification (OQ)
3. Performance qualification (PQ)

Before performing IQ, a prequalification is done to assess the vendor specifications and process and product requirements of the equipment. Once the decision is made to purchase the equipment, preparations are made for IQ in consultation with the vendor and the engineering department. The plant engineering department is responsible for designing the working area as per the manufacturing requirements and the necessary plumbing. As the equipment is installed, each of its components is qualified to perform according to the vendor's specifications. All vital gauges, charts, recorders, and displays are calibrated and appropriate calibration schedules are established. The validation department is responsible for coordinating all the documentation related to the installation, including the operating manuals, technical drawings, calibration requirements, certificates, and standard operating procedures (SOPs). When compiling such documentation, the validation personnel should perform extensive testing of the equipment and should not rely solely on the vendor's claims. The equipment is usually assigned a serial or asset number at this stage. Once the equipment is installed, an OQ is performed using a written protocol to ensure that the equipment performs within the specified limits when operated using approved SOPs. Such OQ studies are usually performed using placebo batches and may involve the combined technical expertise of the production, validation, and engineering departments and also the equipment vendor. PQ on new or existing equipment is done to assure that it is working up to the appropriate level, in reproducing a particular process or product, within predetermined specifications.

2.4.2. Cleaning Validation

Cleaning validation ensures that there is no cross contamination in a multi-product manufacturing plant and also prevents microbial contamination (61). Once a product is manufactured, the equipment is cleaned using appropriate cleaning SOPs established during the IQ of the equipment. Swab or rinse samples from various pieces of equipment are taken as per an approved cleaning validation protocol. These samples are tested using validated analytical methods for drug content. The analytical method should be sensitive enough to detect and quantitate low levels of drug, especially for products containing high potency drugs. Acceptance limits for drug content on equipment surfaces are established by taking into consideration the drug's toxicity, the batch size, and the equipment size or contact surface area. Equipment disassembly, cleaning, and setup must follow SOP. The cleaning validation protocol lists various locations on the equipment, for swab sampling. Several of the swab sampling locations should represent difficult to clean areas. The nature of the drug manufactured and its aqueous solubility dictate the choice of cleaning agents and solvents used. If a waxy matrix is used in the manufacturing process, such as in melt granulation, extra precaution should be taken to remove the wax from the surface of the equipment. A thorough rinse is performed using deionized water or detergent free solvent to wash out the cleaning agent prior to swab. Additional swab samples are to be taken for detergent test. At the end of the cleaning validation study, the data are summarized in a final report. The cleaning program is constantly updated to reflect changes in the manufacturing process or batch size, operator variability, and equipment aging and repair (62).

2.5. Process Demonstration and Technology Transfer

The formulation and process developed at a small scale must be capable of producing the same product using the same process at a larger scale. Manufacturing parameters that affect the quality attributes of the in-process and finished product should be identified. These parameters are to be studied to demonstrate the boundaries of the manufacturing process controls. Statistically designed pilot scale batch experiments may provide valuable information from a limited number of trials to predict the flexibility and constraints to be applied to the scale-up batch.

2.5.1. Process Demonstration

Process demonstration is to demonstrate that the process utilized in the pilot plant is applicable of producing the desired product at a larger scale. The demonstration batch may be an experiential large scale batch or a bio/stability batch that may or may not be the actual production size batch. In a generic industry, several factors such as complexity of the process, in-house expertise, availability of the API, cost, time line, etc., are considered in the planning for a process demonstration batch. Product development personnel in juxtaposition with production and validation personnel manufacture the batch. All important aspects of the process (mixing times, granulation end points, drying curves, moisture contents, compression forces, coating parameters, etc.) are carefully explored and monitored. After completion of the batch, a meeting among the development, manufacturing and validation groups is useful to discuss the process and product performance. Based on the outcome of the batch and input from various experts involved, any changes or modification in the formulation or process can be made before the bio-batch. Production personnel are thus thoroughly aware of critical process steps and successful execution of future batches is well assured.

2.5.2. Technology Transfer

Technology transfer involves transferring the product manufacturing technique and responsibilities from development phase to regular production group. The technology transfer plan and performance vary widely among the generic industries. In many industries, there is no formal technology transfer procedure and in others, it is poorly managed. This may lead to manufacturing problems difficult to correct during the product launch and delays the marketing of the product. Involvement of production personnel in the research batches should start as early as the process demonstration batch as mentioned above. Bio-batch manufacturing in the production floor serves a beneficial step in technology transfer. The process validation/technology transfer group in conjunction with the development, analytical, manufacturing, quality assurance (QA), and packaging groups prepares a technology transfer document. This document should include information on:

1. Formulation development and process optimization studies
2. Relevant analytical data/dissolution data
3. Manufacturing master formula and process flow chart
4. Monographs of all excipients
5. Description of packaging components
6. Cleaning methods and criteria
7. Process validation protocol
8. Resource requirements and time line

It is important for the development team to discuss all aspects of the manufacturing process and resource requirements with relevant departments. The manufacturing process, process controls, in-process sampling and testing specifications, and equipment operation, especially in the case of new technology, are to be explained to the manufacturing personnel. A clear understanding of various steps of the manufacturing process as identified in the manufacturing master batch record is essential. Several critical steps and parameters need to be addressed, e.g., addition of the granulating fluid to a high shear mixer can be done for a fixed time or fixed rate, or by defining granulation end points such as impeller torque or power (kW). Often, the order of addition of a particular ingredient or bulk drug component to the blender is important. In-process sampling procedures, such as granules for moisture content during drying or powder blend for content uniformity, should be clearly stated. The technology transfer completes with the successful completion of three consecutive validation batches. All documents including executed manufacturing masters, test results, out of specification (OOS) values (if any), deviations (if any), and investigations (if any) should be compiled as formal reports. The report must include explanation for any OOS values, and sound corrective action from both technical and compliance points of view.

2.6. Documentation

Documentation is an important aspect of the scale-up, process validation, and technology transfer process. Hence, it becomes imperative that all relevant documents pertaining to the manufacturing, testing, and releasing of the bio/validation batch are compiled and organized prior to a pre-approval inspection (PAI). The documents should be checked for data accuracy and adequacy as required by the FDA's guidelines. Documentation covering the items below should be compiled in a timely manner:

1. Executed masters for the bio/submission batches
2. Test results, including OOS values, repeat testing, etc.
3. Deviation investigations, findings, and conclusions
4. Equipment IQ, OQ, and PQ
5. Equipment cleaning validation
6. Change control documentation
7. Related SOPs
8. Product launch batches (including any scale-up batches)

All documentation relating to active and inactive raw materials, including test methods, vendor's certificates of analysis (COAs), and QC release specifications, are included. The original batch manufacturing records, analytical method validation reports, equipment IQ/OQ, process and product validation documents, production personnel training records, and equipment maintenance records form the main sections of a project documentation file.

2.7. Post-Approval Changes—SUPAC

FDA has issued guidelines to ANDA sponsors who intend to change components or composition, manufacturing site, scale-up/scale-down of manufacturing, and/or manufacturing process and equipment for immediate release (IR) and modified release (MR) solid oral dosage forms during the post-approval period (63,64). These changes are classified under different levels in each of the above categories depending on their effect on final product quality. Depending on the severity of change as listed in the SUPAC guidelines, the ANDA sponsor may have to perform additional in vitro and/or in vivo testing to establish bioequivalence, stability, and similarity to the original bio-batch. The guidelines use a biopharmaceutical classification system of drug solubility/permeability characteristics to determine if additional bio-studies are warranted. In cases where dissolution similarity is required, the use of similarity factor f_2 is recommended for comparing dissolution profiles (65).

3. CONCLUSION

Scale-up, process validation, and technology transfer are conducted at the late phase of product development. However, the performance of these steps is largely dependent on the product composition and process selected in the early phase of development. The technology chosen at an early developmental stage and employed in manufacturing the bio-batch stays with it during its life. During this early phase, the development scientist must consider the future demand of the product in selecting the process and equipment. In reviewing a manufacturing process, it is important to consider the physico-chemical properties of the drug and excipients along with equipment capabilities and limitations. Involvement of production personnel in the manufacturing of a batch prior to the bio-batch often helps in the development of a robust process. All equipment should be qualified for installation, operation, and performance prior to the bio-batch. The equipment should be cleaned and tested as per a cleaning validation protocol. The bio-batch should be evaluated for process performance as per a process validation protocol. All operational documents and test results generated from the bio-batch must be reviewed prior to initiating further scale-up and/or technology transfer. A team effort among formulation, validation, production, analytical, and logistic support groups is crucial to the success of scale-up and technology transfer.

REFERENCES

1. York, P. Solid-state properties of powders in the formulation and processing of solid dosage forms. Int J Pharm 1983; 14:1–28.
2. Lukas, G. Critical manufacturing parameters influencing dissolution. Drug Inf J 1996; 30:1091–1104.
3. Statgraphics Plus. Version 5 Manugistics Inc., Rockville, MD, 2004.
4. Minitab. Version 14 MINITAB, Inc., State College, PA, 2004.
5. Design-Expert. Version 6 Stat-Ease Inc., Minneapolis, MN, 2004.
6. Lewis GA, Mathieu D, Phan-Tan-Luu R. Pharmaceutical Experimental Design. New York: Marcel Dekker, 1999.
7. Bolton S. *Optimization Techniques.* Pharmaceutical Statistics. 3ed New York: Marcel Dekker, 1997:590–626.
8. Cornell JA. Experiments with Mixtures—Designs, Models, and the Analysis of Mixture Data. 2ed New York: Wiley, 1990.

9. Ahmed SU. Development of Oral Sustained Release Tablet Dosage Forms for Sparingly Water Soluble and Highly Water Soluble Drugs: Physicochemical, Biopharmaceutical and Technological Considerations. Ph.D. dissertation, St. John's University, 1989:122–255.
10. Egermann H. Scaling-up and manufacturing site changes mixing. Scale-Up and Manufacturing Site Changes Workshop. Nice, France: Controlled Release Society Workshop, 1994.
11. Luenberger H. Mathematical considerations and the scale-up problem in the field of granulation. Scale-Up and Manufacturing Site Changes Workshop. Nice, France: Controlled Release Society Workshop, 1994.
12. Landin M, York P, Cliff MJ, Rowe RC. Scaleup of a pharmaceutical granulation in planetary mixers. Pharm DevTechnol 1999; 4(2):145–150.
13. Faure, A, Grimsey IM, Rowe RC, York P, Cliff MJ. A methodology for the optimization of wet granulation in a model planetary mixer. Pharm DevTechnol 1998; 3(3):413–422.
14. Schaefer T, Bak HH, Jaegerskou A, Kristensen A, Svensson JR, Holm P, Kristensen HG. Granulation in different types of high speed mixers. Part 1: effect of process variables and up-scaling. Pharm Ind 1986; 48(9):1083–1089.
15. Holm P, Jungensen O, Schaefer T, Kristensen HG. Granulation in high speed mixers. Part 1: effects of process variables during kneading. Pharm Ind 1982; 45(8):806–811.
16. Holm P, Jungensen O, Schaefer T, Kristensen HG. Granulation in high speed mixers. Part 2: effects of process variables during kneading. Pharm Ind 1984; 46(1):97–101.
17. Hlinak T. Granulation and scale-up issues in solid dosage form development. Am Pharm Rev 2000; 3(4):33–36.
18. Faure A, Grimsey IM, Rowe RC, York P, Cliff MJ. Applicability of a scale-up methodology for wet granulation processes in Collette Gral high shear mixer-granulators. Eur J Pharm Sci 1999; 8:85–93.
19. Horsthuis GJB, van Laarhoven JAH, van Rooij RCBM, Vromans H. Studies on upscaling parameters of the Gral high shear granulation process. Int J Pharm 1993; 92:143–150.
20. Levin M. Granulation: endpoint determination and scale-up. www.mcc-online.com. Accessed October 2001.
21. Sirois PJ, Craig GD. Scaleup of a high-shear granulation process using a normalized impeller work parameter. Pharm DevTechnol 2000; 5(3):365–374.
22. Landin M, York P, Cliff MJ, Rowe RC, Wigmore AJ. The effect of batch size on scale-up of a pharmaceutical granulation in a fixed bowl mixer granulator. Int J Pharm 1996; 134:243–246.
23. Rekhi GS, Caricofe RB, Parikh DM, Augsburger LL. A new approach to scale-up of a high-shear granulation process. PharmTech 1996; 20(10):58–67.
24. Parikh DM, Bonck JA, Mogavero M. Batch fluid bed granulation. In: Parikh DM, ed. Handbook of Pharmaceutical Granulation Technology. New York: Marcel Dekker1997:Vol. 81:227–302.

25. Jones DD. Factors to consider in fluid bed processing. Pharm Technol 1985; 9(4):50.
26. Scale up factors in fluid bed processing. www.fluidairinc.com. Accessed October 2001.
27. Adeyeye MC. Roller compaction and milling unit processes: part 1. Am Pharm Rev 2000; 3(4):37–42.
28. Sheskey P, Pacholke K, Sackett G, Maher L, Polli J. Roll compaction granulation of a controlled release matrix formulation containing HPMC: effect of process scale-up on robustness of tablets, tablet stability and predicted in vivo performance. Pharm Technol 2000; 11:30–52.
29. Stahl H. Single-pot systems for drying pharmaceutical granulations. Pharm Tech Yearbook 2000:32–40.
30. Parikh DM. Understanding batch fluid bed drying. Powder Bulk Eng 1992:35–39.
31. Jones DM. Fluidized bed processing and drying. Pharm Eng 1991:1–7.
32. Parrott EL. Milling. Lachman L, Lieberman HA, Kanig JL In: The Theory Practice of Industrial Pharmacy. 3ed. Philadelphia: Lea and Febiger, 1986: 21–46.
33. Hasznos L, Langer I, Gyarmathy M. Some factors influencing pellet characteristics made by an extrusion/spheronization process. Drug Dev Ind Pharm 1992; 18:409–437.
34. Goodhart FW, Draper JR, Ninger FC. Design and use of a laboratory extruder for pharmaceutical granulation. J Pharm Sci 1973; 62:133–136.
35. Malinowsky HJ, Smith WE. Use of factorial design to evaluate granulations prepared by spheronization. J Pharm Sci 1975; 64:1688–1692.
36. Chariot M, Frances J, Lewis GA, Mathieu D, Luu R, Stevens H. A factorial approach to process variables of extrusion spheronization of wet powder masses. Drug Dev Ind Pharm 1987; 13:1639–1649.
37. Hileman GA, Goskonda SR, Spalito AJ, Upadrashta SM. Response surface optimization of high dose pellets by extrusion and spheronization. Int J Pharm 1993; 100:71–79.
38. Levin M. Changing tableting machines in scale-up and production: ramifications for SUPAC. www.mcc-online.com. Accessed October 2001.
39. Levin M, Zlokarnik M. Dimensional analysis of tableting process. AAPS Annual Meeting 2000. Indianapolis, IN: , 2000.
40. Guitard P. Scaling-up of tabletting operation. Scale-Up and Manufacturing Site Changes Workshop. Nice, France: Controlled Release Society Workshop, 1994.
41. Augusburger LL. Scale up of encapsulation. Scale-Up of Solid Dosage Forms— Short Course. University of Maryland–FDA, 1993.
42. Ullah I, Wiley GJ, Agharkar SN. Analysis and simulation of capsule dissolution problem encountered during product scale-up. Drug Dev Ind Pharm 1992; 18:895–910.
43. Campbell RJ, Sackett G. Film coating In: Avis KE, Shukla AJ, Chang R-K, eds. Pharmaceutical Unit Operations: Coating. Drug Manufacturing Technology Series. Buffalo Grove, IL: Interpharm Press1999:Vol. 3:55–176.

44. Sackett G. BASF/Vector coating seminar. www.vectorcorporation.com. Accessed October 2001.
45. Mehta AM. Scale-up considerations in the fluid-bed process for controlled release products. Pharm Technol 1988; 12(2):46–50.
46. Jones DM. Scale-up considerations and troubleshooting for fluidized bed techniques. Process Training Seminar. Ramsey, NJ: Glatt Air Techniques, October 2000.
47. Current Good Manufacturing Practices in Manufacture, Processing, Packaging and Holding of Human and Veterinary Drugs. Federal Register 1978; 43(190):45014–45089.
48. Guidelines on General Principles of Process Validation. Center for Drug Evaluation and Research (CDER-FDA), Rockville, MD, 1987.
49. Avallone H, D'Eramo P. Scale-up and validation of ANDS/NDA products. Pharm Eng 1992; November–December.
50. Nash RA. Process validation: a 17-year retrospective of solid dosage forms. Drug Dev Ind Pharm 1996; 22(1):25–34.
51. Nash RA. The validation of pharmaceutical processes. In: Hynes MD III, ed. Preparing for FDA Pre-Approval Inspections. New York: Marcel Dekker, 1999:161–185.
52. Carstensen JT, Rhodes CT. Sampling in blending validation. Drug Dev Ind Pharm 1993; 19(20):2699–2708.
53. Chowhan ZT. Sampling of particulate systems. Pharm Technol 1994:48–55.
54. Berman J, Planchard JA. Blend uniformity and unit dose sampling. Drug Dev Ind Pharm 1995; 21(11):1257–1283.
55. Carstensen JT, Dali MV, Pudipeddi M. Blending validation of low drug content dosage forms. Pharm Dev Technol 1996; 1(1):113–114.
56. Carstensen JT, Dali MV. Blending validation and content uniformity of low-content, non-cohesive powder blends. Drug Dev Ind Pharm 1996; 22(4):285–290.
57. Garcia TP, Taylor MK, Pande GS. Comparison of the performance of two sample thieves for the determination of the content uniformity of a powder blend. Pharm Dev Technol 1998; 3(1):7–12.
58. Draft Guidance for Industry—ANDA's Blend Content Uniformity Analysis. Office of Generic Drugs (CDER—FDA), Rockville, MD, 1999.
59. Prescott JK, Garcia TP. A solid dosage and blend content uniformity troubleshooting diagram. Pharm Technol 2001; March:68–88.
60. Ferenc BM, Kot L, Thomas R. Equipment validation. In: Berry IR, Nash RA, eds. Pharmaceutical Process Validation. 2nd New York: Marcel Dekker, 1993:351–368.
61. McCormick P, Cullen LF. Cleaning validation. In: Berry IR, Nash RA, eds. Pharmaceutical Process Validation. 2nd New York: Marcel Dekker, 1993: 319–350.
62. Hwang R. How to establish an effective maintenance program for clearing validation. Pharm Technol 2001; April:62–71.

63. Guidance for Industry: Immediate Release Solid Oral Dosage Forms: Scale-Up and Post-Approval Changes. Chemistry and Manufacturing and Controls. Rockville: MD, 1995:In Vitro Dissolution Testing and In Vivo Bioequivalence Documentation. CDER—FDA.

64. Guidance for Industry, SUPAC-MR: Modified Release Solid Oral Dosage Forms. Scale-Up and Post-Approval Changes. In Vitro Dissolution Testing and In Vivo Bioequivalence Documentation. CDER—FDA. Rockville, MD: Chemistry and Manufacturing and Controls, 1997:MD.

65. Liu J, Ma M, Chow S. Statistical evaluation of similarity factor f2 as a criterion for assessment of similarity between dissolution profiles. Drug Inf J 1997; 31:1255–1271.

6

Drug Stability

Pranab K. Bhattacharyya

Eon Labs Inc., Laurelton, New York, U.S.A.

1. INTRODUCTION

In 1984, the Hatch-Waxman Amendment of the Federal Food, Drug, and Cosmetic Act was enacted. This amendment, which is also known as the Drug Price Competition and Patent Term Restoration Act of 1984 (Public Law 98–417), allowed lower priced generic drug equivalents of the off-patent branded drugs in the United States marketplace. In this chapter, the United States Food and Drug Administration (FDA) requirements governing the stability of generic drugs will be discussed. Stimulated by the growth of the generic industry, a comprehensive journal publication (1) devoted exclusively to the development, manufacturing, quality control, and quality assurance of generic drugs is available in print and on the website.

1.1. Why Stability for Generic Drugs?

A generic drug (2) is equivalent to the corresponding branded drug with respect to the active pharmaceutical ingredient (API), strength, dosage form and dose, route of administration, safety, efficacy, and label claim. Generic and branded drugs may, however, differ with respect to inactive ingredients such as lactose, magnesium stearate, etc., which are necessary to formulate the drugs, for example, as tablets and capsules.

When a formula for a generic drug has been finalized for an off-patent branded drug, the generic drug manufacturer is required to conduct certain studies and submit an abbreviated new drug application (ANDA) to the Office of Generic Drugs (OGD) of the FDA to demonstrate its bioequivalency and quality. Proof of bioequivalence is established through an appropriate comparative bioavailability (bioequivalence) study which is discussed in Chapters 10 and 11. Drug quality, on the other hand, is demonstrated through implementation of extensive analytical testing procedures. The analytical testing methodologies and data are described in the Chemistry, Manufacturing, and Controls (i.e., CMC) section of the ANDA application which is covered in Chapters 3 and 9.

A key component of drug quality is its stability profile which is an integral part of the CMC section. Drug stability is characterized by parameters such as identity, assay, degradation profile, and dissolution rate. A drug is stable when these quality characteristics remain within predetermined quality control specifications for at least the duration of the expiration period. A stable generic drug, which has been shown to be bioequivalent to a branded drug, assures that it continues to be safe and efficacious throughout its shelf-life. Assessment of the stability of drugs is also mandated by the Code of Federal Regulations, Title 21, Part 211.166 (usually abbreviated as 21CFR Part 211.166).

1.2. Terminology

In the pharmaceutical industry, the terms active pharmaceutical ingredient or API, drug substance, active ingredient, active substance, or simply active or drug are all used interchangeably. Drug products or drugs or products or finished products are also interchangeable. The term shelf-life is used interchangeably with expiration dating period, expiration period, expiration dating, or expiration date. An excipient is any inactive substance other than the drug substance used in the corresponding drug product.

2. API STABILITY

The development of the stability profile of an API is a prerequisite for approval of an ANDA application. Analytical testing to establish an API's stability profile is usually conducted by its manufacturer. Critical stability parameters include physical appearance (e.g., whether crystalline or amorphous powder for solid APIs), color, assay, degradation profile, and hygroscopic tendency. The API manufacturer's Drug Master File (DMF) submission to the FDA will not be complete without stability data. In practice, the review of the DMF by FDA is triggered upon submission of an ANDA application referencing the DMF.

2.1.   Pharmacopeial and Non-Pharmacopeial APIs

Currently, a large number of APIs are already included in the United States Pharmacopeia (USP) and its supplements. It is known that a vast majority of the pharmacopeial grade API's which are used by generic manufacturers are produced in foreign countries such as Ireland, Italy, India, and China amongst others. It is a requirement that all manufacturers of APIs have modern production facilities which are staffed with well-qualified personnel and have implemented good quality systems which conform to US cGMPs (Current Good Manufacturing Practice) requirements. Over the years, the foreign inspections branch of the FDA has done a truly outstanding job through vigorous inspections in enhancing the cGMP systems to the point that the foreign manufacturers offer high quality APIs and an excellent value for the US as well as for global markets. Through inspectional observations and when/where necessary, warning letters, FDA ensures that only manufacturers who have implemented adequate quality systems and manufacturing technology to comply with cGMP requirements can supply APIs to the US drug product manufacturers.

Many APIs for generic drugs, however, are still not listed in the USP. Various API monographs are currently going through the review process in the Pharmacopeial Forum (PF). cGMP requirements are nevertheless equally applicable regardless of whether the APIs are in the USP or not. The API manufacturers seem to be cognizant that demonstration of stability profiles of APIs are an essential component in meeting these requirements.

2.2.   Specifications and Test Methods

For those APIs with monographs published in the USP, the API manufacturers must ensure that their specifications are not wider than the pharmacopeial specifications. The specifications must be either identical or tighter than the respective pharmacopeial specifications. Historically, third world countries in Asia and Africa have followed the USP. European countries and Japan have their own compendia such as the European Pharmacopeia (EP) and Japanese Pharmacopeia (JP). Since foreign manufacturers are known to produce APIs for international markets, they have focused on developing a single set of specifications with the tightest limits to meet the requirements of the major pharmacopeias (USP, EP, JP). In order to assure that an API meets the stability specifications for international markets, the tightest specifications included in the major pharmacopeias should be selected. For example, if the USP has specifications of 98.0–102.0% for assay and 0.2% for a degradant and other pharmacopeias have specifications of 99.0–101.0% and 0.3%, respectively, the tightest specifications of

99.0–101.0% and 0.2% should normally be set as the stability specifications for the API.

For USP grade APIs, USP test procedures should be followed. If an API manufacturer's test method differs from the USP procedure, crossover studies are required to demonstrate equivalency between these procedures. For example, if a titration procedure is employed by the manufacturer and a high performance liquid chromatographic (HPLC) procedure is described in the USP for an assay, the API sample should be analyzed by both methods. Another possible *scenario* is that an HPLC method may be used for the determination of impurities and degradants by the API manufacturer, which may be different from the HPLC method listed in the USP. Results from the two HPLC methods should be comparable within the experimental errors of the methods. This will allow the use of the titration procedure by the API manufacturer for assay and its HPLC procedure for stability testing, and at the same time permit labeling the API as conforming to USP. The situation becomes complicated if the different pharmacopeiae employ different methods of analysis. In that case, multiple crossover studies should be conducted to allow the use of a single test method by the API manufacturer for the analysis of a given test attribute such as assay.

To harmonize development of specifications for impurities and degradants in ANDAs and DMFs, FDA has published a guidance (3) to provide recommendations on the identification and qualification of impurities in APIs produced by chemical synthesis, which are applicable for both pharmacopeial and non-pharmacopeial APIs.

2.3. FDA and ICH Guidelines

Both FDA and ICH (i.e., International Conference on Harmonization) guidelines (4–8) require stability-indicating assay procedures for analysis of drugs. The HPLC assay procedure is the preferred method for stability testing. For demonstration of stability, an API sample is purposely degraded (6) by stressing it under harsh conditions of temperature, humidity, oxidation, UV light, acidity, and basicity. Evidence for the stability-indicating property of the assay procedure is demonstrated by adequate separation of the degradants from the active ingredient peak. To assure that no degradants are coeluting with the active peak, it is advisable to conduct peak purity studies by multiwavelength scans of the chromatographic peak using a photodiode array (PDA) detector. With this technique, the purity of the main peak can be established only if the UV chromophores of the API and the coeluted degradant are sufficiently different. However, if the UV chromophores are similar, this technique will not succeed in establishing peak purity. In such cases, the more powerful hyphenated technique of HPLC analysis coupled with mass spectrometric detection (known as LC-MS) should be considered.

2.4. Issues for Multisource APIs

Spurred by the growth of the generic industry, multiple manufacturers of APIs have arisen. With time, many more API manufacturers will gain FDA approval and join the ranks of producers of quality APIs. Since they will all compete for essentially the same generic market for a given API, their success will be governed by their ability to deliver quality APIs at the least possible cost. This will require creativity for the API manufacturers to survive and succeed in a highly competitive business. For that to happen, they will have to cut costs in the production of the APIs. The different manufacturers will employ different syntheses for the same API. In all cases, the final product, the API, must be chemically identical. The starting chemicals, intermediates, final intermediates, synthetic pathways, and residual solvents detectable in the API will usually differ from one manufacturer to another. While the API produced by different manufacturers must be chemically indistinguishable, its physical properties such as bulk density, particle size profile, its crystalline or amorphous character, and its rate of degradation may differ. Therefore, in addition to cost, its stability as well as its processing characteristics in the manufacture of finished products should be considered in selecting the manufacturers of the APIs.

2.5. Method Validation

Analytical methods for stability testing of APIs should be validated. USP 27 contains a general chapter ⟨1225⟩ on methods validation (9). FDA has also posted the ICH guidelines, Q2A and Q2B, on validation of analytical procedures on its website (10,11). These and other FDA guidelines (12,13) should be considered in developing and implementing a methods validation protocol for an API. In the USP, validation of an analytical procedure is defined as the testing process by which it is established that certain performance characteristics are achieved. Typical performance characteristics in the USP and ICH for the validation of analytical methods include the following: accuracy, precision, specificity, detection limit, quantitation limit, linearity, and robustness. The definitions for these analytical performance characteristics are provided in the USP and ICH guidelines, and are not covered in this chapter. It should be noted that validation is a dynamic process and should be repeated when an analytical method has been revised or when an API is procured from a different manufacturer or produced by a different synthetic route.

2.6. Shelf-life Development and Assignment

Stability testing should be conducted with the API packaged and stored under the ICH accelerated and long-term stability conditions which are listed below:

accelerated stability condition: $40°C \pm 2°C/75\%RH \pm 5\%RH$;
long-term stability condition: $25°C \pm 2°C/60\%RH \pm 5\%RH$.

For stability testing, samples may be stored in a smaller container/closure system which should be equivalent to the larger container used for storing larger quantities of the API. The smaller container/closure system must have the same composition, closure, and liners, and include desiccants if they are also used in the larger container/closure system.

In a short time of 3 months, the accelerated stability studies provide valuable data on the degradation profile of an API and thus assist in validating a particular container/closure system for storage of the API. However, long-term stability studies are essential in developing a retest period and shelf-life for APIs stored in the warehouse under controlled room temperature conditions which will be defined later in this chapter. A retest period is defined as the period of time during which the API is expected to remain within its specifications. Therefore, it can be used in the manufacture of the corresponding drug product, provided that the API is stored under appropriate environmental conditions. The shelf-life or expiration period for an API is the maximum allowable time period beyond which the API cannot be used in the manufacture of drug products and must be destroyed.

For APIs that exist as solids, a retest period of one year is generally supported by long-term stability data and accepted by the pharmaceutical industry. For stable APIs, a shelf-life of five years or longer derived from long-term stability and retest data is not uncommon. In the absence of an assigned shelf-life, the API can be retested again after one year and assigned a second retest date. This process of retesting can continue as long as the degradation levels and other quality attributes remain well within specifications. Stability studies to justify assigned retest and expiration dates should be repeated by the drug product manufacturer if the API is repackaged in a different container than that used by the API manufacturer.

2.7. Packaging

The FDA guidance (14) entitled "Container Closure Systems for Packaging Human Drugs and Biologics" includes information on container/closure systems for packaging of APIs. In general, APIs are solids; for such APIs, the container/closure system for storage or shipment of APIs usually consists of a fiber drum containing double low density polyethylene liners which are closed with twist ties. For protection from moisture and thus to assure stability, a desiccant may be placed between the bags if necessary. In that event, the stability samples should also contain appropriately placed desiccants to simulate the configuration of the larger container/closure system.

2.8. Shipment

API manufacturers should evaluate test results for critical test attributes such as assay and degradants when they are near specification limits prior to shipment of batches to drug product manufacturers. Existing stability data should be studied to ensure that such batches will remain within specifications, allowing for analytical measurement errors when initially tested at the API manufacturer's site and also at the assigned retest or expiration dates. If stability data are not available for a batch with test results approaching the specification limits, the particular API batch representing the worst case for its closeness to the specification limits should be studied under long-term stability conditions to develop the stability profile in order to justify quality control release and shipment of such batches.

Since the vast majority of APIs are imported from foreign countries, Customs and FDA require verification of the integrity of the container/closure system's labeling information and the manufacturer's analytical documentation to rule out pilferage or tampering. If the container was opened during transit and the API was exposed to the atmosphere, even for a brief duration, the stability profile of the API could be affected and the possibility of contamination could arise. Therefore, at the minimum, assay, impurities, and degradant profile of the API should be determined at the finished product manufacturer's site. The results should be compared with the API manufacturer's certificate of analysis to verify that the quality of the API has not been compromised.

3. INTERMEDIATES FOR DRUG PRODUCTS

In general, the manufacturing process for both immediate release (IR) and modified release (MR) solid oral dosage forms begins with the mixing of the required APIs and excipients, then proceeds through stages of intermediates, and finally ends with the production of finished products such as capsules and tablets. These intermediates are known as blends, intermediate pellets, cores, etc.

3.1. Specifications

Separate specifications are required to verify the quality of the intermediates used in the production of the finished product. Usually the analytical methods for the finished product are also utilized in testing of intermediates.

3.2. Holding Time

21 CFR Part 211.111 requires, where appropriate, time limits for the completion of each phase of production to assure the quality of the drug product. Deviation from established time limits may be acceptable if such deviation does not compromise the quality of the drug product. Such deviation must be justified and documented.

A draft guidance (5) published by the FDA allows an intermediate to be held for a maximum period of 30 days from the date of production without being retested prior to its use in manufacturing. A holding time period of 1 month, instead of 30 days, would also be acceptable, if that is necessary for scheduling convenience. In the guidance, the date of production is defined as the initial date that an API has been added to the inactive ingredients during manufacturing. An intermediate that is held longer than 30 days (or 1 month) should be retested prior to use. The first production batch of the corresponding finished product should be monitored through long-term stability studies. For blends, the purpose of retesting is to ensure that they have remained stable and that no degradation or de-mixing took place during prolonged storage. For intermediate pellets, retesting ensures that the dissolution quality has not been affected. Retesting of cores assures that the assay, degradation, and dissolution results are acceptable.

If a longer holding time, for example 3 months, is necessary to facilitate routine production planning, the quality of an intermediate batch stored in the warehouse under the controlled room temperature condition should be checked for the duration of the holding time. The guidance suggests that at least three test points beyond the initial release should be selected for stability testing. The first finished product batch produced from an intermediate held for the desired duration in the warehouse should be tested. If the test results are found to be satisfactory upon completion of the stability testing of the finished product batch, the holding time of 3 months is deemed to have been qualified and can be routinely used without further stability testing of future batches of the intermediate and the corresponding immediate release or modified release drug products if these intermediate batches are held for not more than 3 months. Since the expiration date of the finished product is assigned from the date of production as defined above, its shelf-life is essentially shortened by the length of a holding time greater than 30 days (or 1 month). Therefore, it is advisable to limit the qualification of the holding time to 3 months or shorter. It should be noted that if an intermediate is not stable for 30 days (or 1 month), its holding time should be appropriately decreased after review of its short-term stability profile.

4. DRUG PRODUCT STABILITY

Stability testing plays a crucial role in the development of generic drug products. It provides valuable information regarding the behavior of drugs when exposed to temperature, humidity, and light. For solid oral generic dosage forms usually packaged in high density polyethylene bottles (HDPE), photostability is not generally considered to be an important contributor to degradation and thus will not be discussed further in this article. The FDA regulations governing drug product stability are stated in 21 CFR 211.166, which require a written testing program to assess the stability characteristics of drug products. The FDA has published guidances (4,5) to harmonize the design and execution of stability testing programs. In addition, ICH guidances (6,15) on stability testing of new drugs are available. Published literature (16) provides further information on designing stability testing programs.

4.1. Pharmacopeial and Non-pharmacopeial Products

With the aim of harmonizing the quality standards for generic drugs, USP 27 has provided many monographs for testing of such drugs. However, with the patent expirations of an increasing number of branded drugs, the corresponding monographs may not be available in the USP 27, its supplements, subsequent editions or Pharmacopeial Forum (PF) for public review, prior to formulation development, ANDA submission, and marketing of generic drugs. Since monographs for these products need to be independently developed by the generic manufactures, additional development and validation resources should be allocated to meet the twin goals of FDA approval and market launch in a timely manner.

4.2. Specifications and Test Methods

Abbreviated new drug applications require inclusion of appropriate and scientifically justifiable specifications and validated test methods for generic products. The cGMP regulations require that each drug product meets the approved specifications when tested by the approved stability-indicating methods. Abbreviated new drug applications also require inclusion of stability specifications for test attributes such as assay, degradants, and dissolution rates. The test results of long-term and accelerated stability samples of each drug product must conform to its stability specifications at least until the approved shelf-life of the product.

For drug products listed in the USP, the pharmacopeial specifications and test methods should be followed. Often, the older pharmacopeial monographs do not include limits for degradants. For such products, the published FDA guidance (17) on the subject of setting specifications for degradants should be followed.

For non-pharmacopeial drug products, the USP, which contains numerous monographs and guidelines titled as general chapters, is a valuable resource in setting templates for specification and testing methodology. The ICH Q6A guidance (18) should also be used as a general guide for ANDA submissions. Quality control and stability results as well as expected manufacturing and analytical variables should be evaluated when setting stability specifications. Valid statistical approaches may be utilized. Data generated from testing of the brand company's reference listed drug product in the FDA publication entitled "Approved Drug Products With Therapeutic Equivalence Evaluations", commonly known as "The Orange Book", can also be used to support the specifications proposed in an ANDA application. As a valuable aid in the development of analytical methods for non-compendial drug products, any information that is globally available from published articles in scientific journals and/or in international pharmacopoeias should be utilized.

In all cases, whether pharmacopeial or non-pharmacopeial analytical procedures, it must be demonstrated that the API and any associated impurities from the synthesis of the API as well as excipients are all separated from the degradation products of the API present in the matrix of the drug product. This is achieved through method validation which is discussed below.

4.3. Method Validation

Stability data serves as a barometer for the shelf-lives of drug products. Stable products are produced from validated production processes which are expected to be in a state of statistical control from one batch to another. It is therefore imperative that every effort be made to ensure that the analytical procedures for measurement of critical stability parameters are fully validated. High performance liquid chromatography (HPLC) has become a universal tool for stability testing because of its demonstrated capability of resolving the main component from degradants and any associated synthesis impurities. The stability-indicating capability of a particular HPLC method is governed by its degree of separation which is established by conducting forced degradation studies of drugs under various stressed conditions of temperature, humidity, oxygen, acid, base, UV light, and visible light. The details of the development of stability-indicating analytical procedures are included in a separate chapter in this book (Chapter 3) and also in several published guidelines (9–13).

An important component of an ANDA application consists of completed analytical method validation reports. During or after approval of an ANDA application, the FDA usually requests samples and test data to conduct regulatory validation. To fulfill this request, the applicant should follow the published FDA guidance on this topic (19). In performing the tests, the FDA laboratories will apply the regulatory methods, which are the analytical methods provided in the ANDA application.

For drugs with published monographs in the current USP, the analytical methods are those legally recognized under Section 501(b) of the Federal Food, Drug, and Cosmetic Act. In this respect, 21 CFR Part 211.194(a) (2) states that the analytical methods described in the USP do not require complete validation. The regulation, however, requires that the suitability of all testing methods must be verified under actual conditions of use. In other words, the pharmacopeial methods should be validated to establish their suitability for specific drug products manufactured by generic companies. This is understandable since stability data are critical attributes of drug products. An important advantage will be gained by conducting method validation consistently for all pharmacopeial and non-pharmacopeial products in raising a company's analytical standard in the eyes of FDA reviewers of ANDA applications as well as FDA investigators during on-site compliance inspections.

4.4. FDA and ICH Guidelines

In 1994, the Center for Drug Evaluation and Research (CDER), FDA, accepted the ICH stability testing conditions (6) for new drugs. In a letter to all ANDA applicants, the Office of Generic Drugs (OGD) of CDER stated that its accelerated stability condition, $40°C \pm 2°C$, $75\%RH \pm 5\%RH$, in support of controlled room temperature tentative expiration dating for ANDA products was identical to the ICH conditions, and would remain unchanged for ANDA submissions (20).

In 1995, the OGD issued a position paper on the conditions required for long-term stability testing of generic drugs, which was posted on the FDA website (20). The long-term stability testing is required to validate the tentative expiration dating derived from accelerated stability studies. The OGD stated that the ICH recommendations of $25°C \pm 2°C$ and $60\%RH \pm 5\%RH$, would be acceptable for long-term stability testing for ANDA applications. Alternatively, the OGD would also continue to accept long-term stability data conducted at the previously allowable conditions of $25°C-30°C$ and at ambient humidity. Even though both sets of conditions have continued to be allowed by the OGD in ANDA submissions, the international generic community has clearly progressed towards harmonization with the ICH conditions.

4.5. Stability Protocol

The stability protocol should be carefully developed by the quality control unit responsible for conducting and monitoring stability studies. The protocol should consist of the stability study design factors such as package sizes, sampling time points, strengths, bracketing, and matrixing. It should specify the environmental conditions for accelerated and long-term stability of packaged products and for bulk stability of unpackaged products. It should also include validated stability-indicating analytical procedures and stability specifications. The protocol must be included in an ANDA submission for approval by the OGD. Subsequently, if any changes are made to the protocol, the revised protocol must also be submitted for approval again by the OGD.

The following lists some key points of a stability protocol for a long-term stability testing program of a solid oral dosage form consisting of one strength and packaged in multiple sizes:

- the first three production lots will be packaged for stability testing;
- a bracketing design will be employed since the container/closure systems of the multiple sizes are chemically equivalent;
- the smallest and largest package sizes only will be stationed in the long-term stability chamber under the ICH storage conditions of $25 \pm 2°C$ and $60 \pm 5\%RH$;
- at least one production batch will be packaged in the smallest and largest package sizes and added annually to the long-term stability testing program;
- testing will be conducted at 0, 3, 6, 9, 12, 18, and 24 months, and annually after 24 months until the expiration date has been reached or longer in order to evaluate the possibility of extending the current expiration period;
- stability testing criteria will include appearance, assay, loss on drying, known and unknown degradation products, and dissolution;
- stability data will be evaluated to justify expiration dating and statistical analysis may be employed if required;
- stability data will be included in the annual report submission to the OGD;
- any batch with non-conforming stability data will be recalled from the market with the required notification to the FDA.

4.6. Shelf-life Development

Shelf-life is the time period during which a drug product is expected to remain within its specifications, provided that it is stored under the conditions defined on the container label. An expiration or expiry date is the date on the container label of a drug product, designating the time period prior to the end of which a batch is expected to remain within the approved shelf-life specification, if stored under the labeled conditions, and after which it must not be used. Regulation 21 CFR Part 211.137 requires that a drug product must bear an expiration date determined by appropriate stability testing in accordance with 21 CFR Part 211.166. The expiration dates must be related to the storage conditions stated on the labeling as determined by the stability studies conducted as described in 21 CFR Part 211.166. If the drug product is to be reconstituted at the time of dispensing, its labeling must bear expiration date information for both the reconstituted and unreconstituted drug products. It should be noted that 21 CFR Part 201.17 requires that the expiration dates must appear on the container labeling.

21 CFR Part 211.166(a) specifies that the results of stability testing must be used in determining appropriate storage conditions and expiration dates. 21 CFR Part 211.166(b) requires testing of an adequate number of batches of each drug product to determine an appropriate expiration date. The regulations allow use of accelerated stability studies to support a tentative expiration date if full shelf-life stability studies are not available at the time of ANDA approval. Where data from accelerated stability studies are used to project a tentative expiration dating period that is beyond a period supported by actual shelf-life studies, long-term stability studies must be conducted, including drug product testing at appropriate intervals until the tentative expiration dating period is verified or the appropriate period is determined. In general, the use of an overage of an API to compensate for degradation during the manufacturing process or a product's shelf-life, or to extend the expiration dating period, is not acceptable (7). Additional information on the subject of shelf-life development has been published (16,21).

Stability data should be developed for the drug product in each type of container/closure system proposed for marketing or bulk storage. Bracketing and matrixing designs, which will be discussed separately in this chapter, may be used if included in the approved stability protocol.

4.7. Action Limits

Long-term stability testing is conducted to assure that the drug product will be within its shelf-life specifications during the expiration period. Action limits tighter than the specification limits should be set to assure that any batch with initial test results close to the action limits is evaluated through an appropriate course of action. By definition, action limits are the maximum or minimum values of a test result that can be considered to be the boundaries of acceptability without requiring further actions. Results less than the minimum or greater than the maximum action limit indicate that an action must be taken. For example, if an assay or degradant, or dissolution result is near, but outside, the action limits, an appropriate action would be to monitor this batch by long-term stability testing to assess whether the batch will meet the shelf-life specifications. Conforming stability results for this batch also builds up a data base in the sense that a future batch with a similar result need not be subjected to stability. That is, a worse case approach can be taken in deciding whether a future batch would require long-term stability testing. From among all of the batches of the product on long-term stability, the worse case batch, which must still conform to specifications, is defined as that batch with results which are outside and farthest from the action limits. If the test results of a future batch are outside the action limits but are superior to the results of the worse case batch, this batch should not require long-term stability studies. However, if the test results pass, but are marginal with respect to the shelf-life specifications with no allowance for analytical variability, that batch should be rejected in order to avoid the risk of a stability failure and consequent recall. It should be noted that anytime an atypical batch is produced, a separate manufacturing investigation should be conducted in order to determine and correct the root causes for the production problem.

4.8. Expiration Date Assignment

The computation of the expiration dating period of a drug product batch should begin not later than the date of the quality control release of that batch and the date of release should not exceed 30 days or 1 month from the date of production, regardless of the packaging date. If the quality control release date of the batch exceeds 30 days or 1 month from the date of production, the expiration date should be calculated from 30 days or 1 month after the date of production. The date of production of a batch is defined as the first date that an API was added to the excipients during manufacturing.

The data generated in support of the assigned expiration dating period should be obtained from stability studies conducted under the long-term stability condition consistent with the storage environment recommended in the labeling. If the expiration date includes only a month and year, the product should meet specifications through the last day of that month.

A stability protocol should also include the statistical methods for analysis of stability data in addition to the design of the stability study. The draft guidance (5) on stability testing contains acceptable statistical approaches for the analysis of stability data and for deriving an expiration dating period. Generally, an expiration dating period should be determined on the basis of statistical analysis of long-term stability data.

If the reworking of a drug product is approved in an application, the expiration dating period of a reprocessed batch should not exceed that of the parent batch and the expiration date should be calculated from the original date of production (7).

4.9. Annual Stability

After the expiration dating has been verified with three production batches, an ongoing stability testing program for an approved drug product should be implemented in accordance with the postapproval stability testing protocol in the ANDA application. The protocol should include the commitment to place at least one batch of every strength in every container/ closure system, such as bottles or blisters, in the annual stability program for the subsequent years. If the manufacturing interval for a drug product is greater than 1 year, a batch of drug product released next year should be added to the stability program. Approved bracketing and matrixing designs should be implemented to reduce the stability testing workload.

Intermediate testing time points may be reduced for annual batches on a case-by-case basis through a prior approval supplement (PAS) (5). The proposed reduction must be justified on the basis of a history of satisfactory long-term stability data. The reduced testing stability protocol should include a minimum of four time points, including the initial and expiration time points, and two time points in between. For example, for an expiration dating period of 36 months or longer, batches should be tested annually. It should be noted that the reduced testing protocol applies only to annual batches and does not apply to batches used to support a postapproval change that requires long-term stability testing at all time points. However, bracketing and matrixing designs may be included in the PAS which will optimize testing efficiency.

4.10. Extension of Expiration Dating Period

An extension of the expiration dating period based on full long-term stability data obtained on at least three production batches in accordance with a protocol approved in the ANDA application may be implemented immediately and does not require prior FDA approval. 21 CFR Part 314.70(d) (5) allows implementation of the extended expiration dating through an annual report submission only if the criteria set forth in the approved stability protocol were met in obtaining and analyzing stability data.

4.11. Bulk Holding

Upon completion of manufacturing, the finished products, such as capsules and tablets for solid oral dosage forms, are usually held for a period of time, often called the bulk holding time, prior to packaging. The length of the bulk holding time is usually governed by scheduling of packaging operations and inventory requirements. In the interest of saving development time during routine production, it is advisable to establish the bulk holding time by monitoring the controlled room temperature stability of a sample of the ANDA submission batch, which is stored in a smaller container equivalent in composition to the larger container used for storage of unpackaged bulk finished tablets. For example, to simulate the larger cardboard containers used for storage in the warehouse, suggested dimensions of the smaller containers would be $4'' \times 4'' \times 4''$ card-board containers, double lined with low-density polyethylene bags which are closed with twist ties. The stability study of samples stationed in the warehouse, maintained at the controlled room temperature condition, should be conducted for the duration of the desired bulk holding time. Typically, this should be not more than 6 months from the date of its quality control release if this date does not exceed 1 month beyond the date that the API was first used in the manufacturing process. For a holding time of 6 months, testing time points of 0, 3, 6 months would be adequate unless dictated otherwise by data. For each product strength, the bulk holding time should be established. The established bulk holding time of one strength would not be transferable to the other strengths of a product line without supportive stability data for these strengths. If the bulk holding time is not established concomitantly with the development of the stability profile of the ANDA batch, it will be necessary to establish the bulk holding time post-ANDA approval. This may create some bottlenecks during prospective validation studies in preparation for a product's launch into the market. Generally, if a bulk holding time of not more than 3 months is desired, stability testing beyond the initial quality release testing is not necessary to accept this time frame routinely as a packaging deadline for solid oral dosage forms.

4.12. Bracketing

The CDER has accepted the ICH recommendations on bracketing designs for stability studies, which are available in published guidances (5,22). In a bracketing design, at any time point for example, only the samples on the extremes of container sizes, fill quantities, and/or dosage strengths are tested. The design assumes that the stability of the samples corresponding to the intermediate conditions is represented by the stability data at the extremes. The guidances that provide extensive details on the principles of various bracketing designs should be studied prior to development of a design for a particular product. The general concepts described in the guidances are equally applicable to both new and generic drugs and will be summarized for solid oral dosage forms.

A bracketing design can be used for most types of drug products, including immediate release and modified release solid oral dosage forms where the drug is available in multiple sizes or strengths. For a range of container sizes/fill quantities for a drug product of the same strength, a bracketing design may be applicable if the material and composition of the container and inner seal of the closure are the same throughout the range. Where either the container size or fill quantity varies while the other remains the same, the bracketing design may be applicable without justification. Where both container size and fill quantity vary, a bracketing design is applicable if appropriate justification is provided. Such justification should demonstrate that the various aspects (e.g., surface area/volume ratio, dead space/volume ratio, container wall thickness, closure geometry) of the intermediate sizes will be adequately bracketed by the extremes selected.

For a range of dosage strengths for a drug product in the same container/closure system with identical material and identical size, a bracketing design may be applicable if the formulation is identical or very closely related with respect to the components/composition. Examples of the former include tablet weights from a common blend made with different compression forces, or capsule weights made by filling a common blend into different size capsule shells. A very closely related formulation means a range of strengths with similar, but not identical, basic composition such that the ratio of the active ingredient to excipients remains relatively constant throughout the range, allowing for addition or deletion of colorant or flavoring, for example. Where the strength and the container size and/or fill quantity of a drug product vary, a bracketing design may be applicable with the necessary justification.

A bracketing design should always include the extremes of the intended commercial sizes and/or strengths. However, if the extremes are not truly the worst case selections on the basis of strengths, container sizes, and/or fill quantities, use of a bracketing design is not appropriate. Where the amount of the active ingredient changes while the amount of each excipient or the total weight of the dosage unit remains constant, bracketing may not be applicable unless justified.

If the market demands require discontinuing either the lowest or the highest bracket extreme and marketing of the intermediate sizes or fill quantities are still needed, the post-ANDA approval commitment to conduct ongoing stability at the extremes of the bracketing should be maintained.

Prior to implementing a bracketing design, its effect on shelf-life verification should be assessed. If the stability of the extremes is shown to be different, the intermediate packages should not be assumed to be more stable than the least stable extreme. In other words, the shelf-life of the intermediate packages should not exceed that for the least stable extreme of the bracket.

A bracketing design from the guidance Q1D is illustrated in the following table to demonstrate the concept behind bracketing (22). This example is based on a product available in three strengths and three container sizes. For the selected combination of batches, the postapproval stability program should require testing at all time points to assure that the results continue to meet all stability related specifications.

Example of a bracketing design:

Batch		Strength								
		50 mg			75 mg			100 mg		
		1	2	3	1	2	3	1	2	3
Container size	15 cc	T	T	T				T	T	T
	100 cc									
	500 cc	T	T	T				T	T	T

T = test sample at all time points specified in the postapproval commitment.

An intended bracketing design should be included in the stability testing protocol of the ANDA application. If the ANDA application does not contain the bracketing design, a supplemental application and approval will be required prior to implementation of the design for stability studies of routine production batches.

4.13. Matrixing

The CDER has also accepted the ICH guidance on matrixing, which is another type of a reduced design based on different principles (5,22). In a matrixing design, a fraction of the total number of samples are tested at any specified time point. At a subsequent time point, different sets of the total number are tested. This design assumes that the stability of the samples tested represents the stability of all samples. The differences in the samples for the same drug product should be identified as, for example, covering different batches, different strengths, different sizes of the same container closure system and, possibly in some cases, different container/closure systems.

Matrixing results in reduced testing when more than one variable is being evaluated. In the matrixing design, each combination of factors should be tested at the specified time points in order to obtain a balanced influence of the factors on the variability of the stability results. While the design will be governed by the factors that would be present in the full stability program, all batches should be tested initially and at the final time point.

The guidances (5,22) provide extensive details on matrixing designs and the important concepts outlined in these guidances are summarized below for solid oral dosage forms.

The factors that can be matrixed include batches, strengths with identical formulation, container sizes, fill quantities, and intermediate time points. Factors that should not be matrixed include initial and final time points, test parameters, dosage forms, strengths with different formulations, i.e., different excipients or different active ingredient/excipient ratios, and storage conditions.

The principles behind a matrixing design can be best explained with the following example reproduced from the ICH Q1D guidance (22).

Matrixing time points and factors for a product with three strengths and three container sizes:

	Strength								
	S1 Container size			S2 Container size			S3 Container size		
	A	B	C	A	B	C	A	B	C
Batch 1	T1	T2		T2		T1		T1	T2
Batch 2		T3	T1	T3	T1		T1		T3
Batch 3	T3		T2		T2	T3	T2	T3	

				Time points (months)				
	0	3	6	9	12	18	24	36
T1	T		T	T	T	T	T	T
T2	T	T		T	T		T	T
T3	T	T	T		T	T		T

S1, S2, S3 are different strengths; A, B, C are different container sizes; T =sample to be tested.

Generally, the matrixing design is applicable if the supportive stability data exhibit small variability and thus can predict product stability accurately. If the supportive data show large variability, a matrixing design should not be used. If a matrixing design is applicable, the extent of reduction from a full design in the number of samples to be tested depends on the factor combinations selected as shown in the above tables. The greater the number of factors and greater the number of levels in each factor, the greater is the extent of reduction in the number of samples to be tested. Any reduced design is justifiable only if it has the ability to accurately predict shelf-life.

An intended matrixing design should be included in the stability testing protocol of the ANDA application. Because of the potential complexity of matrixing designs, it is advisable to discuss a design in advance with the OGD prior to its implementation in the stability program. If the ANDA application does not contain the matrixing design, a supplemental application and approval will be required prior to implementation of the design.

4.14. Controlled Room Temperature

Generally, drug product labeling specifies storage temperature and, in some cases, humidity requirements to maintain product stability. The General Notices section in the USP 27 defines various storage conditions and should be used as a guide to ensure appropriate storage conditions consistent with the product's labeling requirement. The majority of drug products require controlled room temperature (CRT) storage.

In the USP 27, the CRT is defined as a temperature maintained thermostatically that encompasses the usual and customary working environment of 20°C–25°C (68°F–77°F), that results in a mean kinetic temperature (MKT) calculated to be not more than 25°C, and that allows for excursions between 15°C and 30°C (59°F and 86°F) that are experienced in warehouses, pharmacies, and hospitals. Provided that the mean kinetic temperature remains in the allowed range, transient spikes up to 40°C are permitted as long as they do not exceed 24 h. Spikes above 40°C may be permitted if the manufacturer provides data on effects of storage temperature variations. The mean kinetic temperature (MKT) is a calculated value that may be used as an isothermal storage temperature to simulate the nonisothermal effects of storage temperature variations. The procedure for calculation of the MKT is included in the USP 27, General Chapter ⟨1151⟩.

4.15. Stability of Products Containing Iron

In 1997, FDA published the iron regulations requiring label warnings and unit-dose packaging for solid oral drug products that contain 30 mg or more of iron per dosage (23). The regulations were issued to reduce the likelihood of accidental overdose and serious injury to young children through the use of unit-dose packaging. Such packaging was considered to limit the number of doses a child may ingest if the child gained access to the product.

Appropriate expiration dates for drug products in unit-dose packages were required to meet the iron regulations. Accelerated stability testing was not considered to be applicable to drug products containing iron, especially multi-vitamin products, since they were known not to perform well under the unrealistic stressed accelerated conditions. Therefore, long-term stability testing was the only method to determine the expiration date. After publication of the iron regulations which became effective on July 15, 1997, a grace period of 2 years, expiring on July 15, 1999 was provided to allow manufacturers to package products in unit-dose blisters and continue to market the product with reduced expiration dating as defined in the guidance. At the same time, the manufacturers were required to initiate and conduct long-term stability studies to establish anew, the expiration dating for existing products packaged in unit-dose blisters. Notice should be taken that for new products containing 30 mg or more of iron per unit dose, the product must be packaged in unit-dose blisters and set up on long-term stability to develop expiration dating prior to market entry.

4.16. Reprocessing and Reworking

Reprocessing and reworking terminology has been clarified in a recent draft guidance (7). Reprocessing is the introduction of an in-process material or drug product, including the one that does not conform to a standard or specification, back into the process and repeating steps that are part of the approved manufacturing process. Continuation of a process step after a process test has shown that the step is incomplete is considered to be part of the normal process and is not reprocessing. For most drug products, reprocessing does not require to be described in an ANDA application unless it is known that there is a significant potential for the reprocessing operation to adversely affect the quality attributes of the drug product. Generally, a reprocessed drug product does not require stability testing unless warranted otherwise because of quality concerns.

Reworking is subjecting an in-process material or drug product that does not conform to a standard or specification to one or more processing steps that are different from the manufacturing process described in the ANDA application to obtain acceptable quality in-process material or drug product. In general, reworking operations should be generated postapproval and the ANDA application should be updated through the submission of a prior approval supplement, unless reworking operations are anticipated and included at the time of the original ANDA application. Reworking of drug products should be justified by monitoring at least one batch representative of the reworked process under accelerated and/or long-term stability testing (7).

4.17. Packaging

Section 505(b)(1)(D) of the Federal Food, Drug, and Cosmetic Act (the Act) requires a full description of the facilities and controls used in the packaging of a drug product. Essentially, the Act mandates that the integrity of the container/closure system used in the packaging of a drug product must be maintained during routine packaging operations for marketed products. By definition, the container/closure system means the sum of all packaging components that together protect and contain the drug product. For control of the quality of the container/closure system, the USP has established requirements in the General Chapters ⟨661⟩ Containers and ⟨671⟩ Containers - Permeation. For solid oral dosage forms such as capsules and tablets, the USP requirements essentially relate to moisture permeability, oxygen permeability, and light transmission properties of the container/closure systems. Ultimately, proof of the suitability of the container/closure system and the packaging process is obtained from shelf-life stability studies.

4.18. Shipment

Package sizes and the corresponding container/closure systems intended for marketing must be included in the ANDA application with the necessary accelerated and long-term stability data for approval by OGD. A container/closure system, i.e., shipping containers, used for the transportation of bulk drug products to contract packaging companies should be described in the application (5). The container/closure system should be adequate to protect the dosage form, be constructed with materials that are compatible with the product being stored, and be suitable for the intended use. The protective properties of the shipping container are verified by the practice of annual stability studies.

   If a container closure/system is specifically intended for the transportation of a large quantity of a drug product to a repackaging company, it is considered to be a market package. Usually, such package sizes are well outside the range of the package sizes used in shelf-life stability testing and are not monitored in the annual stability program. For example, the large container closure/system used for bulk holding of capsules or tablets is not usually supported by shelf-life stability data and thus is not usually included in the application as a package to be marketed. It should be noted that such packages cannot be sold to repackagers.

5. CONTROLLED DRUGS

The Drug Enforcement Administration (DEA) is the US agency which is responsible for enforcement of the regulations of the Controlled Substances

Act. The regulations that are described in 21 CFR Parts 1300–1316 define the controls relating to the manufacture, distribution, and dispensing of controlled substances. The controlled substances have been divided into five different classes or schedules. Controlled substances under Schedule I and Schedule II require the greatest degree of security and controls. The substances under Schedule III, Schedule IV, and Schedule V require lesser degrees of control and security. Examples of drug product classifications are: heroin (Schedule I), oxycodone hydrochloride tablets, (Schedule II), phendimetrazine tartrate tablets (Schedule III), diazepam tablets (Schedule IV), and diphenoxylate hydrochloride and atropine sulfate tablets (Schedule V). To facilitate the use of abbreviations for the different schedules, 21 CFR Part 1302.03(c) has designated the following symbols: CI or C-I for Schedule I, CII or C-II for Schedule II, CIII or C-III for Schedule III, CIV or C-IV for Schedule IV, and CV or C-V for Schedule V.

5.1. Storage Requirements for CI to CV Drugs

The FDA regulations require accelerated and long-term stability testing for all drug products regardless of their classification as controlled substances. For such substances, pharmaceutical companies have employed additional controls to assure security during short-term and long-term storage of stability samples. As an example, the chamber used for long-term stability studies may allocate space for a locked cage for Schedule I and Schedule II drugs, which should be situated within the confines of the larger locked cage for Schedule III, Schedule IV, and Schedule V drugs. The chamber also provides a level of security with its own lock. For Schedule III, Schedule IV, and Schedule V drugs, the larger locked cage situated within the chamber provides a second level of security. For Schedule I and Schedule II drugs, the smaller locked cage situated within the larger locked cage provides the highest level of security. In all cases, a limited number of personnel should be authorized to access the chamber and the cages containing the controlled drugs for long-term stability testing. For accelerated stability testing of drugs, a small commercially available chamber is traditionally used for the short-term studies. This chamber should allow limited access and be located in a secure area. It should be noted that the general storage requirements of stability samples are also covered in 21 CFR Part 1301.75(b) and 21 CFR Part 1301.75(c), which allow dispersing controlled substances throughout the stock of non-controlled substances in such a manner as to prevent the theft or diversion of the controlled substances from the stability chamber. Prior to designing and implementing procedures for securing controlled drugs in the accelerated and long-term stability chambers, it is essential to consult with the DEA and seek their approval.

6. SUBMISSION REQUIREMENTS

Considering that a significant body of stability data is usually available on the branded drugs at the time of their patent expirations and well before an ANDA can be submitted, the ANDA submission requirements for stability data are less extensive than the new drug application (NDA) requirements for such data. Thus, valuable time is saved by the generic industry and also in the regulatory review by OGD, which contributes to the process of quick introduction of cheaper generic products into the market for the benefit of all patients.

6.1. ANDA Submission

6.1.1. General Requirements for ANDA Submissions for Generic
        Products

Accelerated stability data at 0, 1, 2, and 3 months on a minimum of one batch which can be a pilot scale batch with a minimum batch size of 100,000 capsules or tablets are required (24). For multiple sizes and strengths, scientifically justifiable bracketing and matrixing designs can be employed. The tentative expiration dating period of up to 24 months may be granted on the basis of satisfactory stability data unless not supported by the available long-term stability data. Available long-term stability data should be included in the original ANDA application and subsequent amendments.

Additional stability studies (12 months at the intermediate conditions or long-term stability data through the proposed expiration date) are required if "significant change" is seen after 3 months during accelerated stability. The tentative expiration dating will be determined on the basis of available data from the additional study.

Where "significant change" occurs under accelerated testing, additional testing at an intermediate condition, $30°C \pm 2°C/60\%RH \pm 5\%RH$ should be conducted. "Significant change" at the accelerated condition is defined as (5,6):

- a 5% potency loss from the initial assay value of a batch;
- any specified degradant exceeding its specification limit;
- the product exceeding its pH limits;
- dissolution results exceeding the specification limits for 12 capsules or tablets;
- failure to meet specifications for appearance and physical properties, e.g., color, caking, hardness, etc.

Should significant change occur at $40°C/75\%RH$, the ANDA applications should include a minimum of 6 months stability data at $30°C/60\%RH$; the same significant change criteria will then apply. The long-term testing should be continued beyond 12 months to derive shelf-life data.

6.2. Postapproval Changes

21 CFR Part 314.70(a) requires applicants to notify the FDA when there are any changes to an approved ANDA application. To facilitate less burdensome postapproval changes within the meaning of this regulation, the FDA has published three guidances (25–27) on postapproval changes, including two separate SUPAC guidances on IR and MR products, where SUPAC is an abbreviation for scale-up and postapproval changes, IR for immediate release, and MR for modified release. These guidances provide recommendations on the following categories of postapproval changes:

- changes in the components and composition;
- changes in the site of manufacture;
- changes in batch size (scale-up/scale-down);
- changes in manufacturing equipment and manufacturing process.

The guidances have defined levels of changes and, for each level of change, specified the requirements for stability data in support of the change. Because of the increasing necessity for site transfers in the pharmaceutical industry, stability documentation requirements for site changes are discussed below. The stability documentation requirements outlined in SUPAC-IR and SUPAC-MR for the other categories of changes are not included in this discussion.

6.3. Site Transfer

Site transfer usually consists of relocating manufacturing, packaging, and/or laboratory testing operations to a different site or to an alternate site. With increasing competition and consolidation in the generic pharmaceutical industry, site transfer of products has become popular in order to increase operational flexibility and speed and, at the same time, decrease cost of marketing products.

To facilitate the site transfer process, the FDA has published guidances (25–27) on the requirements for postapproval site transfer of products from the originally approved location to a different location.

In this section, the stability testing requirements and submission categories for the three levels of site transfer of solid oral dosage forms defined in SUPAC-IR and SUPAC-MR are summarized. For detailed information on the chemistry documentation, dissolution, bioequivalence, stability, and reporting requirements, the above-noted guidances should be studied.

An IR solid oral drug product is defined as a product that allows the drug to dissolve in the gastrointestinal contents, with no intention of delaying or prolonging the dissolution or absorption of the drug. An MR drug product is defined as a product whose drug content is released as a function of predetermined time points. Modified release solid oral dosage forms include both delayed and extended release drug products.

Level 1: Level 1 changes are defined as site changes within a single facility where the same equipment, standard operating procedures (SOPs), environmental conditions and controls of temperature and humidity, and personnel common to both manufacturing sites are used, and where no changes are made to the manufacturing batch records, except for administrative information and the location of the facility.

The Level 1 site change requires an Annual Report (AR) submission. No additional accelerated or additional long-term stability data from the different location are required.

Level 2: Level 2 changes are defined as site changes within a contiguous campus, or between facilities in adjacent city blocks, where the same equipment, SOPs, environmental conditions and controls of temperature and humidity, and personnel common to both manufacturing sites are used, and where no changes are made to the manufacturing batch records, except for administrative information and the location of the facility.

The Level 2 site change requires a changes being effected (CBE) supplement. For IR products, no accelerated stability data are required in the CBE submission. The first production batch produced at the different site should be monitored under long-term stability and the data should be submitted in an AR. For MR products, one batch with 3 months' accelerated stability data should be included in an CBE supplement and long-term stability data of the first production batch should be reported in an AR.

It should be noted that if the different site does not have a satisfactory cGMP inspection for the type of products being transferred, a PAS should be submitted instead of a CBE submission.

Level 3: Level 3 changes consist of a change in the manufacturing site to a different campus. A different campus is defined as one that is not on the same original contiguous site or where the facilities are not in adjacent city blocks. To qualify as a Level 3 change, the same equipment, SOPs, environmental conditions and controls should be used in the manufacturing process at the new site, and no changes should be made to the manufacturing batch records except for administrative information, location, and language translation, where needed.

In the SUPAC guidances, a significant body of information on the stability is defined as that which is likely to exist after five years of commercial experience for new molecular entities, or three years of commercial experience for new drugs. The scenario which provides for the following simpler submission requirements is applicable to generic drugs which are marketed after twenty or more years following initial marketing of the corresponding branded drugs.

For Level 3 site transfer of generic IR drugs, 3 months' accelerated stability data from one batch should be included in the CBE supplement and long-term stability data from the first production batch should be included in ARs.

For MR products, the Level 3 change requires a PAS. For site transfer of generic MR drugs, 3 months accelerated stability data on one batch should be included in the PAS and long-term stability data of the first three production batches should be included in ARs.

7. COMPLIANCE ISSUES

Regulatory implications governing stability testing needs to be clearly understood and communicated throughout an organization to assure compliance with regulations and guidances. It should not be forgotten that contract testing laboratories and drug substance manufacturers constitute an extension of the organization with respect to the need for prompt communication and compliance with regulations.

7.1. Drug Substance (API) Stability

Stability testing of the generic drug substance (API) is conducted following a protocol included in a DMF submission. Usually, the DMF is referenced in the ANDA application submitted by drug product manufacturers and its review is triggered by the submission of the ANDA. The DMF needs to be updated with new annual stability data as they become available. If accelerated stability testing was conducted to justify process change(s), such information should be provided via amendment of the DMF in a timely manner. Failure to update the DMF may adversely affect the compliance status of the drug substance as well as the corresponding drug product especially in the event of unreported significant process changes and unavailability of stability data. Significant changes in the manufacturing process and/or equipment and/or site of manufacture for a drug substance may require separate stability evaluation and supplemental submissions to the FDA in ARs, CBEs, or PASs. Therefore, it is imperative that the drug substance manufacturers keep the drug product manufacturers in the loop to ensure timely supplemental submissions on drug products. Theoretically, in the absence of timely submissions on significant process changes, the drug substances and drug products may both be considered to be out of compliance with the FDA regulations.

7.2. Drug Product Stability

Stability testing of the generic drug product is also conducted following a protocol included in an approved ANDA application. The protocol specifies time points for "pulling" stability samples for analysis. A log of "pull" dates for all stability samples should be maintained. It may be advantageous to initiate testing by performing the assay first and recording this date as the appropriate time point in the stability records and reports. It is important to complete testing of the samples in a timely manner. Delays in completion of testing should not exceed 30 days or 1 month from the dates when samples were collected from the stability chamber. Every attempt should be made to avoid omission of testing time points. Missing time points in stability reports have been cited by FDA investigators on the Notice of Inspectional Observations, FDA Form 483.

7.3. cGMP Considerations

21 CFR Part 211.166 requires a written testing program to assess the stability characteristics of drug products. To comply with this requirement, SOPs should be written to define the details of the stability program, such as container sizes/fill quantities, testing time points, temperature, and humidity conditions for the accelerated and long-term stability chambers.

The chambers used for accelerated and long-term stability studies should be validated. A validation protocol describing the requirements for installation qualification (IQ), operational qualification (OQ), and performance qualification (PQ) should be prepared and executed. The installation qualification essentially verifies that the chamber was properly installed as specified by its manufacturer and provides controlled access to selected personnel only. The operation qualification should verify conformance of the chamber's performance to specifications for temperature, humidity, air flow, and water pressure. The performance qualification study should be conducted over several days to ensure long-term reliability of the chamber. Temperature and humidity mapping studies should be incorporated in the performance qualification to ensure that temperature and humidity gradients are acceptable. The completed validation report should be approved by the quality assurance (QA) department. Upon approval of the validation report, the chamber can be used for stability studies. For continued quality assurance, temperature and humidity data for both accelerated and long-term stability chambers must be recorded continuously and these records must be archived for future audits by the QA personnel and FDA investigators.

7.4. FDA Inspection

Stability testing methodology and data constitute an integral part of an ANDA application on a specific product and provide the foundation for continued demonstration of the validity of the expiration dates of all products manufactured. This information is subject to inspections by FDA investigators, usually from a local district office. The FDA evaluates the integrity of stability data during pre-approval inspections (PAI) related to one or more ANDA applications, and during cGMP inspections to assess the company's compliance with regulations. During these inspections, the method validation reports in support of the stability-indicating analytical procedures, stability data, and the temperature and humidity records for the accelerated and long-term stability chambers must survive the close scrutiny of the investigators to succeed in the process of obtaining FDA approval of the ANDA applications and maintaining the facility's cGMP status. Examples of typical issues that may delay FDA approval of applications and adversely affect acceptable cGMP status are:

- inadequate resolution of impurities and degradants from the main peak in the HPLC analysis;
- inability to detect and accurately quantify small impurities in the 0.1% range;
- unsatisfactory investigations of out of specification stability data;
- failure to follow stability testing procedures submitted in the application;
- inadequate method validation;
- inadequacy of the SOPs for stability testing;
- omission of testing time points;
- missing temperature and humidity charts for the stability chambers;
- lack of periodic calibration of the chambers.

7.5. Documentation

21 CFR Part 211.180, which contains regulations on general requirements for records and reports, requires that all records must be retained for at least 1 year after the expiration date of the batch. The regulations require that all records must be readily available for FDA inspections during the retention period at the establishment where the activities described in such records occurred. It is important to interpret this regulation correctly for retention of stability data. It is essential that the original accelerated and long-term stability data in support of the shelf-life of a product are maintained indefinitely since such data provided the foundation for the established expiration

date assigned to all lots of the product. For a product, the particular lot introduced into the ongoing annual stability testing program also represents the continued validity of the expiration dates assigned to all lots of the product manufactured in that year. Therefore, annual stability data for a given year should be retained for at least 1 year past the expiration date of the last lot manufactured in that year. Complete records must be maintained of all stability testing performed as required by 21 CFR Part 211.194(e).

7.6. Training

21 CFR Part 211.25 on personnel qualifications is also applicable to personnel engaged in stability testing. The regulation requires that each person shall have education, training and experience or an appropriate combination thereof, to enable that person to perform the assigned functions. In addition to hiring personnel with the necessary academic background and skills, it is important to certify the newly hired personnel in the analytical procedures employed by the company. The certification process should be formalized in an SOP and should be based on having the new employee and an experienced person conduct the same critical tests, such as assay, impurities, and dissolution on selected lots of the product. The results obtained by the new and experienced employees should be compared. If the new employee's results are unsatisfactory, the certification process should be repeated until satisfactory results are obtained. In the case of demonstrated poor analytical understanding and accuracy, the employee should not be assigned analytical testing duties.

It is important from the cGMP perspective as well as for laboratory efficiency that training on analytical procedures, laboratory SOPs, applicable cGMP regulations for laboratory operations and record keeping requirements, and new analytical technology, should be a periodic process and formalized in an SOP on training. Trainers should not be limited to laboratory experts only. Instrument manufacturers, technical seminars, and scientific meetings are valuable external training resources which should be sought, when necessary, in enhancing employees' analytical expertise especially on new technology such as computerized and networked HPLC and GC systems, multi-wavelength photodiode array detection in HPLC analysis, particle size measurement based on laser diffraction, and Fourier Transform Infrared Spectrometry (FTIR). For training on USP monographs and general chapters and dissolution technology, USP experts provide onsite training. Essentially, periodic training demonstrates a company's commitment to continuing improvements in laboratory quality. All certification and training records on all employees should be maintained by the QA Department and presented on request to FDA investigators.

7.7. Out of Specification (OOS) Investigation

The procedure for investigation of out of specification (OOS) test results varies within the pharmaceutical industry. With the objective of developing a harmonized approach for investigation of OOS test results, the FDA published a draft guidance in September, 1998 (28). The term, OOS results, includes all suspect results that fall outside the specifications submitted in ANDA applications. For products with monographs in the USP, the ANDA specifications would usually correspond to the USP specifications.

Even though the guidance is still in the draft stage, it represents FDA's current thinking on evaluation of OOS results and should be viewed as an important resource in evaluating and validating or invalidating OOS stability data. To meet FDA's requirement, an investigation should be conducted whenever an OOS stability test result is obtained. The guidance requires that the investigation should be thorough, timely, unbiased, well-documented, and scientifically defensible. Since the particular annual stability batch with an OOS result represents all batches of the product manufactured in a given year, it is necessary to evaluate all batches manufactured in the year in order to determine whether or not the OOS result was limited to this batch only. If only one batch is affected by the OOS result and other batches are not, the investigation must show the unique circumstances responsible for the failure of the particular batch to meet specifications and at the same time, demonstrate clearly that the annual stability program was not compromised.

7.8. Annual Product Review

Annual product reviews are mandated in 21 CFR Part 211.180(e) which states that written records must be maintained so that data therein can be used for evaluating, at least annually, the quality standards of each drug product to determine the need for changes in drug product specifications or manufacturing or control procedures. As an important objective of the annual product review program, the results of ongoing annual stability batches must be reviewed for continued justification of the shelf-lives of all products manufactured. If stability results cast any doubt with respect to the validity of the shelf-life of a particular product, the situation should be investigated in a timely manner to determine the assignable reasons for the stability problem. If warranted by the investigation, the shelf- life should be reduced until the problems, for example, marginally acceptable assay results with respect to specifications, have been identified and addressed.

7.9. Field Complaint

21 CFR Part 211.180(e) (2) requires a review of field complaints and investigations conducted for each drug product. The complaints may provide clues

to the product's performance in the field and should be studied to show whether they relate to any physical or chemical changes in the product's specifications. Such changes can be caused by contamination in the plant or the field or can be caused by the packaged product's physical and chemical stability characteristics. For example, chemical discoloration of capsules or tablets due to moisture, caking of tablets, or ineffective product may indicate compromised integrity of the particular lot of the container/closure system and/or the need to tighten up on batch manufacturing parameters.

7.10. Recall

The failure of any annual stability batch to meet any specification needs to be promptly and thoroughly investigated to ascertain the reason(s) for the OOS result and to ascertain whether other batches which were not included in the annual stability program are affected. Examples of failures during annual stability would be nonconforming assay, degradant, or dissolution results. The unacceptable batches identified in the investigation should be withdrawn from the market. The FDA should be informed and a prompt voluntary recall of all affected batches should be conducted with the consent of the FDA. This will avoid possible product seizures by FDA and/or court injunctions. In addition, 21 CFR Part 314.81(b) (1) requires submission of a Field Alert Report to the local FDA district office within 3 working days of the occurrence of the OOS result.

8. STABILITY SOFTWARE

For over a decade, it has been a common practice by the drug manufacturers to rely on stability software to store, organize, retrieve, and analyze the vast amount of stability data generated by laboratory testing. Stability software may either be developed in-house or procured from vendors.

8.1. Computer Validation

The stability software must be validated according to the commonly accepted principles of computer software validation. If the stability software is developed in-house, it is important that internal experts are available for validation. If it is decided to outsource validation, the process will be costly since external experts will have to fully understand the software in order to develop and execute an appropriate validation protocol. Stability software supplied by vendors is usually accompanied by a validation package for on-site execution. Regardless of whether validation is conducted by internal or external validation specialists, the QA Department's approval will be required prior to use of the software. To facilitate the approval process, QA personnel will require computer software validation training, whether provided by vendors or through various computer validation seminars, to develop the necessary expertise to assess the validation report prior to sign off.

8.2. CFR Part 11

21 CFR Part 11 (commonly referred to as 'Part 11') states the regulatory requirements for electronic records and electronic signatures. In the regulation, electronic records are defined as records in electronic form that are created, modified, maintained, archived, retrieved, or transmitted electronically. The regulations also define electronic signatures that can be used instead of manual signatures and require complex controls to assure the security and integrity of electronic signatures. By definition, all stability software and stability data maintained and processed by the software are electronic records. In many companies, manual signatures may still be employed which will obviate the need to adhere to the additional and complex requirements for electronic signatures. To clarify the requirements for complying with Part 11, the FDA initially published a guidance which was subsequently withdrawn because of objections from the industry. Recently, to facilitate the process of compliance for electronic records and electronic signatures, the FDA has published a simpler draft guidance(29). It is important for stability testing laboratories to understand and utilize the guidance for compliance with Part 11.

9. VALUE OF STABILITY

Long-term stability studies assure, on an ongoing basis, that the products continue to conform to quality control specifications and thus maintain their safety and efficacy requirements throughout their shelf-lives. The studies consistently build up a long-term track record of stability data. Stable results continue to demonstrate that raw materials, manufacturing processes, packaging components, and packaging processes have all been in a state of control and have resulted in stable products until at least their expiration periods. The ongoing stability studies also serve as an invaluable tool in the quality control system to detect any unexpected spikes in the test result(s) during the shelf-life of a product and allow for implementation of corrective actions after investigating and ascertaining the root causes of the problem.

10. COST OF STABILITY

Annual stability studies assure that production processes continue to be in a state of control to produce stable drug products. Regulations require that, for each marketed product, one lot produced per year must be set up on long-term stability studies for at least the duration of the expiration period of the product. Thus, for a given number of marketed products, the cost of ongoing stability studies is independent of the number of batches produced in a given year. If only one batch is produced in a given year, that batch still must go on annual stability. If one hundred batches are produced for a certain product, only one batch needs to be set up for stability testing. Clearly, the cost of stability is proportionately greater for low volume products. There is no regulation requiring that the first lot produced in a particular year needs to be on stability. Since the stability workload can be substantial, it is important to spread the workload throughout the year to prevent overloading the first few months of a year with stability testing. This will also spread the cost of stability testing evenly throughout the year.

With the growth of the generic industry, the stability testing workload and thus its cost are destined to grow as well. Ultimately, the cost is borne by the consumers, i.e., patients. Creativity will be required to control the cost of stability. Usually, the stability protocol requires testing at 0, 3, 6, 9, 12, and 18 months and yearly thereafter until the expiry period. For stable products with a documented history of at least 5 years, the stability workload can be reduced significantly through deletion of the intermediate short-term test points of 3, 6, 9, and 18 months. For products with multiple strengths and package sizes, the stability protocol should be amended to reduce testing requirements via justifiable reduction of intermediate time points and appropriate bracketing and matrixing designs. Of course, the amended protocol needs to be submitted to the FDA as a prior approval supplement. Upon approval, the reduced time points can be immediately implemented which will reduce the cost of stability testing and also bring down the price of generic drugs. To further control costs, the stability samples for a given product should be set up in a manner to allow batch processing for laboratory testing.

11. CONCLUSIONS

Patients depend on high quality and affordable generic drugs which are safe and efficacious. The generic drug industry must make every attempt to lower the cost of drugs without compromising their quality, safety, or efficacy. Raw material, research and development, production, quality control and stability testing, storage and distribution costs all contribute to the cost of medicines. Creativity will be required to control these costs, which include the significant costs of stability testing.

It is common knowledge that brand companies, faced with an ever-increasing prospect of many drugs losing their patent protection have been resorting to court actions to gain one or more 30-month stays of FDA approvals for many generic drug products. Often, just prior to patent expirations, these companies have employed the tactic of filing pediatric clinical studies to gain an additional 6 months' patent extension, which has effectively blocked FDA approvals of generic equivalents during this period. Meanwhile, the generic industry continues to bear the cost of product development and ongoing stability testing during the exclusivity periods, which ultimately increases the cost of sale.

On the generic side, there is an ongoing battle to obtain the coveted 180-day exclusivity granted by FDA to the first-to-file company of a generic drug product. Also, because of increasing competition among generic manufacturers for market share, monopolistic tendencies have been developing through mergers and locking-in raw material sources through acquisitions or special contracts. A generic company awarded marketing exclusivity by the FDA for a product, can market this drug without competition from the other generic companies for 6 months after its patent expiration. As a result, other generic companies cannot recover their development, stability testing and other costs during this period. These factors are also conducive to increasing the price of generic drugs.

REFERENCES

1. Jeremy D. Block, ed. International Journal of Generic Drugs. LOCUM Publishing House. www.locumusa.com.
2. Generic Drugs: Questions and Answers. www.fda.gov/cder/consumerinfo/generics_q&a.htm.
3. Guidance for Industry, ANDAs: Impurities in Drug Substances. FDA, CDER, November, 1999.
4. Guideline for Submitting Documentation for the Stability of Human Drugs and Biologics. FDA, CDER, February 1987.
5. Draft Guidance on Stability Testing of Drug Substances and Drug Products. FDA, CDER, June 1998.
6. Guidance for Industry, Stability Testing of New Drug Substances and Drug Products. ICH, Q1A, September 1994.
7. Draft Guidance for Industry: Drug Product, Chemistry, Manufacturing, and Controls Documentation. FDA, CDER, January 2003.
8. Guideline for the Format and Content of the Chemistry, Manufacturing, and Controls Section of an Application. FDA, CDER, February 1987.
9. USP 27/NF 22 General Chapter ⟨1225⟩: Validation of Compendial Methods.
10. Guideline for Industry: Text on Validation of Analytical Procedures. ICH, Q2A, March 1995.
11. Guidance for Industry, Q2B Validation of Analytical Procedures: Methodology. ICH, November, 1996.
12. Reviewer Guidance: Validation of Chromatographic Methods. FDA, CDER, November, 1994.

13. Draft Guidance for Industry: Bioanalytical Methods Validation for Human Studies. FDA, CDER, December 1998.

14. Guidance for Industry, Container Closure Systems for Packaging Human Drugs and Biologics, Chemistry, Manufacturing, and Controls Documentation. FDA, CDER, May 1999.

15. Guidance for Industry, Q1C Stability Testing for New Dosage Forms. ICH, November 1996.

16. Grimm W, Krummen K, eds. Stability Testing in the EC, Japan and the USA, Scientific and Regulatory Requirements. Stuttgart: Wissenschaftliche Verlagsgesellschaft mbH, 1993.

17. Guidance for Industry, ANDAs: Impurities in Drug Products. CDER, FDA, December 1998.

18. Guidance on Q6A Specifications: Test Procedures and Acceptance Criteria for New Drug Substances and New Drug Products: Chemical Substances. ICH, Federal Register. December 29, 2000; 65 (251):83041–83063.

19. Guidelines for Submitting Samples and Analytical Data for Methods Validation. FDA, CDER, February 1987.

20. Letter to All ANDA and AADA Applicants from the Office of Generic Drugs. CDER, FDA, August 18, 1995.

21. Drug Stability Testing and Shelf-Life Determination According to International Guidelines. Saranjit Singh, Pharmaceutical Technology, June 1999: 68–88.

22. Guidance for Industry, Q1D Bracketing and Matrixing Designs for Stability Testing of New Drug Substances and Products. CDER, FDA, January 2003.

23. Guidance for Industry, Expiration Dating and Stability Testing of Solid Oral Dosage Form Drugs Containing Iron. FDA, CDER, June, 1997.

24. Guidance On The Packaging of Test Batches, Policy and Procedure Guide # 41–95. Office of Generic Drugs. FDA, February 8, 1995.

25. Guidance for Industry, Changes to an Approved NDA or ANDA, FDA, CDER, November, 1999.

26. Guidance for Industry, SUPAC-IR: Immediate Release Solid Oral Dosage Forms; Scale-up and Postapproval Changes: Chemistry, Manufacturing, and Controls: In Vitro Dissolution Testing and In Vivo Bioequivalence Documentation, FDA, CDER, November, 1995.

27. Guidance for Industry, SUPAC-MR: Modified Release Solid Oral Dosage Forms; Scale-up and Postapproval Changes: Chemistry, Manufacturing, and Controls: In Vitro Dissolution Testing and In Vivo Bioequivalence Documentation. FDA, CDER, September, 1997.

28. Draft Guidance for Industry, Investigating Out of Specification (OOS) Test Results for Pharmaceutical Production. FDA, CDER, September, 1998.

29. Draft Guidance for Industry, Part 11, Electronic Records; Electronic Signatures — Scope and Application. FDA, CDER, February 2003.

7

Quality Control and Quality Assurance

Loren Gelber

Andrx Pharmaceuticals, LLC, Davie, Florida, U.S.A.

Joan Janulis

Able Laboratories, Inc., Cranbury, New Jersey, U.S.A.

1. INTRODUCTION

In August of 1989, the FDA made it clear to members of the generic drug industry that many aspects of cGMPs apply to the product development process. The unfortunate problems uncovered at that time led Agency Investigators to request, for the first time, records showing how formulations were developed. Disappointingly, many firms had little documentation related to product development activities.

In the past, the process of formulation development has often had an almost mystical quality. We have seen a formulator listen to the sound of a listed reference tablet breaking, watch its behavior in 5 mL of water, close his eyes, commune with the laws of the universe, and then write down a formulation and manufacturing process. At times, he was so confident that the firm proceeded to produce the ANDA batch directly thereafter. Such ex nihilo batches passed FDA bioequivalence requirements more frequently than one would expect.

Unfortunately, the product development process described in the previous paragraph does not lend itself to acceptable record keeping. In today's regulatory environment, this form of development has become

173

essentially obsolete. Sponsors are well aware that their developmental records are subject to extensive scrutiny during pre-approval inspections. Given that satisfactory completion of a pre-approval inspection is a prerequisite for ANDA approval, it is in the best interest of sponsors to ensure that formulation and process development follow a logical sequence. This is accomplished by way of the production of a series of "pilot" or "experimental" batches that ultimately lead to formulation and method of manufacture that will be documented in the ANDA. Experimental batches are usually quite small. They are manufactured in bench-top scale production equipment and are used to do preliminary formulation work. Once a tentative formulation has been established, pilot batches may be manufactured in batch sizes between the experimental batch size and that required by FDA for ANDA batches. Smaller versions of the production equipment to be used for commercial manufacturing are often used. If a pilot batch will be used for a pilot biostudy (a small study to determine if the formulation is promising), it must be manufactured using all appropriate cGMP controls.

The rationale for the chosen formulation and manufacturing process must be clear, and the sponsor must ensure that raw data from all pilot, experimental and ANDA batches are preserved and maintained throughout the process. Although not required by FDA, formal development reports are recommended to assist the investigator during the pre-approval inspection. Through narrative and presentation of data, these reports afford the ANDA sponsor the opportunity to guide the FDA investigator through the process that was followed during development, and define the key milestones that led to chosen formulation and method of manufacture.

Once the formulation and method of manufacture have been identified, it is advisable that the sponsor produce a confirmatory batch at the same scale as the exhibit batch that is intended to support the ANDA submission. This confirmatory batch enables the sponsor to identify and implement minor adjustments in processing parameters and controls before producing the batch that will be evaluated by FDA's Office of Generic Drugs in determining the approvability of the ANDA.

The batches whose documentation is part of the ANDA may be called ANDA batches, submission batches, or exhibit batches. Throughout this chapter, we use these words as synonyms. Some of these batches are also biobatches, that is, the batches used in the pivotal biostudy or biostudies. However, not all submission batches are biobatches, because FDA may grant a waiver, permitting the biostudy data from one strength of a product to be applied to a different strength of the same product. Even though a waiver is granted, a batch must be produced and its documentation included in the ANDA.

This chapter will discuss the Quality Assurance and Quality Control requirements for pre-ANDA (commonly referred to as experimental, pilot, confirmatory batches) and ANDA batches. They include equipment, its qualification and calibration, documentation, optimization of process parameters, and justification of in-process specifications. We will also discuss Development Reports or Logs and FDA Pre-Approval Inspections. Several regulatory requirements that vary according to scale and purpose of the batch are summarized in Table 1. They are discussed in more detail in the following pages.

2. EQUIPMENT

Often R&D personnel will argue that since the experimental batch will not be used in any biostudy or other human testing, and since the records and results will not be submitted to FDA in the ANDA, the experimental batch does not need to be made using calibrated equipment. This can lead to problems further in the development sequence. The results obtained with the experimental batch will be used to make decisions about how to produce the pilot biostudy batch(es), if needed, and the ANDA submission batch(es). Use of unqualified or uncalibrated equipment may lead to erroneous conclusions and the establishment of process parameters that ultimately may not work. The purpose of Installation Qualification (IQ), Operational Qualification (OQ), Process Qualification (PQ), and calibration are to ensure that the equipment is doing exactly what it is supposed to do. Hence, the essential elements of these processes must be performed on the equipment used to make experimental batches. By essential element, we mean all those functions that are part of the critical processing parameters, such as mixing speed or temperature, whose value has a substantial effect on the quality of the product. For equipment used to manufacture pilot batches to be used in pilot biostudies, complete qualification and calibration are required.

Requirements for prevention of cross-contamination are not the same for experimental batches as for later batches. For batches intended to be administered to humans (research subjects or patients), the sponsor must take steps to ensure that the level of cross-contamination is minimal. Acceptable levels are normally determined by the toxicity of the compound in question. Because both equipment qualification and contamination control requirements for pilot biostudy batches approach those of submission and commercial batches, these types of batches are usually manufactured in production equipment. Larger firms may have a GMP Research and Development manufacturing facility for making these batches.

For experimental batches, cross-contamination must be low enough so that it does not alter the results of any measurements or tests performed on

TABLE 1 Regulatory Requirements for ANDA and Pre-ANDA Batches

Batch type	Experimental batch	Batch		
		Pilot/confirmatory batch	ANDA batch ('Biobatch')	
Batch use	Research and development only	Pilot biostudies/trial run before ANDA batch	Submission and any required biostudies	
Equipment qualification or calibration	Essential elements (critical processing parameters)	Full	Full	
Prevent cross contamination	Limited	Yes	Yes	
Documentation	Abbreviated batch record or laboratory notebook	Full batch record	Full batch record	
Batch size	Smallest possible with equipment used	Intermediate for pilot/not less than 100,000 dosage units for confirmatory	Not less than 100,000 dosage units for ANDA pivotal bioequivalence study	

the batch. Since this level is usually many times higher than the threshold for batches administered to humans, equipment for experimental batches does not require isolation or stringent dust control. Many firms have a separate area for making such batches. This "pilot laboratory" has small versions of production equipment, usually contained within a single room. It is necessary to keep records of the cleaning of such equipment; however, QA sign off is not required.

3. DOCUMENTATION

Product development groups are strongly encouraged to have SOPs that define how all activities are documented. Some firms use abbreviated batch records for experimental batches. These records may be completely or partially hand written. They do not require QA or regulatory approval. Other firms prefer to document the preparation of an experimental batch in a laboratory notebook.

No matter which type of documentation the firm chooses, the records must clearly reflect what was done to produce the batch, all observations and test results, and a conclusion drawn from the results. The last item has, at times, been neglected by R&D Departments. However, it is essential for reconstructing product development during an FDA Pre-approval Inspection.

Pilot biostudy and submission batches must be manufactured under production conditions and cGMPs, with complete documentation. Complete documentation includes inventory records, batch records documenting every step in batch production, packaging records, analytical laboratory records (including retention of all raw data), and a certificate of analysis or analytical report. QA review and sign off are required. Firms should develop procedures that define pre-requisite steps and requirements for release of such batches for biostudy testing.

4. OPTIMIZATION OF PROCESS PARAMETERS AND JUSTIFICATION OF IN-PROCESS SPECIFICATIONS

Since 1989, FDA investigators and reviewers have become more interested in optimization of process parameters and justification of in-process specifications. It is strongly advised that such activities be completed before ANDA submission batch manufacture. If the process is optimized at a later time, it will be necessary to amend master batch documentation to encompass the associated adjustments. This often leads to additional ANDA review cycles, which delay approval.

Due to Agency concerns about blend uniformity and for maximum efficiencies in manufacturing, blending times should be optimized. For example, if the R&D staff believes that 15 min of mixing is likely to work at a given step in the process, the best way to test this is to manufacture several experimental batches with different mixing times at that step, for example 5, 10, 15, and 20 min. If there are several mixing steps in the process, testing all steps this way is not practical. FDA will accept testing at the most critical mixing steps as a means of demonstrating uniform distribution of the drug. For solid dosage form manufacture, this is often the last mixing step, in which the lubricant is added. Many firms choose to use only one batch for mixing time studies, stopping the mixer every 5–10 min to sample the blend. While in theory a batch mixed for four periods of 5 min is not the same as one mixed continuously for 20 min, the difference is usually insignificant. However, if there is any indication that the blend is prone to segregation or otherwise less than rugged, use of one batch is not advisable. In extreme cases it may be necessary to test large numbers of finished dosage units in order to correlate blend uniformity to dosage form uniformity and optimize mixing times.

Experiments to establish the best method of sampling a given product blend for uniformity should be conducted early in the experimental batch process. If this is not done, errors due to sampling bias may confound conclusions about the effect of various process parameters on blend uniformity. A blend sample of adequate size should be taken using various techniques. The technique giving results that correlate with finished dosage uniformity should be selected (1–4).

In-process specifications such as unit weight and tablet hardness are justified by manufacturing product at or just outside the desired specification ranges. This material is tested for those attributes most likely to be affected by any deviation from specifications. For tablets, hardness is a parameter that may affect product quality, by altering dissolution behavior. In most cases, dissolution decreases with increasing hardness. Therefore, tablets manufactured at the extremes of the desired hardness range are tested for dissolution profile. For a liquid product, or for solid products manufactured by processes including one or more solution steps, the pH of the solution may affect stability. For example, if the active ingredient is acid labile and the liquid product contains a buffer to keep the pH over 7, change in the buffer over time may lead to a decrease in the pH. The pH specification must take into account the maximum possible change in the buffer system. Samples manufactured at the pH extremes can be subject to accelerated stability conditions and tested for assay to confirm the specification limits. A similar approach can be used for processing and drying times of wet granulations.

It is not unusual for specifications and process parameters that work for a very small batch to be unsuitable for manufacture of a larger batch. Experiments to determine the effect of scale up are advisable for all but the simplest formulations. Scaling up in smaller increments, rather than from a few thousand dosage units directly to 100,000 is advisable.

The results of the testing described in the previous paragraphs and the conclusions drawn from these results should be presented in a report that is reviewed by Regulatory Affairs and Quality Assurance. It is also advisable that firms include their manufacturing department in the review process, as it will ultimately inherit and be responsible for executing the chosen method of manufacture on an ongoing basis to supply commercial need.

5. BATCH SIZE

Since 1990, FDA has required that exhibit batches intended to support an ANDA submission comprise a minimum of 100,000 finished dosage units or 10% of the batch size intended for commercial production, whichever is greater (5). The original basis for establishment of this standard was somewhat arbitrary, however, it has since proven to be an appropriate benchmark for scale-up operations.

6. DEVELOPMENT REPORTS OR LOGS

Many generic firms prepare formal development reports for each product. Development reports usually outline the rationale for formulation development, summarize all the experimental batches made and what was concluded from the results obtained on them, explain what changes were made in the formulation during development and list the processing parameters that were used for each batch. These reports are very useful, especially if prepared at the time of ANDA submission or before. However, CGMPs do not require such reports, as long as the information is readily available from other documentation.

A possible alternative to the process of preparing a Development Report is the use of a Development Log. A log is maintained for each project, showing the receipt of all raw materials, including samples for preliminary testing, testing done, experimental batches made, conclusions drawn, manufacturing and testing of the submission batches, biostudy sampling, etc. References to laboratory notebooks and other documentation are included. An example of a idealized Product Development Log is shown in Table 2. In larger R&D groups, which may have several projects ongoing at the same time, maintaining these logs is an ideal task for Project Managers separate from those individuals who make or test experimental or submission batches. Investment of a few minutes each day to make sure that the logs are complete and up-to-date will reap substantial benefits during the Pre-Approval Inspection.

TABLE 2 Product Development Log for Profitabilamine Tablets, 1 mg Code Number: P0022

Date	Action	Notebook references
01/07/97	Received raw material sample from Cornucopia Fine Chemicals	
01/14/97	Received technical dossier from Cornucopia Fine Chemicals	
01/28/97	Completed sample testing; material acceptable	RDP0022-1 pp. 1–10
01/31/97	Ordered 1.0 kg raw material from Cornucopia	
02/18/97	Material received from Cornucopia-receiving number 97B055-P	
02/19/97	QA sample of 97B055-P received by lab	
02/20/97	Preliminary raw material analytical method approved	
03/06/97	97B055-P released by R&D Lab	RDP0022-1 pp. 11–20
03/07/97	Experimental batch X005-C prepared in pilot lab; samples to R&D Lab	
03/21/97	Dissolution of batch X005-C profile similar to brand batch 97XYZ09; uniformity and all other tests acceptable	RDP0022-1 pp 25–35
03/25/97	Hardness. Thickness and weight specification report approved	
04/02/97	Master #P0022-1 for 100,000 tablet batch size approved	

7. PRE-APPROVAL INSPECTIONS

According to the FDA's Pre-Approval Inspection Compliance Guide, FDA will always conduct a Pre-Approval Inspection (PAI) for the first ANDA (or NDA) submitted by a firm. The compliance program also requires an inspection for the first submission of a given product and for all submissions whose reference listed drug is one of the top 200 sellers in the US. While the firm's FDA District will almost always choose to do an inspection in the former case, it is somewhat less likely to do so in the latter. This may be because the Compliance Program does not specify which top 200 list to use, or because the lists change from year to year (6). For submissions that do not meet any of these criteria, the FDA District may choose not to inspect, if the firm has had an acceptable cGMP inspection in the last two years, and has demonstrated successful pre-approval inspection history over the same time period. The District will simply tell CDER Compliance (Food and Drug Administration, Center for Drug and Research, Office of Compliance) that it has no objection to the approval.

What will FDA look for during a Pre-approval Inspection? FDA Investigators will verify the accuracy and completeness of key information in an ANDA submission during the inspection. They will examine bulk active ingredient purchase orders, invoices, and packing slips to ensure that the material was actually available to make the batch on the dates recorded in the batch record. If any of the inactive ingredients were not previously used by the firm, receiving records may be checked as well. FDA investigators will compare the batch records in the submission to the use and cleaning logs for the equipment used, to determine if the dates (and times, if recorded) match. Both of these activities are intended to rule out the possibility of falsified batch records.

The FDA Investigators will also determine whether the firm has the equipment designated in the master batch records for commercial-size batches intended for manufacture after approval. This provision of the Pre-Approval Inspection program has historically generated the greatest number of recommendations to withhold ANDA approval among the various categories of required inspectional elements. In FDA summaries of reasons for a District not recommending ANDA or NDA approval, this deficiency is included in the failure category "plant not ready".

What is causing this problem? In many cases, a firm does not wish to purchase any equipment that will be unique to the commercial process of a submitted product until it is needed to start commercial production. The Pre-Approval Inspection generally occurs months, or, in some cases years, before the ANDA is approved.

Fortunately for industry, FDA now has Scale-Up and Post Approval Changes (SUPAC) Guidances for various types of dosage forms (7) and a general guidance to changes permitted under the FDA Modernization Act of 1997 (8). Firms may use these Guidances to scale up a process without prior approval from FDA. When a firm is introducing a new type of equipment in a submission, it is recommended that the scale-up information in the ANDA reflect the largest size batch that can be made on the equipment used to make the submission batch, or other existing equipment, but not more than 10 times the size of the submission batch in dosage units. After ANDA approval, the firm can purchase and qualify larger equipment and use SUPAC to implement the production of larger batch sizes.

FDA Investigators will spend a lot of time during the Pre-Approval Inspection comparing the analytical data in the ANDA to that in the laboratory notebooks or other records. They often focus on any data that was rejected. Since the analytical methods used to test ANDA batches are generally new to the firm, unexpected method problems or chemist errors are not uncommon. The FDA is concerned that firms will reject valid data. Doing so may give an unrealistically favorable profile of the product. (The dilemma of when to properly reject laboratory data was one of the basic issues addressed in the "Barr Decision (9)). Over the past two years, laboratory controls have become a very key element of pre-approval inspections. Much focus is placed on the handling of out-of-specification (OOS) test results. It is imperative that firms have written procedures in place regarding the investigation and ultimate disposition of OOS and other anomalous data. Often, a "decision tree" approach is used as the process can become complicated and the outcome can be dependent on a number of pre-requisite steps including, but not limited to, sample reinjection, re-prepping and repeat testing, or, in extreme cases, batch resampling (Fig. 1). Error simulation may be used as a means of confirming the cause of a suspect result, and can add substantial weight to the overall quality of the investigation.

The ultimate disposition of a suspect result must be approved by the firm's quality assurance unit after reviewing the associated investigation report. Thus, the investigating parties must ensure that the rationale for the proposed action is well documented and follows a logical sequence, and that the data supporting the conclusions are referenced in the appropriate sections of the report.

On occasion, FDA investigators have taken the position that the ANDA submission should contain reference to the existence of rejected data. Opinions among Investigators vary on whether this is required for the submission to be complete or just something that makes the pre-approval inspection easier. A firm should feel confident defending the exclusion of such references in its ANDA submission as long as the rationale for rejecting data is well justified, in compliance with its SOPs and has obtained quality assurance approval. With this approach, the appropriateness of the firm's

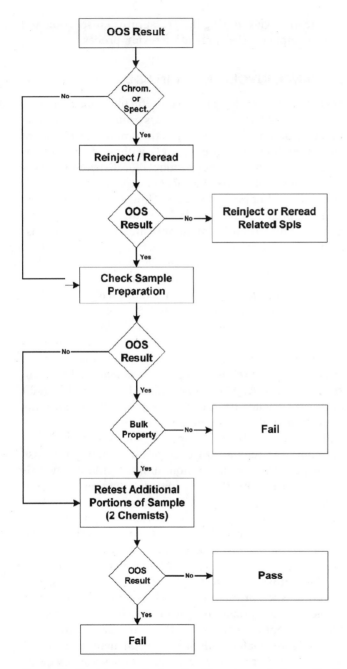

FIGURE 1 Decision tree for handling laboratory out of specification results.

action becomes an issue for review during the pre-approval inspection and does not unnecessarily complicate the application review process.

8. QUALITY ASSURANCE INVOLVEMENT IN R&D

Several generic drug manufacturers have found it useful to create a separate Quality Assurance group for R&D. Members of this group receive special training so that they have a better understanding of the product development process. They are also free to concentrate on R&D without distraction or competition from the need to release other products for distribution. This practice can create efficiencies that have the effect of expediting the overall development, submission, and approval process. However, firms must be cautious in taking this approach. Firstly, it is imperative to structure the reporting relationship such that a conflict of interest situation does not exist (i.e., this dedicated unit should report into the existing quality assurance unit). Secondly, the policies and procedures of the dedicated unit should be consistent with those employed by the main quality unit.

Whether or not a firm chooses to establish a dedicated quality unit for R&D, the QA discipline must be involved in key activities of product development. Support for this involvement must come from the highest levels of management. Management needs to take concrete steps to make this commitment clear to all. An QA audit of all relevant documentation while an ANDA submission is being prepared is strongly recommended if the firm wishes to have a successful Pre-Approval Inspection. However, this audit will be prone to problems and delays if QA has not been involved in checking the key elements of product development documentation on a regular basis. The audit will be most useful if it is performed by staff members who were not those doing the regular QA checks. Firms may opt to use outside consultants to perform pre-submission audits. While costly, this approach can often be justified by the anticipated reduction in overall approval time.

An issue related to those discussed in the previous paragraphs is the nature and timing of analytical method transfer from the R&D method development laboratory to the Quality Control laboratory responsible for releasing approved products for marketing. The normal mechanism for this transfer is to have QC laboratory staff test samples of active ingredients, process intermediates, and finished product previously tested by R&D. Some firms opt to use samples that are prepared by R&D specifically for method transfer with known amounts of all analytes. This is a "safe harbor" approach intended to avoid the risks associated with practicing an analytical technique on an actual submission batch. If the prepared samples are powdered (made by accurately weighing all ingredients) while the dosage form is a tablet, a key step in the method is not tested. Extraction of the analyte can cause problems when the matrix is not sufficiently disintegrated. Preparation of compressed tablets from a small batch may be appropriate for simpler formulations, but not for more complex ones. The use of submission batch samples for the method transfer experiments avoids these issues but introduces the risk of OOS results from the QC laboratory. Even though the procedure is essentially a training exercise, FDA investigators have been known to later question OOS results obtained during method transfer. If a firm opts to use submission batch samples for method transfer, it must ensure that any OOS results produced during the exercise are investigated in accordance with procedures previously discussed in this chapter (Fig. 1).

Timing of method transfer often depends on available QC resources. A firm may choose to perform the transfer after ANDA approval, and may even use the first scale-up batch as transfer testing material. The degree of risk assumed with this approach increases with the complexity of the product and/or the analytical method.

Some firms have chosen to transfer the methods to QC before manufacture of the submission batch. An experimental or pilot batch with the same formulation and manufacturing process as anticipated for the submission batch is used as testing material. This approach enables the resolution of method-related issues prior to the generation of supporting data for the submission batch. Here, a firm can reduce the time to approval by avoiding additional review cycles otherwise warranted by method revisions identified later in the process.

A large number of firms choose a middle course. When Regulatory Affairs declares that all major FDA observations related to the submission have been resolved, plans are made to manufacture commercial batches and validate the scaled-up process. Method transfer is conducted while the materials needed for the scale-up are on order, so that the QC laboratory is ready to test the process validation samples for the commercial batches when they are available. Firms that opt to take this approach must have a substantial degree of confidence in the robustness of their methods. Otherwise, late fixes may be required and the ANDA submission will have to be amended.

9. CONCLUSION

As the information in this chapter demonstrates, QA and QC oversight are an essential part of generic drug development. Firms that establish and follow sound procedures and practices for drug development and ensure proper quality oversight throughout the process will reap the benefits of successful pre-approval inspections and timely ANDA approvals. While resource-intensive, this approach can provide substantial commercial advantage and significant contribution to the "bottom line".

The authors would like to thank Elsa Gomez, David Cohen, Carla Hedrick, Suzanne Yu, and Izzy Kanfer for their assistance.

REFERENCES

1. Berman J, Planchard J. A blend uniformity and unit dose sampling. Drug Develop Indust Pharm 1995; 21(11):1257–1283.
2. Berman J, Schoeneman A, Shelton JT. Unit dose sampling: a tale of two thieves. Drug Develop Indust Pharm 1996; 22(11):1121–1132.
3. FDA's Guide to Inspections of Oral Solid Dosage Forms, January 1994.
4. Technical Report No. 25: Blend uniformity analysis: validation and in-process testing. J Pharmaceut Sci Technol 1997;51(53): 51–599. Supplement published by the Parenteral Drug Association and FDA's response to it, 8/29/97 (by Pat Beers Block, Special Assistant to the Director, Division of Manufacturing and Product Quality, Office of Compliance, CDER).
5. Manual of Policies and Procedures 5223.3 (formerly Office of Generic Drugs Policy and Procedure Guide 22–90), Center for Drug Evaluation and Research, Food and Drug Administration.
6. The Pharmacy Times Web Site Top 200 list at www.pharmacytimes.com.
7. SUPAC-IR: Immediate-Release Solid Oral Dosage Forms: Scale-Up and Post-Approval Changes: Chemistry, Manufacturing and Controls, InVitro Dissolution Testing and In Vivo Bioequivalence Documentation; Center for Drug Evaluation and Research, Food and Drug Administration, November 1995. Other SUPAC documents are available on the FDA web site, http://www.fda.gov/cder/guidance/index.htm.
8. Guidance for Industry, Changes to an Approved NDA or ANDA, Center for Drug Evaluation and Research, Food and Drug Administration, November 1999. Guidance for Industry, Changes to an Approved NDA or ANDA, Questions and Answers, Center for Drug Evaluation and Research, Food and Drug Administration, January 2001.
9. United States of America, Plaintiff, v. Barr Laboratories, Inc., et al., Defendants, Civil Action No. 92–1744, US District Court for the District of New Jersey, February 4, 1993.

8

Drug Product Performance, In Vitro*

Pradeep M. Sathe, Andre S. Raw,
Larry A. Ouderkirk, Lawrence X. Yu, and
Ajaz S. Hussain
Center for Drug Evaluation and Research,
U.S. Food and Drug Administration, Rockville, Maryland, U.S.A.

1. INTRODUCTION

This chapter examines the issues related to the in vitro characterization of solid oral dosage forms. The importance and utility of in vitro characterization are discussed in relation to the factors influencing in vitro drug release, including those intrinsic to the drug substance, the drug product and manufacturing process, and relevant dissolution test methodology. A discussion is also provided on practical issues that may be faced during the conduct and evaluation of in vitro dissolution testing and the application of in vitro drug product performance testing.

2. IMPORTANCE OF IN VITRO DRUG PRODUCT CHARACTERIZATION

Modern solid oral dosage forms are expected to be of high quality and exhibit reliable performance characteristics. This is achieved by careful selection

---

*Opinions expressed in this chapter are those of the authors and do not necessarily reflect the views or policies of the FDA.

and quality control of various ingredients and a well-defined manufacturing process, giving careful thought to different variables that may influence product appearance, potency, stability, and dissolution. In modern pharmaceutics, as the complexity of materials, instruments, equipment, and techniques have increased, it has become imperative to apply up-to-date research methods, techniques, and tools to manufacture and monitor these dosage forms. In vitro characterization of solid oral dosage forms is important from the perspective that it provides us with information regarding active ingredient potency and uniformity, as well as information regarding the rate at which the active ingredient is released from the dosage form. This characterization is vital for formulation development, comparability assessment, and for quality assurance and control.

In vitro testing to characterize the potency and release rate of the active ingredient(s) in solid oral dosage forms is based on the monographs and general chapters in the United States Pharmacopoeia/National Formulary (USP/NF) (1) and on various guidance documents of the Food and Drug Administration/Center for Drug Evaluation and Research (FDA/CDER) (2–4).

Tests and requirements for content and consistency of the dosage form include assay or potency of the active ingredient(s) and content uniformity/weight variation of dosage units. Tests for in vitro release of active ingredient(s) from the dosage form include dissolution and disintegration.

Following oral administration of a solid oral dosage form, the critical elements of drug absorption are (1) disintegration, dissolution, and solubilization and (2) permeability across the membranes of the gastrointestinal tract. Due to the critical nature of the first of these steps, in vitro dissolution is often relevant to the prediction of in vivo drug product performance. This is particularly true for low-solubility drugs and for modified-release dosage forms, for which dissolution/drug release is usually the rate-limiting step in the in vivo absorption of the active drug.

3. TYPES OF SOLID ORAL DOSAGE FORMS

Among the different types of solid oral dosage forms available, tablets and capsules are the most popular and constitute a major share of the market. Tablets are often variously categorized as regular (oral), effervescent, chewable, orally disintegrating, etc. Capsules may be of either the soft- or hard-gelatin variety. Examples of less-common solid oral dosage forms are powders, granules, chewing gum, troches, and wafers.

The solid oral dosage forms may also be categorized by their release characteristics. The two types are immediate-release and modified-release. The immediate-release drug products are designed to release their active ingredient(s) promptly following administration. Modified-release drug products comprise delayed-release (enteric-coated) and extended-release dosage forms (also referred to as controlled-release, sustained-release, etc.).

Delayed-release (DR) products are formulated to retard release of the active ingredient until the dosage form leaves the stomach. This is done to protect the gastric mucosa from drug irritation, or to limit exposure of acid-labile drugs to stomach acid, or to target release of the active ingredient to the lower intestinal tract in order to enhance in vivo absorption. Often, delayed-release dosage forms have an enteric polymeric coating with characteristic pH-dependent solubility (or stability) to prevent release of the active ingredient in the stomach at low acidic pH. Once the delayed-release product leaves the stomach, the enteric coating dissolves (or is degraded); subsequent in vivo drug release then generally follows the same course as for an immediate-release product.

Extended-release (ER) products are formulated to make the active ingredient available over an extended period of time. These extended-release products which comprise sustained-release, controlled-release and repeat-action varieties are expected to lengthen the dosing interval and reduce the dosing frequency as compared to the corresponding immediate-release product (5,6). This is achieved to enhance patient convenience/compliance, increase therapeutic effectiveness, and/or to help minimize toxicity or side effects, especially in those products for which a rapidly released dose, or for which drug level fluctuations might not be desirable.

4. FACTORS AFFECTING IN VITRO DRUG PRODUCT DISSOLUTION

The process of drug product dissolution can be viewed as proceeding through several discrete steps. The first of these involves the wetting and penetration of the dissolution medium into the dosage unit. The second step, which generally occurs in many conventional dosage forms, but certainly not a prerequisite for dissolution, involves disintegration and/or de-aggregation into granules or fine particles of the drug substance. The third step involves solubilization of the drug substance into solution. These steps need not proceed in a stepwise manner, but can occur simultaneously during the dissolution process.

In vitro drug product dissolution can be affected by various factors including those intrinsic to the drug substance, the drug product formulation, the manufacturing process, and the dissolution testing methodology, as individually discussed below.

4.1. Factors Related to Drug Substance

Dissolution refers to the process of solubilization of the drug into the dissolution medium. As a fundamental process, dissolution is controlled by the affinity between the solid and the dissolution medium (7), and can be modeled as the diffusion of the drug into the bulk liquid media. Noyes and Whitney (8) in 1897 proposed a fundamental equation for dissolution:

$$dm/dt = K \times (C_s - C_t) \tag{1}$$

Here dm/dt is the mass rate of dissolution, K is the proportionality constant called the dissolution constant, C_s is the concentration at saturation or maximum solubility and C_t is the concentration at time t. The term $C_s - C_t$ in the above equation represents the concentration gradient between the diffusion layer and the bulk solution. In 1900 Brunner and Tolloczko (9) modified the above equation by incorporating the surface area, S

$$dm/dt = K' \times S \times (C_s - C_t) \tag{2}$$

Here K' is a constant unique to the chemical substance and varies widely from drug to drug.

Brunner expanded the scope of the above equation to include Nernst's (1904) theory (10) of a saturated and stagnant liquid film diffusion layer of thickness h around the drug particle, having a diffusion coefficient D in a bulk dissolution volume V

$$dC/dt = [DS/Vh] \times (C_s - C_t) \tag{3}$$

From these theoretical principles, it is quite apparent that drug dissolution is influenced by solubility, diffusivity, surface area, and solution hydrodynamics.

4.1.1. Solubility of the Drug Substance

The dissolution rate of a drug is closely associated with drug substance solubility. Compounds with high solubility generally exhibit significantly higher dissolution rates as shown in Eq. (3) . The solubility of compounds containing "ionizable groups" is a function of the pH of the dissolution media and the pK_a of the compound. Solubility of a drug is traditionally determined using an equilibrium solubility method and involves suspending an excess amount of solid drug in a selected aqueous medium. In some cases, it may not be feasible to measure the equilibrium solubility of a compound, such as for a metastable polymorph which undergoes conversion during the time frame of the solubility measurement. In this instance, a dynamic method may be used to estimate the solubility of the compound. This is referred to as kinetic solubility and is generally determined by measuring the intrinsic dissolution rate (11).

The "dose/solubility" ratio of the drug provides an estimate of the volume of fluids required to dissolve an individual dose. When this volume exceeds about 1 L, in vivo dissolution is often considered problematic (12). For example, griseofulvin has an aqueous solubility of 15 μg/mL and at a dose of 500 mg, has a dose/solubility ratio of 33.3 L. This therefore exhibits a dissolution/solubility limited oral absorption.

4.1.2. Polymorphism

The drug substance may also exist in different physical forms and exhibit solid-state polymorphism. Polymorphism refers to a drug substance:

1. existing in two or more crystalline phases that have different arrangements and/or conformations of the molecules in the crystal lattice,
2. having differing hydrate (or other solvate) forms, and
3. having amorphous phases which do not possess a distinguishable crystal lattice (13,14).

Difference in the lattice energies of these polymorphs results in differences in the solubilities and hence in the dissolution rates of these various polymorphic forms (15). The solubility differences between different crystalline polymorphs will typically be less than several-fold and in the case of hydrates, these generally exhibit lower solubilities than the anhydrous form. In the case of amorphous forms, these can have solubilities several hundred times that of the corresponding crystalline counterparts (16). Polymorphism in chloramphenicol palmitate provides a classic example illustrating the significance of this phenomenon. Chloramphenicol palmitate can exist in two polymorphic forms: Form A and Form B. Form B is shown to exhibit greater oral absorption than Form A, due to enhanced solubility (17).

4.1.3. Salt Factor and 'pH' of the Diffusion Layer

In general, organic salts are more water-soluble than the corresponding unionized molecule and this offers a simple means of increasing dissolution rate. It is for this reason that sodium and potassium salts of weak acids, as well as hydrochloride or other strong acid salts of weak bases, are frequently selected during drug development. A multi-tier approach to select salts for achieving optimal product performance is discussed in the literature (18).

In addition, even if the equilibrium solubility of the parent drug and the salt in the dissolution medium may be alike, the dissolution rate of the salt of the weak acid or base will often be enhanced. This effect can be explained on the basis of differences in the pH of the thin diffusion layer surrounding the drug particle (19). In the case of salts of free acids, the pH of the diffusion layer will be greater than the pH of the diffusion layer for the acid. Analogously, in the case of salts of the free base, the pH of the diffusion layer will be less than the pH of the diffusion layer for the free base. This will result in higher effective solubilities of these salts in the diffusion layer as compared to their parent unionized compounds, and in an increased dissolution rate. The salt occasionally may be useful for another therapeutic indication. For example, the non-steroidal anti-inflammatory drug naproxen (20) was originally marketed as a free acid for the treatment of rheumatoid or osteo-arthritis. However, the sodium salt, which is absorbed faster than the acid, was found to be more effective in post-partum pain than the parent compound.

4.1.4.   Surface Area and Particle Size

The dissolution rate of a compound is also directly related to its exposed surface area (as is evident from Eq. (3)). Therefore, drug particle size reduction, which results in an increased surface area exposed to the dissolution medium, would be expected to increase the dissolution rate. Hence, micronized formulations of poorly soluble drugs may exhibit markedly increased rates of dissolution compared to non-micronized formulations (19). This is evidenced in marketed formulations of products such as glyburide tablets. The micronized formulations (e.g., Glynase® tablets) dissolve much faster than the non-micronized formulations (e.g., Micronase® tablets).

4.2.   Formulation Factors

The inactive ingredients (excipients) used in the formulation may also have an important effect on drug product dissolution. In the case of immediate-release dosage forms, excipients are often used to enhance dissolution rates. For example, disintegrants such as crosscarmellose sodium and sodium starch glycolate are used to facilitate breakup of the tablet dosage form and promote deaggregation into granules or fine particles (21). The effect of the disintegrant is to promote tablet deaggregation and expose a greater drug particle surface area, thereby facilitating dissolution. Surfactants such as sodium laurel sulfate and polysorbate may also be used to accelerate dissolution rates. This effect of the surfactant is achieved by increasing the aqueous solubility of hydrophobic drugs by micelle formation, and/or by facilitating drug wetting, by decreasing the surface tension of the hydrophobic drug particle with the dissolution media and thereby creating a larger drug–solvent surface interface for dissolution to occur (22,23). Hydrophilic binders and fillers may also be incorporated into the formulation to promote wetting of hydrophobic drug particles in order to enhance dissolution rates (22).

Conversely, excipients may sometimes have an inadvertent retarding effect upon drug dissolution. For example, during formulation development, care must be taken to ensure that the drug does not bind to an excipient, such as in the formation of an insoluble metal chelate which may alter the drug dissolution profile. Lubricants such as the stearates, which are commonly used to decrease friction in the die wall cavity, are generally hydrophobic in nature and at high concentrations (>1%), these may have the effect of reducing drug wettability (22,24). This will have the effect of prolonging disintegration times or in diminishing the effective interface of drug particles with the solvent medium, resulting in reduced dissolution rates. Gelatin capsule shells are prone to cross-linking in the presence of free aldehydes or keto groups. This may result in pellicle formation and a greatly reduced dissolution rate. This type of phenomenon has been attributed to the dissolution failures seen with gelatin capsules and gelatin coated tablets packaged with rayon fillers (25).

For modified-release drug products, the excipients are chosen to have a controlled effect on the rate of drug release from the dosage form, in order to target the delivery to certain sites along the gastrointestinal tract, commonly referred to as the "absorption windows". This can be achieved by dispersing or incorporating the active ingredient into a hydrophilic or hydrophobic matrix, ion-exchange resin, osmotic pump, or by coating the drug particles or the dosage unit with a polymeric or wax film. These modified-release dosage forms are formulated by a complex process that must take into consideration the properties of the active ingredient, the type of release device that is to be used, the characteristics of modifying release excipients that may be chosen, and the desired drug release profile that is to be achieved (26).

4.3. Manufacturing Process Factors

Several manufacturing variables can affect the drug product dissolution characteristics. Here, manufacturing strategies may be employed to enhance dissolution rates. For example, spray drying or melt extrusion of the active ingredient with excipients such as polyvinylpyrrolidine (PVP) can be used to generate stabilized amorphous dispersions, which have greatly accelerated dissolution rates (19,27). Improved wetting of hydrophobic drug surfaces and enhanced dissolution rates are sometimes achieved by employing wet granulation vs. dry granulation processes, during product manufacture (28). Direct compression may also be chosen over granulation for enhancing dissolution, based upon the propensity for directly compressed tablets to de-aggregate into finer drug particles (29).

Conversely, manufacturing variables may also have a retarding effect upon dissolution. For example, over-mixing with lubricants may have an adverse effect on drug wettability, and hence upon drug disintegration and dissolution (19). Tablet punch pressures must also be optimized to achieve acceptable disintegration rates (30). At low punch pressure, liquid penetration in the tablet will be facile, but disintegrant swelling may not result in tablet de-aggregation due to its high porosity; on the other hand, excessive punch pressure may hinder the penetration of liquid into the tablet and result in slower disintegration rates.

For modified-release products, the manufacturing process must be well defined and be highly robust to assure reproducible drug release from batch to batch. Here, the process of dispersing the drug into the matrix or of coating the drug with modified-release excipients must be tightly controlled. The manufacturing process must have well-defined "endpoints" and must distribute the modified-release excipients uniformly around the active ingredient; otherwise this will be reflected in variable dissolution performance (31).

4.4. Dissolution/Drug Release Test Conditions

Dissolution test parameters such as apparatus type and rotation speed (32), and dissolution medium pH and volume (22) can also significantly influence the dissolution rate of a solid oral dosage form. The dissolution test conditions are discussed in greater detail in Sections 5.2 and 5.3. The dissolution assay method and adequate instrumentation are important to generate valid measurements of the dissolution process.

5.   IN VITRO DRUG PRODUCT PERFORMANCE EVALUATION

5.1. Disintegration Test

The disintegration test is described in the USP General Chapter ⟨701⟩ *Disintegration*. Disintegration testing is considered appropriate when a relationship to dissolution has been established or when disintegration is shown to be more discriminating than dissolution. It is a qualitative test and does not quantify drug dissolution. An official disintegration apparatus, the USP basket–rack assembly, is used to perform the test, which is generally applicable only to immediate-release products. The International Conference on Harmonization (ICH) Q6A Guidance document (33) has proposed a decision tree for the application of the disintegration test. When product dissolution is rapid (defined by ICH as dissolution NLT 80% in 15 min at pH 1.2, 4.0, and 6.8) and the dosage form contains drugs that are highly soluble throughout the physiological range, disintegration testing may be meaningful. The ICH Guidance considers a drug substance to be *highly soluble* when the highest dose strength is soluble in 250 mL or less of aqueous media over the pH range of 1.2–6.8. The volume estimate of 250 mL is derived from a typical bioequivalence study protocol that prescribes administration of a drug product to fasting human volunteers with a glass (about 8 oz) of water.

5.2. Dissolution Test—Immediate-Release Solid Oral Dosage Forms

The dissolution test is referenced in USP General Chapter ⟨711⟩ *Dissolution*. The test quantitatively measures the amount of active drug that dissolves from the dosage form in a liquid dissolution medium using standard dissolution apparatus and procedures. The FDA's general recommendations regarding dissolution testing are given in the Agency's Guidance *Dissolution Testing of Immediate-Release Solid Oral Dosage Forms* (2). The dissolution test is required for virtually all solid oral dosage forms as a condition of product approval. The International Conference on Harmonization (ICH) Q6A Guidance document (33) provides three decision trees for assisting in the development of suitable dissolution test conditions and tolerances. The dissolution test conditions are generally selected to ensure a sensitive and discriminatory measure of drug product performance (34). As discussed later in the chapter, dissolution data can also be used to support certain post-approval changes in manufacturing and/or formulation, as well as to waive the requirement to conduct in vivo bioequivalence studies under certain conditions.

5.2.1. Apparatus

USP General Chapter ⟨711⟩ *Dissolution* establishes equipment specifications and operational standards for the Apparatus 1 (basket) and 2 (paddle), the apparatus most commonly used for studying the dissolution of solid oral dosage forms. The basket at 100 rpm is commonly used for testing capsules, and the paddle at 50 rpm for tablets. The dissolution rate generally increases as the stirring rate or dissolution speed is increased. This increase, however, may not necessarily follow a simple mathematical relationship (32). The USP Apparatus 3 (see USP General Chapter ⟨724⟩ *Drug Release*) is also sometimes used for dissolution testing of immediate-release drug products, in addition to extended-release products (35). Apparatus 4 and 7 are used exclusively for extended-release dosage forms, including oral tablets and capsules. For convenience, the official USP apparatus used for dissolution/drug release testing of solid oral dosage forms, along with their recommended operational parameters and target drug products are given in the following table:

USP apparatus	Description	Rotational speed	Dosage form
1	Basket	50–120 rpm	IR[a], DR[b], ER[c]
2	Paddle	25–00 rpm	IR, DR, ER
3	Reciprocating cylinder	6–35 dpm[d]	IR, ER
4	Flow-though cell[e]	N/A	ER and poorly soluble active pharmaceutical ingredient/s in IR
7	Reciprocating disk	30 cpm[f]	ER

[a]IR = immediate-release
[b]DR = delayed-release
[c]ER = extended-release
[d]Six to thirty-five dips per minute currently in approved USP monographs; other speeds may also be acceptable.
[e]USP Apparatus 4 currently not used in any USP monograph Dissolution or Drug Release test.
[f]Thirty cycles per minute currently in approved USP monographs; other speeds may also be acceptable.

5.2.2. Media

The selection of a dissolution test medium is based on the physico-chemical properties of the drug substance and characteristics of the dosage form. In selecting the medium, an attempt should be made to emulate physiologic conditions. Thus, media with pHs ranging from 1.2 (gastric pH) to 6.8 (intestinal pH) are generally preferred. The most common media used in dissolution testing are water, 0.1 N hydrochloric acid, pH 4.5 acetate buffer, and pH 6.8 phosphate buffer. For drugs that are weak acids, the dissolution rate increases with increasing pH; while for weak bases, dissolution rate decreases with increasing pH. Selection of appropriate medium volume (generally 500–1000 mL, with 900 mL being the most common) is primarily based on drug solubility. For drugs with poor aqueous solubility, a larger volume may be necessary to achieve sink conditions and effect complete drug dissolution in a reasonable time. Alternatively, surfactants may be added to the dissolution medium. The incorporation of surfactants into the dissolution medium generally enhances solubility and dissolution rate through reduction of the interfacial tension and induction of micellar formation. Addition of ionic salts to the dissolution medium also may increase the dissolution rate, but the use of hydroalcoholic or any other media containing organic solvents is discouraged. For hard- and soft-gelatin capsules and gelatin-coated tablets, specified quantities of enzymes may be added to the dissolution medium to prevent the formation of pellicles that may result from cross-linking of gelatin (1). Also, tiny air bubbles can circulate in the medium and affect the uniformity of hydrodynamics of the test. The air can be removed from the medium by the deaeration method described in USP ⟨711⟩ *Dissolution* or another validated method. The temperature of the dissolution bath is usually maintained at 37 ± 0.5°C to reflect human body temperature. Currently, new research efforts are being made on the use of "bio-relevant" media to predict the dissolution of poorly soluble drugs and to predict plasma levels of lipophilic drugs (36,37).

5.2.3. Tolerance

The dissolution test acceptance criterion, or *tolerance*, is specified in terms of the quantity ("Q") that is dissolved within a specified time interval. The quantity is expressed as a percentage of the *labeled claim* (and not the assayed amount) of active ingredient in the dosage form. Typically, for most immediate-release oral dosage forms, 75% or 80% ("Q") of the labeled amount of the active drug ingredient is specified to be dissolved within a set time duration (test times between 15 and 60 min are most common). The dissolution test results are evaluated using the Acceptance Table in USP ⟨711⟩, which describes criteria for mean and individual sample dissolution results through three progressive stages of testing (S_1, S_2, and S_3, specifying 6, 12, and 24 samples tested, respectively). The value specified for "Q" should be used "as is" and should not be confused with the "Q + 5%" value specified for the S_1 stage of testing. Drug products may meet the dissolution requirement at any stage of testing; however, for bioequivalence purposes, the stage S_2 testing (12 units tested) is recommended. The dissolution tolerances are initially established based on the dissolution profiles obtained from the drug product lot(s) upon which the in vivo bio-availability/equivalence study was performed. The initial specifications can be revised later, if necessary, as more data become available. A generic immediate-release drug product should generally meet the dissolution requirements specified in the USP monograph. If no USP requirements are established, the product should be formulated to meet or exceed the in vitro dissolution performance of the Reference Listed Drug (RLD), as identified in the FDA "Orange Book" (6). Characteristics such as drug solubility, permeability, dissolution rate, and pharmacokinetics should be considered in setting dissolution test specifications, in order for the test to be useful in ensuring product similarity/equivalence.

5.3. Drug Release Test—Modified-Release Solid Oral Dosage Forms

The drug release test is referenced in the USP General Chapter ⟨724⟩ *Drug Release*. The drug release test is analogous to the dissolution test, except that it is applied to modified-release drug products rather than to immediate-release drug products. The FDA's general recommendations regarding drug release testing are given in its Guidances: *Bioavailability and Bioequivalence Studies for Orally Administered Drug Products—General Considerations* and *Extended release Oral Dosage Forms: Development, Evaluation, and Application of In vitro/in vivo Correlation*. As in the dissolution test, the test for drug release is conducted on sample sizes of 6–24 individual dosage units (12 dosage units are required for bioequivalence testing). Owing to differences in release mechanisms among extended-release drug products, the products for a given drug type made by different manufacturers are allowed to have unique drug release tests and do not necessarily have to use the tests approved for the RLD or other manufacturers. However, unjustified proliferation of tests should be avoided. The recommended test apparatus, media, and tolerances are discussed in detail below.

5.3.1. Apparatus

For modified-release oral dosage forms, the USP General Chapter ⟨724⟩ *Drug Release* provides equipment specifications and operational standards for the Apparatus 3, 4, and 7 in addition to Apparatus 1 and 2 (see the table in Section 5.2.1). Use of Apparatus 1 and 2 is usually preferred, however, for solid oral dosage forms unless there is a demonstrated advantage in using another official Apparatus. The use of non-official Apparatus is generally discouraged.

5.3.2. Media

The media are generally the same as those recommended for testing immediate-release products, except that there is no provision for the addition of enzymes (two-tiered testing) . For delayed-release (enteric-coated) solid oral dosage forms, a two-stage procedure is followed—first, testing in 0.1 N HCl for 2 h to demonstrate acid resistance, followed by testing in pH 6.8 buffer. The acid-stage and buffer-stage tests each have their own Acceptance Table in the USP General Chapter ⟨724⟩.

5.3.3. Tolerances

Release tolerances are proposed based on the in vitro drug release performance of the bio-study lot or lots. The tolerances should include a minimum of three time points selected from within the labeled dosing interval.

The first tolerance range is generally set at one hour to ensure against "dose-dumping". Subsequent time points are also established as ranges and the final time point is set as a minimum value of labeled amount released [for example NLT 80% (Q)]. The tolerances are generally interpreted according to the Acceptance Table 4 in the USP General Chapter ⟨724⟩. Three levels of testing are described, similar to those for the immediate-release drug products.

5.4. Dissolution/Drug Release Profile Comparisons

For adequate and complete characterization of dissolution, several FDA "Guidances" request submission of comparative multi-time point dissolution profile data in addition to meeting a single-point tolerance ("Q") requirement (2,3,38,39). Several different profile comparison approaches (such as model-dependent, model-independent-multivariate, and model-independent-index) have been developed and evaluated by the Agency (40–43). These approaches are useful for comparing the dissolution profiles of drug product lots, especially to evaluate the effects of scale-up and post-approval changes.

In the model-dependent approach, the profile similarity is evaluated using a suitable mathematical model function to describe the dissolution data. The approach is recommended for a dissolution "data rich" scenario. After selecting a model, the dissolution profiles are evaluated in terms of model parameters. The approach is exercised through the following steps:

1. Select a suitable mathematical function (model) to describe the dissolution data at hand (say, coming from a few production-size pre-change lots).
2. Fit the individual unit dissolution data from different standardized production-size lots to the selected model and estimate the inter- and intra-lot variability of the model parameters.
3. Define a "similarity region" or criterion on the basis of the inter- and intra-lot parameter variance.
4. Fit the dissolution data from "N" units of the reference (say, pre-change) and test (say, post-change) lots using the same mathematical function to generate model parameters.
5. Calculate a "statistical distance" between parameter means of the test and Reference lots.
6. Compute a 90% "confidence region" around the statistical distance.
7. Compare the "confidence region" with the "similarity region" calculated in step (iii) to assess the similarity or dissimilarity of the profiles.

If the confidence region computed from step (6) falls within the bounds of the similarity region generated in step (3), the profiles are considered similar, else they are considered dissimilar. A comprehensive discussion of this approach is beyond the scope of this chapter. For a detailed and hands-on discussion of this approach, the readers are directed to references 40 and 41.

In the model-independent "Multivariate" approach, the dissolution values are compared directly without assuming a model or creating parameters. Each dissolution measurement, coming from the multiple dissolution time points, is considered as a variable, correlated to adjacent time points. First a "statistical distance" is computed which accounts for the mean dissolution differences as well as their variance, covariance matrix. A confidence region is then computed around the statistical distance. The statistical distance often used for this type of (multivariate) analysis is known as "Mahalanobis Distance" or "M-Distance". It is given by the formula

$$D_M = \text{SQRT}\{(X_2 - X_1)'S_{\text{pooled}}^{-1}(X_2 - X_1)\} \tag{4}$$

where D_M = "Mahalanobis" distance, SQRT = square root of the entire term, $S_{\text{pooled}} = (S_1 + S_2)/2$ is the sample variance–covariance matrix pooled across both the test and reference batches where S_1 and S_2 are the individual sample-lot variance–covariance matrix, X_1 = vector of mean dissolution of Reference and X_2 = vector of mean dissolution of Test. For a detailed discussion of the approach, readers are directed to Ref. 42.

In the index approach, profiles are compared with respect to a particular a priori defined index. Several indices have been proposed, such as "Rescigno" in 1992 (44), fit factors "f_1" and "f_2" by Moore and Flanner in 1996 (45), and Rho, Rho-m, Delta-a and Delta-s by Seo et al.(46). Various FDA "Guidances" recommend the "f_2" index, re-named "similarity factor" (38), for mean dissolution profiles comparison, due to simplicity and ease. The f_1 and f_2 indices, which measure the overall difference and similarity between the two profiles are defined as follows:

$$f_1 = \{[\Sigma_{i=1}^{P}|\mu_{t_i} - \mu_{r_i}|]/[\Sigma_{i=1}^{P}\mu_{r_i}]\} \times 100 \tag{5}$$

and

$$f_2 = 50 \times \log\{[1 + (1/P)\Sigma_{i=1}^{P}(\mu_{t_i} - \mu_{r_i})^2]^{-2} \times 100\} \tag{6}$$

In the above expressions, μ_{t_i} and μ_{r_i} are the test and reference assays at ith time point, and P is the number of sample points. The "f_1" index is the cumulative absolute mean difference of the dissolution points normalized to the cumulative reference. It is thus a measure of relative error between the two curves. The "f_2" index is a function of reciprocal of mean square root transform of sum of squared differences at all points. Essentially, it is the sum of squared error arranged on a logarithmic scale. When the two profiles are exactly identical, $f_1 = 0$ and $f_2 = 50 \times \log(100) = 100$. When one product dissolves completely before the dissolution begins for another product, $f_1 = 100$ and f_2 becomes $= 50 \times \log\{[1 + (1/P)\Sigma_{i=1}^{P}(100)^2]^{-2} \times 100\}$ $= -0.001$, which can be approximated to 0. The f_1 and f_2 indices therefore can be considered as scaled between approximately 0 and 100. A relationship of average global percent difference and corresponding f_1 and f_2 index values is plotted in Figure 1.

As seen from the graph, the greater the value of "f_2" or smaller the value of "f_1", more similar are the two profiles. An "f_2" value between 50 and 100 suggests a less than 10% global or overall difference between the two dissolution profiles. Due to its global nature, the "f_2" index acquires certain advantages and disadvantages. The advantages include simplicity, ease of calculation, and unbiased estimate irrespective of the position of test sample points to reference points. The limitations include omission of inter- or intra-lot variability, as well as covariance estimation, non-consideration of positional or directional differences and a bias with respect to the number of sample points and their selection. Also though useful to a great extent for evaluating scale-up and post-approval product changes, "f_2" index is of limited value for products having a permeability-limited absorption. In these cases "f_2" profile comparison failure (value less than 50) becomes meaningless. In 1998, Shah et al. (43) evaluated "f_2" as a population measure and discussed the statistical properties of the estimate based on sample means. It was pointed out that the commonly calculated and used "f_2" of sample means is a biased and conservative estimate of the population "f_2".

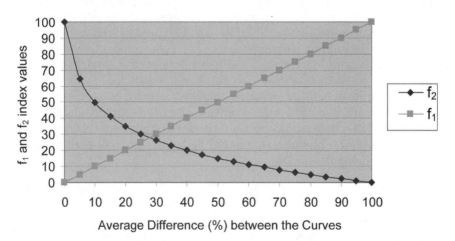

FIGURE 1 Relationship of fit factors and percent average difference.

6. APPLICATIONS OF IN VITRO DISSOLUTION

6.1. Product Development

In vitro dissolution is an important and useful tool during the development of a dosage form. In vitro dissolution often aids in guiding the selection of prototype formulations and for determining optimum levels of ingredients to achieve drug release profiles, particularly for extended-release formulations. In vitro testing also guides in the selection of a "market-image" product to be used in the pivotal in vivo bioavailability or bioequivalence studies.

6.2. Quality Assurance

A dosage form must possess acceptable in vivo bioavailability or bioequivalence performance characteristics. Following pivotal in vivo studies, in vitro dissolution testing methodology and acceptance criteria are devised on the basis of dissolution testing of these bio-lots, as well as upon the current knowledge of drug solubility, permeability, dissolution, and pharmacokinetics. This in vitro dissolution testing is then performed on future production lots, and is used to assess the lot-to-lot performance characteristics of the drug product, and provide continued assurance of product integrity/similarity.

6.3. Product Stability

In vitro dissolution is also used to assess drug product quality with respect to stability and shelf life. As products age, physicochemical changes to the dosage form may alter the dissolution characteristics of the drug product over time. For example, as the moisture level increases or decreases over time, this can result in altered tablet hardness and subsequent possible changes in dissolution characteristics. For some products, polymorph transformations to more stable, and hence less soluble crystalline forms may result in reduced dissolution rates. As mentioned previously, for gelatin-encapsulated drug products, aldehyde-amino cross-linking over time may result in pellicle formation that also slows the dissolution rate (47). As the in vitro dissolution testing is performed for products throughout their shelf life, this provides assurance of adequate product performance, throughout the expiry period.

6.4. Comparability Assessment

In vitro dissolution is also useful for assessing the impact of pre- or post-approval changes to the drug product, such as changes to the formulation or manufacturing process. Various "SUPAC Guidances", depending on the nature and extent of these changes, describe the use of either a single point or dissolution profile comparison(s) approach to evaluate the effect of these changes. This type of in vitro comparability assessment is critical to ensure continued performance equivalency and product similarity.

6.5. Waivers of In Vivo Bioequivalence Requirements

In vitro dissolution testing or drug release testing may be used for seeking waiver of the requirement to conduct in vivo bioavailability or bioequivalence studies in conjunction with the following.

6.5.1. Formulation Proportionality

In situations where an in vivo bioavailability and bioequivalence study is conducted on one-strength of the drug product, in vivo bioavailability and bioequivalence testing on other lower strength(s) of the same dosage form may be waived, provided that the lower strength(s) are proportionally similar in their active and inactive ingredients and that their dissolution profiles have sufficient similarity (3,48). Two types of formulation proportionalities are seen. One is a constant proportion, where active and inactive ingredients are changed proportionately across the strengths and another is constant weight, seen especially with products with small quantities of active drug, where the total weight rather than proportion is held constant across strengths.

6.5.2. Biopharmaceutics Classification System

The Biopharmaceutics Classification System (BCS) (49) categorizes drug substances into four classes; High Solubility/High Permeability, Class I; Low Solubility/High Permeability, Class II; High Solubility/Low Permeability, Class III; and Low Solubility/Low Permeability, Class IV. A drug substance is considered highly soluble when the highest dose strength is soluble in less than or equal to 250 mL in aqueous media over a pH range of 1–7.5 (49) or the more physiologic pH 6.8. A drug is considered highly permeable when extent of absorption (as measured by the area under the plasma concentration time curve) in humans is determined to be greater than 90% of an administered dose. An immediate-release drug product is also characterized as a *rapidly dissolving* product when not less than 85% of the labeled amount of the drug substance dissolves within 30 min using USP Apparatus I at 100 rpm or USP Apparatus II at 50 rpm in a volume of 900 mL or less of each of the following media: (a) acidic media, such as 0.1 N HCl or USP simulated gastric fluid without enzymes (SGF); (b) a pH 4.5 buffer; and (c) a pH 6.8 buffer or USP simulated intestinal fluid without enzymes (SIF) . If the drug product meets the BCS criteria for Class I, meaning that the drug substance is highly soluble and highly permeable, and the drug product is rapidly dissolving, it is quite likely that the rate-limiting step for drug absorption is gastric emptying. In this instance, the requirements for in vivo bioavailability or bioequivalence studies for this product can be waived (48). The BCS (49) thus far is an attractive approach in its formative stage. Attempts have been made (50) to ascertain the maximum absorbable dose using information such as solubility, trans-intestinal absorption rate constant, small intestine water volume, and transit time.

6.5.3. In Vitro/In Vivo Correlations

After a formulation is developed, meaningful in vitro dissolution in conjunction with techniques such as de-convolution can be used to predict in vivo dissolution and absorption and establish an in vitro/in vivo relationship. These relationships between in vitro drug release and in vivo absorption (level "A", "B", or "C" correlation) are generally more likely for drugs exhibiting low solubility and high permeability (BCS Class II) and for extended-release products. When these in vitro/in vivo correlations have been established, in vivo bioavailability or bioequivalence studies, which are normally required may be waived (4). Polli (51) recently suggested development of an objective criterion to identify models a priori to in vitro/in vivo correlation analysis.

7. LIMITATIONS OF IN VITRO DISSOLUTION

The chapter thus far focused on the general utility of dissolution testing. Nonetheless, the limitations of this methodology cannot be overlooked. The precision and accuracy of dissolution testing often depends upon several subtle operational controls, including stirring element eccentricity, agitation alignment, torsional vibration, dosage form position, sampling position, dissolved gases, flow patterns, and heat transfer amongst other factors, which if overlooked, may have a large effect upon the dissolution measurement. This is exemplified by a recent study demonstrating dramatically different dissolution rates as a result of different tablet positions. The dissolution rate differences are attributed to the segregation of solution hydrodynamics in the dissolution testing apparatus (52). A strict control of these many subtle factors is therefore essential to assure reliable and reproducible test results.

Relevance is another dissolution limitation. In the absence of a suitable in vitro/in vivo correlation, dissolution testing may not be particularly relevant to drug product performance. In case of IR products containing BCS Class I and Class III drugs, dissolution testing may be "over-discriminating" since oral absorption is likely to be limited by gastric emptying or intestinal permeation. In the case of IR products containing BCS Class II and IV drugs, on the other hand, single point dissolution testing may be "non-discriminating" and may not be able to detect lots having poor in vivo performance. Additionally, even when an in vitro/in vivo correlation has been developed for a product, it is likely to be of limited value for other products, since such correlations are often "product specific".

Despite these limitations, dissolution testing remains one of the most important and useful in vitro tests for assuring product quality. It is only by recognizing these limitations that one can make judicious conclusions about the significance or insignificance of a dissolution test result as it pertains to product performance. Recognizing these limitations may also help us develop a more meaningful and useful dissolution testing methodology.

8. SUMMARY

From the product quality perspective and for adequate assurance of in vivo performance of a solid dosage form, a detailed in vitro characterization is essential. In vitro dissolution testing of the solid oral dosage form can be conducted using various tests and techniques. This type of evaluation is useful during product development, for quality assurance and control, product stability testing, and during assessment of comparability. In vitro dissolution testing may also be useful for getting waivers of in vivo bioavailability or bioequivalence studies, particularly when the dosage form exhibits formulation proportionality to the bio-studied lot, or when the drug meets the criteria for BCS Class I and exhibits rapid dissolution, or when a meaningful in vitro/in vivo relationship has been established. The modern frontiers in developing efficient in vitro performance testing include areas such as fiber optics for monitoring the drug concentration in the dissolution medium (53), application of artificial neural network for dissolution prediction (54), and Process Analytical Technology (PAT) (55).

9. WEBSITES

1. http://www.fda.gov/cder/: FDA Center for Drug Evaluation and Research (CDER) Homepage.
2. http://www.fda.gov/cder/ob/default.htm: FDA/CDER "Orange Book".
3. http://www.fda.gov/cder/approval/index.htm: CDER New and Generic Drug Approvals Listings for 1998–2002.
4. http://www.fda.gov/cder/guidance/index.htm: CDER Guidance Documents.

5. http://www.fda.gov/cder/ogd/: CDER Office of Generic Drugs Homepage.
6. http://www.accessdata.fda.gov/scripts/cder/iig/index.cfm: Inactive Ingredient Guide 12/30/02.
7. http://www.webmd.com/: WEB-MD.
8. http://www.usp.org/: United States Pharmacopeial Convention Inc. (USP).

REFERENCES

1. The US Pharmacopeia/National Formulary, USP 26-NF 21. Rockville, MD: United States Pharmacopeial Convention Inc., 2002.
2. Guidance for Industry: Dissolution Testing of Immediate Release Solid Oral Dosage Forms. Rockville, MD: Food and Drug Administration/Center for Drug Evaluation and Research, 1997.
3. Guidance for Industry: Bioavailability and Bioequivalence Studies for Orally Administered Drug Products—General Considerations. Rockville, MD: Food and Drug Administration/Center for Drug Evaluation and Research, 2003.
4. Guidance for Industry: Extended Release Oral Dosage Forms: Development, Evaluation and Application of In vitro/In vivo Correlations. Rockville, MD: Food and Drug Administration/Center for Drug Evaluation and Research, 1997.
5. Food and Drug Administration/Center for Drug Evaluation and Research Data Standards Manual. Rockville, MD: Food and Drug Administration/Center for Drug Evaluation and Research, 1992:18.
6. Approved Drug Products with Therapeutic Equivalence Evaluations (Orange Book). 23rd ed. Rockville, MD: US Department of Health and Human Services/Food and Drug Administration, 2003.
7. Abdou HM. Evolution of Dissolution Testing, Theory of Dissolution, Theoretical Concepts for the Release of a Drug from Dosage Forms and Factors Affecting Rate of Dissolution. Dissolution Bioavailability & Bioequivalence. Easton, PA: Mack Publishing Company, 1989:1–105.
8. Noyes A, Whitney W. The rate of solution of solid substances in their own solutions. J Amer Chem Soc 1897; 19(12):930–934.
9. Brunner L, Tolloczko S. Über die auflösungsgeschwindingkeit fester körper. Zeitschrifft für Physiologische Chemie 1900; 35(3):283–290.
10. Nernst W. Theorie der reaktionsgeschwindigkeit in heterogenen Systemen. Zeitschrifft für Physiologische Chemie 1904; 47(1):52–55.
11. Yu LX, Amidon GL. Analytical solutions to mass transfer In: Amidon GL, Lee PI, Topp EM, eds. Transport Processes in Pharmaceutical Systems, New York: Marcel Dekker, Inc., 1999:23–54.
12. Horter D, Dressman JB. Influence of physicochemical properties on dissolution of drugs in the gastrointestinal tract. Adv Drug Del Rev 2001; 46(1–3):75–87.
13. Byrn S, Pfeiffer R, Ganey M, Hoiberg C, Poochikian G. Pharmaceutical solids: a strategic approach to regulatory considerations. Pharm Res 1995; 12(7): 945–954.

14. Yu LX, Furness MS, Raw A, Woodland Outlaw KP, Nashed NE, Ramos E, Miller SPF, Adams RC, Fang F, Patel RM, Holcombe FO Jr, Chiu Y, Hussain AS, Scientific considerations of pharmaceutical solid polymorphism in abbreviated new drug applications. Pharm Res 2003; 20(4):531–536.

15. Grant DJW, Higuchi T. Solubility Behavior of Organic Compounds, New York: John Wiley & Sons, 1990.

16. Hancock BC, Parks M. What is the true solubility advantage for amorphous pharmaceuticals? Pharm Res 2000; 17(4):397–404.

17. Aguiar AJ, Krc J, Kinkel AW, Samyn JC. Effect of polymorphism on the absorption of chloramphenicol from chloramphenicol palmitate. J Pharm Sci 1967; 56(7):847–853.

18. Morris KR, Fakes MG, Thakur AB, Newman AW, Singh AK, Venit JJ, Spagnualo CJ, Abu TM. An integrated approach to the selection of optimal salt form for a new drug candidate. Int J of Pharm 1994; 105: 209–217.

19. Stavchansky R, McGinity J. Bioavailability and tablet technology. In: Lieberman HA, Lachman L, Schwartz JB, eds. Pharmaceutical Dosage Forms: Tablets. Vol. 2. New York: Marcel Dekker 1989; 2:349–553.

20. Sevelius H, Runkel R, Segre E, Bloomfield SS. Bioavailability of naproxen sodium and its relationship to clinical analgesic effects. Br J Clin Pharmacol 1980; 10(3):259–263.

21. Peck GE, Baley GJ, McCurdy VE, Banker GS. Tablet formulation and design In: Lieberman HA, Lachman L, Schwartz JB, eds. Pharmaceutical Dosage Forms: Tablets Vol. 1. New York: Marcel Dekker Inc. 1989; 1:73–130.

22. Banaker UV. Pharmaceutical Dissolution Testing. New York: Marcel Dekker, Inc., 1991:133–187.

23. Solvang S, Finholt P. Effect of tablet processing and formulation factors on dissolution rate of the active ingredient in human gastric juice. J Pharm Sci 1970; 59(1):49–52.

24. Pinnamaneni S, Das NG, Das SK. Formulation approaches for orally administered poorly soluble drugs. Pharmazie 2002; 54:291–300.

25. Schwier JB, Cooke GG, Hartauer KJ, Yu L. Rayon: A source of fural—a reactive aldehyde capable of insolubilizing gelatin capsules. Pharm Technol 1993:78–80.

26. Lee TWY, Robinson JR. Controlled-Release Drug Delivery Systems. In: Gennaro AR, ed. Remington: The Science and Practice of Pharmacy. Philadelphia. Vol. 20. Lippincott Williams & Wilkins 2000; 20:903–929.

27. Yi L. Amorphous pharmaceutical solids: preparation characterization and stabilization. Adv Drug Del Rev 2001; 48:27–42.

28. Bandelin FJ. Compressed tablets by wet granulation. In: Lieberman HA, Lachman L, Schwartz JB, eds. Pharmaceutical Dosage Forms: Tablets. New York: Marcel Dekker, Inc. 1990; 1:199–302.

29. Shangraw RF. Compressed tablets by direct compression. Lieberman HA, Lachman L, Schwartz JB, eds. Pharmaceutical Dosage Forms: Tablets. New York: Marcel Dekker, Inc. 1990; I:195–246.

30. Carstensen JT. Advanced Pharmaceutical Solids. New York: Marcel Dekker, Inc., 2001:427–438.

31. Chang RK, Robinson JR. Sustained Release from Tablets and Particles through Coating. In: Lieberman HA, Lachman L, Schwartz JB, eds. Pharmaceutical Dosage Forms: Tablets. New York: Marcel Dekker, Inc. 1990; 3:199–302.

32. Levy G. Effect of certain tablet formulation factors on dissolution rate of the active ingredient I. importance of using appropriate agitation intensities for In vitro dissolution rate measurements to reflect In vivo conditions. J Pharm Sci 1963; 52:1039–1046.

33. International Conference on Harmonisation, pp. 83041–83063; Guidance on Q6A Specifications: Test Procedures and Acceptance Criteria for New Drug Substances and New Drug Products: Chemical Substance, Federal Register 65 (251), December 29, 2000, pp. 83059–83061.

34. Hanson WA. Handbook of Dissolution Testing. 2nd ed. Eugene, OR: Aster Publishing Corporation, 1991.

35. Yu L, Wang J, Hussain A. Evaluation of USP Apparatus 3 for dissolution testing of immediate-release products. AAPS PharmSci 2002; 4(1):1–7.

36. Kostewicz ES, Brauns U, Becker R, Dressman JB. Forecasting the oral absorption behavior of poorly soluble weak bases using solubility and dissolution studies in biorelevant media. Pharm Res 2002; 19(3):345–349.

37. Nicolaides E, Symillides M, Dressman JB, Reppas C. Biorelevant dissolution testing to predict the plasma profile of lipophilic drugs after oral administration. Pharm Res 2001; 18(3):380–388.

38. Guidance for Industry: SUPAC-IR: Immediate Release Solid Oral Dosage Forms Scale Up and Post Approval Changes: Chemistry Manufacturing and Controls In vitro Dissolution Testing and In vivo Bioequivalence Documentation Rockville, MD: Food and Drug Administration/Center for Drug Evaluation and Research, 1995.

39. Guidance for Industry: SUPAC-MR: Modified Release Solid Oral Dosage Forms—Scale-Up and Post-Approval Changes: Chemistry, Manufacturing and Controls—In vitro Dissolution and In vivo Bioequivalence Documentation, Rockville, MD: Food and Drug Administration/Center for Drug Evaluation and Research, 1997.

40. Sathe P, Tsong YI, Shah V. In vitro dissolution profile comparison: statistics and analysis model dependent approach. Pharm Res 1996; 13(12):1799–1803.

41. Sathe P, Tsong Yi, Shah, V. In vitro dissolution profile comparison and IVIVR—carbamazepine case. In: Young D, DeVane JG, Butler J, eds. In vitro In vivo Correlations, New York: Plenum Press, 1997; 31–42.

42. Tsong Yi, Sathe P, Hammerstrom T, Shah V. Statistical assessment of mean differences between two dissolution data sets. Drug Information J 1996; 30(4):1105–1112.

43. Shah V, Tsong Yi, Sathe P, Liu J-P. In vitro dissolution profile comparison: statistics and analysis of the similarity factor f2. Pharm Res 1998; 15(6):889–896.

44. Rescigno A. Bioequivalence. Pharm Res 1992; 9(7):925–928.

45. Moore JW, Flanner HH. Mathematical comparison of dissolution profiles. Pharm Technol June 1996:64–74.

46. Seo PR, Shah VP, Polli JP. Novel metrics to compare dissolution Profiles. Pharm Dev Technol 2002; 7(2):257–265.

47. Digenis GA, Gold TB, Shah VP. Crosslinking of gelatin capsules and its relevance to their in vitro/in vivo Performance. J Pharm Sci 1994; 83(7):915–921.

48. Code of Federal Regulations—Title 21 Food and Drugs—Parts 300 to 499, Office of the Federal Register/National Archives and Records Administration: Washington DC 2003:181–182.

49. Guidance for Industry: Waiver of In vivo Bioavailability and Bioequivalence Studies for Immediate Release Dosage Forms Based on a Biopharmaceutics Classification System; Rockville, MD: Food and Drug Administration/Center for Drug Evaluation and Research, 2000.

50. Johnson KC, Swindell AC. Guidance in the Setting of Drug Particle Size Specifications to Minimize Variability in Absorption. Pharm Res 1996; 13(12):1795–1798.

51. Polli JE. Dependence of in vitro-in vivo correlation analysis acceptability model selections. Pharm Dev Technol 1999; 4(1):89–96.

52. Kukura J, Arratia PE, Szalai ES, Muzzio FJ. Engineering tools for understanding the hydrodynamics of dissolution tests. Drug Dev Industrial Pharm 2003; 29(2):231–239.

53. Rainbow Dynamic Dissolution Monitor™ System Manual, Northvale, NJ: Delphian Technology Inc., 2002; 1–8.

54. Sathe P, Venitz J. Comparison of neural network (NN) and multiple linear regression (MLR) as dissolution predictors. Drug Dev Industrial Pharm 2003; 29(3):349–355.

55. Workman J Jr, Creasy KE, Dohertyl S, Bond L, Koch M, Ullman A, Veltkamp DJ. Process analytical chemistry. Anal Chem 2001; 73(12):2705–2718.

9

ANDA Regulatory Approval Process

Timothy W. Ames, Karen A. Bernard,
Beth Fabian Fritsch, Koung Lee,
Aida L. Sanchez, Krista M. Scardina, and
Martin Shimer
U.S. Food and Drug Administration Center for Drug Evaluation and
Research, Rockville, MD, U.S.A.

The Food and Drug Administration (FDA) is organized into eight offices/centers, the Center for Drug Evaluation and Research (CDER), the Center for Biologics Evaluation and Research (CBER), the Center for Devices and Radiological Health (CDRH), the Center for Food Safety and Applied Nutrition (CFSAN), the Center for Veterinary Medicine (CVM), the National Center for Toxicological Research (NCTR), the Office of the Commissioner (OC), and the Office of Regulatory Affairs (ORA).

The CDER reviews the safety and efficacy of drug products. The Center Director oversees 11 offices which include, the Office of Pharmaceutical Science, the Office of New Drugs, the Office of Executive Programs, the Office of Pharmacoepidemiology and Statistical Science, Office of Management, the Office of Regulatory Policy, the Office of Medical Policy, the Office of Counter-Terrorism and Pediatric Drug Development, the Office of Training and Communications, the Office of Compliance, and the Office of Information Technology. Additional information about the organization of the CDER can be found on the FDA website at www.fda.gov/cder.

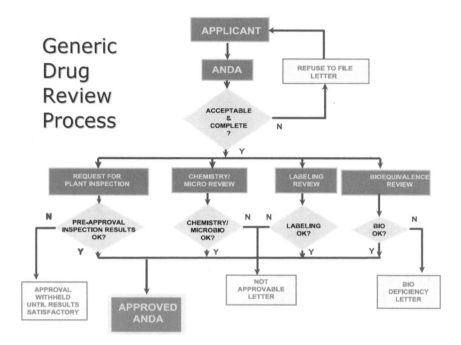

FIGURE 1 Generic drug review process.

Organizationally, the Office of Generic Drugs (OGD) is located within the CDER under the Office of Pharmaceutical Science. It consists of the following divisions: Chemistry, Bioequivalence, and Labeling and Program Support. The following will provide a brief overview of the history of the OGD.

Nearly 20 years after its enactment, The Drug Price Competition and Patent Term Restoration Act of 1984, commonly known as the Hatch–Waxman Amendments (HWA), has proven to be an effective piece of legislation. One outcome of this legislation is the increased availability of less-expensive medications to millions of Americans. The HWA to the Federal Food, Drug and Cosmetic Act (FD&C) gave clear statutory authority to submit Abbreviated New Drug Applications (ANDAs) for all approved innovator drugs. With the passage of the HWA, firms who sought to market a generic version of a drug were not required to repeat the costly preclinical and clinical testing associated with a New Drug Application (NDA).

The OGD had its origins in the early 1970s and was known as the Office of Drug Monographs. After the passage of the HWA in 1984, the Office of Drug Monographs became the Office of Drug Standards. The Office of Drug

Standards contained the Division of Generic Drugs (DGD) and the Division of Bioequivalence. The OGD as we know it today was established in 1990 as part of the Office of Pharmaceutical Science (OPS). Its mission is to ensure that safe and effective generic drugs are available for the American people. The OGD ensures the safety and efficacy of generic drugs by employing a review process that is similar to the NDA process. The primary difference between the Generic Drug Review process and the NDA review process is the study requirements. For example, an ANDA generally requires a bioequivalence study between the generic product and the reference listed drug (RLD) product. The safety and efficacy of the RLD product were established previously through animal studies, clinical studies and bioavailabilty studies. Thus, these studies need not be repeated for the ANDA.

The economic impact of the HWA is best demonstrated by the increased market share of generic medications. In 1984, just 14% of all prescriptions dispensed were for generic drugs. In contrast, 17 years later in 2001, approximately 48% of all prescriptions dispensed were for generic drugs. Furthermore, for each 1% increase in the use of generic drugs, consumers save an additional $1.32 billion per year.

The goal of this chapter is to provide an overview of the generic drug review process for solid oral dosage forms. Each step of the review process will be discussed from the initial submission of the application to its final approval. As one reads through the chapter, it may be useful to refer to the flow diagram given in Figure 1. Since the discussion is limited to the review of solid oral dosage forms, the microbiology review is omitted.

1. FILING REVIEW OF ABBREVIATED NEW DRUG APPLICATIONS (ANDA)

The ANDA process begins when an applicant submits an ANDA to the OGD. The document room staff processes the ANDA, assigns it an ANDA number, and stamps a received date on the cover letter of the ANDA. The ANDA is then sent to a consumer safety technician, who reviews the preliminary sections of the ANDA Checklist.

Within the first 60 days following the submission of an ANDA, a filing review is completed. The Regulatory Support Branch (RSB) is responsible for the filing review. This group, organized under the Division of Labeling and Program Support (DLPS), consists of project managers and a support staff including technical information assistant(s), legal instruments examiner(s), and consumer safety technician(s). The branch chief who reports to the Division Director of DLPS supervises the branch.

The RSB ensures that the ANDAs contain the information necessary to merit a technical review. To determine whether an application is acceptable for filing, an RSB project manager (RPM) compares the contents of each section of the application (see Appendix A) against a list of regulatory requirements. An applicant may receive a "refuse to receive" letter when an inactive ingredient level exceeds the level previously used in an approved drug product via the same route of administration. Other common reasons that a "refuse to receive" letter may be issued to the applicant include but are not limited to; incomplete bioequivalence studies, incomplete stability data, incomplete packaging, and incorrect basis for submission. The filing date of an application is critical since it may determine the eligibility for exclusivity. The RSB verifies that all applications contain a patent certification and exclusivity statement. The patent certification and exclusivity statement must address all existing patents and exclusivities for the RLD published in the "Approved Drug Products with Therapeutic Equivalence Evaluations", commonly known as the "Orange Book". If an RLD has expired patents, an applicant may certify that no relevant patents remain. The review of patents and exclusivities is an ongoing process throughout the review cycle, as new patents and exclusivities may become listed in the "Orange Book". An explanation of patent certifications with their corresponding definitions may be found in 21 CFR 314.94(a)(12).

Once the RSB completes the filing review of the ANDA and verifies that the application contains all the necessary regulatory requirements, an "acknowledgment" letter is issued to the applicant indicating its acceptance for filing and the official filing date. The application is then assigned to the technical reviewers. If the ANDA does not meet the criteria for filing, a "refuse-to-receive" letter is issued to the applicant with a list of deficiencies.

Upon filing an ANDA, the RPM forwards an Establishment Evaluation Request (EER) to the Office of Compliance. The Office of Compliance then determines if the drug product manufacturer, the drug substance manufacturer and the outside testing facilities are operating in compliance with current Good Manufacturing Practice (cGMP) regulations as outlined in 21 CFR Parts 210 and 211. Each facility listed on the request is evaluated individually and the Office of Compliance makes an overall evaluation of all facilities listed in the application. Furthermore, a pre-approval inspection may be performed to assure the data integrity of the application.

Currently, ANDAs can be submitted entirely electronically. Applicants can also submit electronic submissions of bioequivalence data along with the traditional paper application. The electronic document room staff processes the electronic files, so that the reviewers can access them. The data contained in the electronic submission are copied onto CDER's computer network. Additional processing may occur to populate the electronic tools used by the reviewers.

All applicants who plan to submit ANDAs electronically should consult CDER's website for electronic submissions at www.fda.gov/cder/regulatory/rsr/default.htm.

2. COORDINATION OF THE GENERIC DRUG REVIEW PROCESS

Once the ANDA is accepted for filing, the application enters the review queue. This means that the application is assigned to a bioequivalence reviewer, a chemist, and a labeling reviewer.

Each chemistry team consists of a team leader, a project manager, and several reviewers. In this section, the emphasis will be placed on the chemistry project manager's role in the generic drug review process.

The chemistry project manager serves as the "Application" Project Manager (APM). While APMs are located within the Chemistry review teams, they are actually a part of the Review Support Branch within the DLPS. Specifically, they plan, organize, and coordinate all of the review activities for the applications that they manage. This requires the coordination of all discipline reviews which include chemistry, bioequivalence, and labeling.

The APMs serve as co-leaders for the chemistry review teams. They assure timely resolution of scientific and regulatory conflicts to prevent delays in the review process. The APMs also make every effort to meet the review goals set by the OGD management.

The APMs manage and coordinate the work of the review teams to assure that reviews are performed in a timely manner. In addition, the APMs identify and resolve potential problems such as the inequality of individual workload and regulatory issues. The OGD makes a concerted effort to comply with the statutory 180 day review cycle mandated by the Federal FD&C Act. The APMs play a key role in coordinating the various disciplines to review the applications within 180 days from the submission date. In attempt to achieve OGD's management goals, the APMs may recommend redistribution of work according to the policies and procedures within the OGD.

The APMs enter key information about their applications into a project management database. This database allows the OGD staff to access the status and outcome of discipline reviews and the status of the field and compliance inspection reports. The APMs use the information to provide applicants and OGD management the status of applications.

Since communication plays a large role in the generic drug review process, the APMs are designated as the primary contacts for all issues relating to the review of the application. As such, they communicate the status of all aspects of the applications that they manage. The APMs attempt to address all applicant inquiries within 2 working days of receiving a request. If the questions from the applicant are of a technical nature and require further evaluation by a reviewer and/or team leader, the APMs make the appropriate arrangements for either a telephone conference and/or a meeting. The APMs generally request applicants to submit a proposed agenda prior to the telephone conference or meeting. The APMs and the review teams work with the applicants to resolve scientific issues that may delay the approval of applications.

3. BIOEQUIVALENCE REVIEW PROCESS

After an ANDA is accepted for filing by the RSB, the bioequivalence section is assigned to the Division of Bioequivalence to review. The Bioequivalence Project Managers (BPM) access a list of pending ANDAs and assign them to individual reviewers according to the "first-in, first-reviewed" policy. The BPMs also randomly assign other review documents such as Bio-INDs, protocols, and correspondence.

The DBE's responsibilities include the review of the bioequivalence section of ANDAs, supplemental ANDAs, Bio-Investigational New Drug Applications (Bio-INDs), protocols, and controlled correspondence. It is worth mentioning that more than half of all correspondence submitted to the OGD requests guidance from the DBE.

Structurally, the DBE is organized into three review branches; each branch consists of approximately six reviewers, who are supervised by a team leader. The team leaders complete a secondary review of all bioequivalence submissions assigned to their branch. In addition, they ensure the consistency of the recommendations provided to the applicants. A BPM is assigned to each branch and is responsible for processing all reviews and managing the bioequivalence review process. A statistician is also available to resolve statistical issues.

The bioequivalence review process establishes bioequivalence between a proposed generic drug and the RLD. Bioequivalence is established when the ratio of the means of the test product compared to the reference product (T/R) of the pharmacokinetic parameters for rate (C_{max}) and extent of absorption (AUC) of log transformed data meet the 90% confidence intervals of 80–125%. Refer to Chapters 10 and 11 for a more detailed discussion of bioequivalence testing requirements and statistical considerations.

The BPMs provide regulatory guidance on bioequivalence issues through correspondence and teleconferences. In addition, the BPMs coordinate the resolution of all regulatory and scientific issues regarding the bioequivalence of drug products submitted for marketing approval. All meetings and teleconferences regarding bioequivalence issues are scheduled and documented by the BPM.

The BPMs request and track inspections of the clinical and analytical sites through the Division of Scientific Investigations (DSI). Inspection requests to the DSI are sent immediately after the ANDA is assigned to a reviewer. The clinical and analytical sites are inspected for two reasons: (1) to verify the quality and integrity of the scientific data submitted in bioequivalence studies and (2) to ensure that the rights and welfare of human subjects participating in the studies are protected in accordance with the regulations (21 CFR 312, 320, 50, and 56). Significant problems, such as research misconduct or fraud (see MaPP 5210.7) are promptly acted upon. One of the most common findings on an DSI inspection is the absence of retention samples by the testing facility (refer to 21 CFR 320.38 and 320.63 and the draft guidance "Handling and Retention of BA and BE Testing Samples" for more information). If problems are discovered during these inspections, additional studies from the applicant may be requested.

If a bioequivalence reviewer requires additional information to complete their review, they will first consult with their team leader and then request the BPM to obtain the information from the applicant. If an issue can be resolved within 10 working days, a teleconference with the applicant is initiated by the BPM. The BPM maintains a record of all teleconferences with the applicants. The applicant's response to the teleconference is labeled as a "Bioequivalence Telephone Amendment". A deficiency letter is issued to the applicant when a review contains numerous deficiencies that require more than 10 days to resolve.

The reviewer prepares a draft or primary review, which is then forwarded to the team leader for a secondary review and/or revisions. During the secondary review, the team leader provides comments on the primary review, discusses regulatory or scientific issues with the Division Director and assesses the need for additional data from the applicant. Once all unresolved or outstanding issues are addressed, the team leader sends the review back to the reviewer with his comments. The reviewer then finalizes the review and forwards it to the Division Director. The Division Director performs a tertiary review and documents his concurrence.

Once the bioequivalence review is completed and all bioequivalence requirements are addressed, the DBE forwards an acceptable letter that states that there are no further questions at this time. The bioequivalence review is then forwarded to the APM. If the bioequivalence review indicates deficiencies, a deficiency letter is issued to the applicant.

Bioequivalence studies with clinical endpoints are often recommended to establish bioequivalence between dosage forms intended to deliver the active ingredient(s) locally, (i.e., topical creams and ointments) and between dosage forms that are not intended to be absorbed (i.e., Sucralfate)(21 CFR 320.24(b)(4)). The OGD's Associate Director of Medical Affairs (ADMA) and the clinical team review these studies for the DBE. The ADMA also forwards all comments and recommendations to the Director of the DBE for concurrence. The ADMA consults with the Office of New Drugs for input on the appropriateness of clinical endpoints (see MaPP 5210.4). For this reason, it is strongly advised that applicants submit protocols or Bio-INDs prior to the initiation of bioequivalence studies to ensure the appropriateness of study designs and endpoints (see MaPP 5240.4).

4. CHEMISTRY REVIEW PROCESS

After an ANDA has been accepted for filing by the RSB, the Chemistry, Manufacturing and Controls (CMC) section of the application is assigned to the appropriate Chemistry Division and Team, based on the therapeutic category of the drug product. Once the application is assigned to the team, the application is designated as "random" and placed on the team leader's queue. The team leader assigns the application to a reviewer on his or her team according to the "first-in, first reviewed policy". The Chemistry Divisions review the CMC section of ANDAs, Drug Master Files, Supplemental ANDAs, Annual Reports, and Controlled Correspondence.

The Chemistry Divisions are organized into review teams consisting of five or six reviewers and a team leader. Team leaders perform a secondary review of all chemistry submissions. An APM assigned to each team coordinates the entire review process and acts as the primary point of contact for the application. Each division is led by a Division Director and Deputy Director. A tertiary review is often performed by the Deputy Director, but may be performed by the Division Director, to ensure consistent recommendations to applicants. Inter-divisional consistency is also emphasized through regular meetings between the Chemistry Divisions and the OGD management.

The goal of the chemistry review process is to assure that the generic drug will be manufactured in a reproducible manner under controlled conditions. Areas such as the applicant's manufacturing procedures, raw material specifications and controls, sterilization process, container and closure systems, and stability data are reviewed to assure that the drug will perform in an acceptable manner.

The chemistry reviewer drafts a primary review that is forwarded to the team leader for secondary review. The secondary review may require little or no revision from the first draft or it may require major revision. Team leaders provide comments and corrections to the primary reviewer. The APM also assists in the correction process. Once the team resolves the issues internally, the review is finalized and signed by the team leader, primary reviewer and APM. The finalized review, including a list of deficiencies, is forwarded to the Deputy Director for concurrence. The Deputy Director, or in some cases the Division Director, completes the tertiary review. If the application is a "first generic drug product", the Associate Director for Chemistry performs a quality control audit. This function is completed outside of the Chemistry Divisions at the Office level.

After all issues are resolved within the Chemistry Divisions, it is the responsibility of the APM to communicate the status of the application to the applicant. After designating the chemistry deficiencies as "Minor" or "Major," the APM faxes them to the applicant. When the application is ready for final approval, the approval package is processed through the immediate office and the applicant is contacted. The Chemistry Divisions coordinate with all of the disciplines for each application prior to full approval. Since the Chemistry Divisions generate the final approval letter for the Office Director, the other disciplines must be found acceptable with respect to the approval of the application.

5. LABELING REVIEW PROCESS

After an ANDA has been accepted for filing by the RSB, the Labeling section of the application is assigned to the appropriate labeling reviewer based on the therapeutic category of the drug product. The Labeling Review Branch is part of the DLPS. A team leader oversees the work of 4–6 reviewers.

The basis for the labeling review is to ensure that the generic drug labeling is the "same as" the RLD labeling. There are several exceptions to the "same as" regulation. Exceptions are allowed for: differences due to changes in the manufacturer or distributor, unexpired patents, or exclusivities and other characteristics inherent to the generic drug product, such as tablet size, shape, or color.

The labeling reviewer also identifies and resolves concerns that may contribute to medication errors. For example, the labeling reviewer may identify drug names that are similar or that sound alike. In addition, the labeling reviewer may address concerns associated with the prominence and/or legibility of drug names on a container label. To ensure that the proposed labeling in an ANDA is the "same as" the RLD, the labeling reviewer must first identify the RLD. The next step is to find the most recently approved labeling for the RLD. If the RLD labeling is not the most recently approved, it is considered discontinued labeling. Hence, it is not acceptable for the labeling review. It is very important to monitor FDA's database and website on a regular basis to determine the most recent labeling approvals.

One allowed difference between the generic and the RLD labeling is the omission of information protected by patents and exclusivity. The labeling reviewer ensures that the applicant properly addresses all patents and exclusivities by verifying the information in the "Orange Book." The applicant's patent certification and exclusivity statement determines the way the proposed labeling will be drafted.

The applicant may submit four copies of draft labeling or 12 copies of final printed labeling as proposed labeling. Draft copies may also be submitted for tentative approval. The labeling branch supports the submission of electronic labeling. This practice is preferred and strongly encouraged.

For USP products, the labeling reviewer uses the United States Pharmacopeia (USP) to evaluate the established name, molecular structure, molecular weight, structural formula, chemical name, and the storage conditions of the proposed drug product.

As the container label or carton label is reviewed, the labeling reviewer decides if the labeling is easy to read and positioned in accordance with the regulations. In addition, the labeling reviewer encourages applicants to revise their labeling to decrease the likelihood of confusion with other drug products.

After completing the review of the proposed labeling, the labeling reviewer drafts a review that either identifies labeling deficiencies or recommends approval. A tentative approval may be issued for an application with outstanding patent and exclusivity issues. The team leader completes a secondary review of the application. If he or she is in agreement with the review, the review is sent back to the labeling reviewer to finalize. The labeling reviewer then forwards the review back to the team leader for concurrence.

If the proposed labeling is deficient, the APM or the labeling reviewer communicates the deficiencies to the applicant. If the proposed labeling is acceptable, an approval or tentative approval summary is forwarded to the APM.

6. PUTTING IT ALL TOGETHER

After the final Office level administrative review and individual disciplines have resolved their deficiencies, the application will either receive a full approval or a tentative approval letter (See ANDA Approval Chart).

The APMs are instrumental in assembling an approval package. This package includes all reviews supporting final or tentative approval. When the review of an ANDA is completed, the APMs draft the appropriate approval letter and circulate it with the reviews and application for concurrence. The APMs communicate with the OGD management on a weekly basis to update them on the progress of reviews.

A full approval letter details the conditions of approval and allows the applicant to market the generic drug product. A tentative approval letter is issued if there are unexpired patents or exclusivities accorded to the RLD. The tentative approval letter details the circumstances associated with the tentative approval and delays the marketing of the product until all patents and/or exclusivities expire. Once the Office Director or his designee has signed the final approval letter, the APM calls and faxes a copy of the approval letter to the applicant. The document room staff then mails the final approval letter to the applicant.

As one can see, the generic drug review process incorporates a series of checks and balances to ensure the integrity of the reviews. The OGD is comprised of bioequivalence reviewers, chemists, labeling reviewers, and project managers. These individuals work together as a team to accomplish the OGD's mission of providing safe and effective generic drugs to the American People.

APPENDIX A

ANDA CHECKLIST FOR COMPLETENESS and ACCEPTABILITY of an APPLICATION

ANDA # _____   FIRM NAME _____

RELATED APPLICATION(S) _____   FIRST GENERIC? _____

DRUG NAME: _____
DOSAGE FORM: _____

Electronic Submission: E-mail notification sent: Comments: _____
Random Assignment Queue: Chem Team Leader: PM: _____
Labeling Reviewer: _____ Micro Review: _____ PD study (Med Ofcr): _____

	Letter Date		Received Date
Comments		On Cards	Therapeutic Code
Methods Validation Package (3 copies)			
(Required for Non-USP drugs)			
Archival, and Review copies Field Copy			
Certification (Original Signature)			
Cover Letter			
Table of Contents			

ACCEPTABLE

Sec. I	Signed and Completed Application Form (356h) (Statement regarding Rx/OTC Status)	☐
Sec. II	Basis for Submission NDA: RLD: Firm: ANDA suitability petition required? If yes, consult needed for pediatric study requirement.	☐
Sec. III	Patent Certification 1. Paragraph: 2. Expiration of Patent: A. Pediatric Exclusivity Submitted? B. Pediatric Exclusivity Tracking System checked? Exclusivity Statement	☐
Sec. IV	Comparison between Generic Drug and RLD- 505(j)(2)(A) 1. Conditions of use 2. Active ingredients 3. Route of administration 4. Dosage Form 5. Strength	☐
Sec.V	Labeling 1. 4 copies of draft (each strength and container) or 12 copies of FPL 2. 1 RLD label and 1 RLD container label 3. 1 side by side labeling comparison with all differences annotated and explained	☐
Sec. VI	Bioavailability/Bioequivalence 1. Financial Certification (Form FDA 3454) and Disclosure Statement (Form 3455) 2. Request for Waiver of In-Vivo Study (ies): 3. Formulation data same? (Comparison of all Strengths) (Ophthalmics, Otics, Topicals Perenterals) 4. Lot Numbers of Products used in BE Study (ies): 5. Study Type: (Continue with the appropriate study type box below)	☐
Study Type	IN-VIVO PK STUDY (IES) (i.e., fasting/fed/sprinkle) a. Study (ies) meets BE criteria (90% CI or 80–125, Cmax, AUC) b. Data Files (Computer Media) Submitted c. In-Vitro Dissolution	☐
Study Type	IN-VIVO BE STUDY with CLINICAL ENDPOINTS a. Properly defined BE endpoints (eval. by Clinical Team) b. Summary results meet BE criteria (90% CI within $\pm$ 20% or 80–120)	☐

| | c. Summary results indicate superiority of active treatments (test & reference) over vehicle/placebo ($p < 0.05$) (eval. by Clinical Team) |
| | d. Data Files (Computer Media) Submitted |

Study Type   TRANSDERMAL DELIVERY SYSTEMS   □

    a. In-Vivo PK Study

        1. Study(ies) meet BE Criteria (90% CI or 80–125, Cmax, AUC)

        2. In-Vitro Dissolution

        3. Data Files (Computer Media) Submitted

    b. Adhesion Study

    c. Skin Irritation/Sensitization Study

Study Type   NASALLY ADMINISTERED DRUG PRODUCTS   □

    a. Solutions (Q1/Q2 sameness):

        1. In-Vitro Studies (Dose/Spray Content Uniformity, Droplet/Drug Particle Size Distrib., Spray Pattern, Plume Geometry, Priming & Repriming, Tail Off Profile)

    b. Suspensions (Q1/Q2 sameness):

        1. In-Vivo PK Study

            a. Study(ies) meets BE Criteria (90% CI or 80–125, C_{max}, AUC)

            b. Data Files (Computer Media) Submitted

        2. In-Vivo BE Study with Clinical EndPoints

            a. Properly defined BE endpoints (eval. by Clinical Team)

            b. Summary results meet BE criteria (90% CI within +/- 20% or 80–120)

            c. Summary results indicate superiority of active treatments (test & reference) over vehicle/placebo ($p < 0.05$) (eval. by Clinical Team)

            d. Data Files (Computer Media) Submitted

        3. In-Vitro Studies (Dose/Spray Content Uniformity, Droplet/Drug Particle Size Distrib., Spray Pattern, Plume Geometry, Priming & Repriming, Tail Off Profile)

Study Type   TOPICAL CORTICOSTEROIDS (VASOCONSTRICTOR STUDIES)   □

    a. Pilot Study (determination of ED50)

    b. Pivotal Study (study meets BE criteria 90%–CI or 80–125)

Sec. VII   Components and Composition Statements   □

    1. Unit composition and batch formulation

    2. Inactive ingredients as appropriate

Sec. VIII   Raw Materials Controls   □

    1. Active Ingredients

        a. Addresses of bulk manufacturers

        b. Type II DMF authorization letters or synthesis

        c. COA(s) specifications and test results from drug
           substance mfgr(s)
        d. Applicant certificate of analysis
        e. Testing specifications and data from drug product
           manufacturer(s)
        f. Spectra and chromatograms for reference standards
           and test samples
        g. CFN numbers
      2. Inactive Ingredients
        a. Source of inactive ingredients identified
        b. Testing specifications (including identification and
           characterization)
        c. Suppliers' COA (specifications and test results)
        d. Applicant certificate of analysis

Sec. IX   Description of Manufacturing Facility   ☐
      1. Full Address(es) of the Facility(ies)
      2. CGMP Certification
      3. CFN numbers

Sec. X   Outside Firms Including Contract Testing Laboratories   ☐
      1. Full Address
      2. Functions
      3. CGMP Certification/GLP
      4. CFN numbers

Sec. XI   Manufacturing and Processing Instructions   ☐
      1. Description of the Manufacturing Process (including
        Microbiological Validation, if Appropriate)
      2. Master Production Batch Record(s) for largest
        intended production runs (no more than 10x pilot
        batch) with equipment specified
      3. If sterile product: Aseptic fill/Terminal sterilization
      4. Filter validation (if aseptic fill)
      5. Reprocessing Statement

Sec. XII   In-Process Controls   ☐
      1. Copy of Executed Batch Record (Antibiotics/3
        Batches if bulk product produced by fermentation)
        with Equipment Specified, including Packaging
        Records (Packaging and Labeling Procedures), Batch
        Reconciliation and Label Reconciliation
      2. In-process Controls - Specifications and data

Sec. XIII   Container   ☐
      1. Summary of Container/Closure System (if new resin,
        provide data)
      2. Components Specification and Test Data (Type III DMF
        References)
      3. Packaging Configuration and Sizes

	4. Container/Closure Testing	
	5. Source of supply and suppliers address	
Sec. XIV	Controls for the Finished Dosage Form	☐
	1. Testing Specifications and Data	
	2. Certificate of Analysis for Finished Dosage Form	
Sec. XV	Stability of Finished Dosage Form	☐
	1. Protocol submitted	
	2. Post Approval Commitments	
	3. Expiration Dating Period	
	4. Stability Data Submitted	
	a. 3 month accelerated stability data	
	b. Batch numbers on stability records the same as the test batch	
Sec. XVI	Samples—Statement of Availability and Identification of:	☐
	1. Drug Substance	
	2. Finished Dosage Form	
	3. Same lot numbers	
Sec. XVII	Environmental Impact Analysis Statement	☐
Sec. XVIII	GDEA (Generic Drug Enforcement Act)/Other:	☐
	1. Letter of Authorization (U.S. Agent [if needed, countersignature on 356h])	
	2. Debarment Certification (original signature)	
	3. List of Convictions statement (original signature)	

Reviewing
CSO/CST
Date
Supervisory Concurrence/Date: _____
Duplicate copy sent to bio:
(Hold if RF and send when acceptable)
Duplicate copy to HFD- for consult: Type:

Recommendation:

☐ FILE   ☐ REFUSE to RECEIVE
Date: _____

10

Bioequivalence and Drug Product Assessment, In Vivo

Dale P. Conner and Barbara M. Davit

Center for Drug Evaluation and Research,
US Food and Drug Administration, Rockville, MD, U.S.A.

1. INTRODUCTION

No topic seems so simple but stimulates such intense controversy and misunderstanding as the topic of bioequivalence. The apparent simplicity of comparing in vivo performance of two drug products is an illusion that is quickly dispelled when one considers the difficulties and general public misunderstanding of the accepted regulatory methodology. In the US one often hears members of the public and medical experts alike stating various opinions on the unacceptability of approved generic drug products based on misconceptions regarding the determination of therapeutic equivalence of these products to the approved reference. These misconceptions include the belief that the US Food and Drug Administration (FDA) approves generic products that have mean differences from the reference product of 20–25% and that generic products can differ from each other by as much as 45%. In addition, some incorrectly assume that, since most bioequivalence testing is carried out in normal volunteers, it does not adequately reflect bioequivalence and therefore therapeutic equivalence in patients. When the current bioequivalence methods and statistical criteria are clearly understood it becomes apparent that these methods constitute a strict and robust system that provides assurance of therapeutic equivalence. In this chapter we will discuss the history, rationale and methods utilized for the demonstration of bioequivalence for regulatory purposes in the US as well as briefly reviewing the bioequivalence requirements in other countries. In addition, we will touch on some of the controversial issues and difficulties in demonstrating bioequivalence for locally acting drug products.

2. OBJECTIVES OF BIOEQUIVALENCE STUDIES

The most important concept in the understanding of bioequivalence is that the sole objective is to measure and compare formulation performance between two or more pharmaceutically equivalent drug products. Formulation performance is defined as the release of the drug substance from the drug product leading to bioavailability of the drug substance and eventually leading to one or more pharmacologic effects, both desirable and undesirable. If equivalent formulation performance from two products can be established then the clinical effects, within the range of normal clinical variability, should also be equivalent. This is the same principle that leads to an equivalent response from different lots of the brand-name product.

When generic drugs are submitted for approval through the Abbreviated New Drug Application (ANDA) process in the US, they must be both pharmaceutically equivalent and bioequivalent to be considered therapeutically equivalent and therefore approvable. To be considered pharmaceutically equivalent, two products must contain the same amount of the same drug substance and be of the same dosage form with the same indications and uses. Thus, an immediate release tablet would not be considered pharmaceutically equivalent to an oral liquid suspension, capsule or modified release tablet. Bioequivalence means the absence of a significant difference in the rate and extent to which the active ingredient becomes available at the site of drug action when administered at the same molar dose under similar conditions in an appropriately designed study. Two drug products are considered therapeutically equivalent if they are pharmaceutical equivalents and if they can be expected to have the same clinical effect and safety profile when administered to patients under the conditions specified in the labeling. The FDA believes that products classified as therapeutically equivalent can be substituted for each other with the full expectation that the substituted product will produce equivalent clinical effects and safety profile as the original product.

3. HISTORY OF BIOEQUIVALENCE EVALUATION OF GENERIC DRUG PRODUCTS

In 1938, the Federal Food Drug and Cosmetic Act was signed into law. The new law required, among other things, that a "new drug" product would need to provide proof of safety before it could be marketed. The New Drug Application (NDA) was established to provide a mechanism for proof of safety of drugs to be submitted to the FDA. Regulations were promulgated as to the form and content of the data to be submitted for an NDA. Originally only toxicity studies were required along with informative labeling and adequate manufacturing data. These early requirements have since evolved into the comprehensive regulations found in Title 21 of the Code of Federal Regulations Part 300, Subchapter D: Drugs for Human Use (21 CFR Part 300).

In 1962, The Kefauver–Harris Amendment to the Food Drug and Cosmetic Act mandated that all new drug products subsequently approved for marketing must have adequate evidence of effectiveness, as well as safety (1). The FDA was assigned the responsibility for receiving, reviewing, and evaluating required data submissions, and enforcing compliance with the law. An applicant submitting an NDA was now required to submit "substantial evidence" in the form of "adequate and well-controlled studies" to demonstrate the effectiveness of the drug product under the conditions of use described in its labeling. The new drug effectiveness provision of the law also applied retrospectively to all drugs approved between 1938 and 1962 on the basis of safety only. The FDA contracted with the National Academy of Sciences/National Research Council (NAS/NRC) to review this group of drugs for effectiveness. The NAS/NRC appointed 30 panels of experts and initiated the Drug Efficacy Study. The panels reviewed approximately 3400 drug formulations and classified them either effective or less than effective (2). The FDA reviewed the reports and any supporting data, and published its conclusions in the Federal Register as Drug Efficacy Study Implementation (DESI) notices. The DESI notices contained the acceptable marketing conditions for the class of drug products covered by this notice.

Many drug products had active ingredients and indications that were identical or very similar to those of drug products found to be effective in the DESI review but lacked NDA's themselves. Initially, in implementing the DESI program, the FDA required that each of these duplicate drug products should have its own approved NDA before it could be legally marketed. Later, the FDA concluded that a simpler and shorter drug application was adequate for approving duplicate DESI drugs for marketing, and, in 1970, created the ANDA procedure for the approval of duplicate DESI drug products (3–5). The FDA believed that it was not necessary for firms seeking approval of duplicate DESI drug products to establish the safety and efficacy of each new product identical in active ingredient and dosage form with a drug product previously approved as safe and effective. However, many of the DESI notices included, as a requirement for approval of the duplicate drug application, presentation of evidence that the "biologic availability" of the test product was similar to that of the innovator's product.

Introduction in the late 1960s and early 1970s of sophisticated bioanalytical techniques made possible measurements of drugs and metabolites in biological fluids at concentrations as low as a few nanograms per milliliter. Using these methods, the disposition of drugs in the human body could be characterized by determining pharmacokinetic profiles. The rate processes of drug absorption, distribution, metabolism, and excretion could now be quantified and related to formulation factors and pharmacodynamic effects. As these techniques were applied to investigate the relative bioavailability of various marketed drug products, it became apparent that many generic formulations were more bioavailable than the innovator products, while others were less bioavailable.

In the late 1960s and early 1970s, many published studies documented differences in the bioavailability of chemically equivalent drug products, notably chloramphenicol (6), tetracycline (7), phenylbutazone (8), and oxytetracycline (9). In addition, a number of cases of therapeutic failure occurred in patients taking digoxin. These patients required unusually high maintenance doses and were subsequently found to have low plasma digoxin concentrations (10). A crossover study conducted on four digoxin formulations available in the same hospital at the same time revealed striking differences in bioavailability. The peak plasma concentrations following a single dose varied by as much as seven-fold among the four formulations. These findings caused considerable concern because the margin of safety for digoxin is sufficiently narrow that serious toxicity or even lethality can result if the systemically available dose is as little as twice that needed to achieve the therapeutic effect.

To address this problem of bioinequivalence among duplicate drug products, the US Congress in 1974 created a special Office of Technology Assessment (OTA) to provide advice on scientific issues, among which was the bioequivalence of drug products. The OTA formed the Drug Bioequivalence Study Panel. The basic charge to the panel was to examine the relationships between chemical and therapeutic equivalence of drug products, and to assess whether existing technological capability could assure that drug products with the same physical and chemical composition would produce comparable therapeutic effects. Following an extensive investigation of the issues, the panel published its findings to the US Congress in a report, dated July 15, 1974, entitled Drug Bioequivalence (11,12). Notably, the panel concluded that variations in drug bioavailability were responsible for some instances of therapeutic failures and that analytical methodology was available for conducting bioavailability studies in man. Several recommendations pertained to in vivo bioequivalence evaluation. The panel recommended that efforts should be made to identify classes of drugs for which evidence of bioequivalence is critical, that current law requiring manufacturers to make bioavailability information available to the FDA should be strengthened, and that additional research aimed at improving the assessment and prediction of bioequivalence was needed.

In 1977, the FDA published its *Bioavailability and Bioequivalence* regulations under 21 CFR. The regulations were divided into Subpart A—*General Provisions*, Subpart B—*Procedures for Determining the Bioavailability of Drug Products*, and Subpart C—*Bioequivalence Requirements* (13). The regulations greatly aided the rational development of dosage forms of generic drugs, as well as the subsequent evaluation of their performance. With the publication of these regulations, a generic firm could file an ANDA that provided demonstration of bioequivalence to an approved drug product in lieu of clinical trials. Subpart B defined bioavailability in terms of rate and extent of drug absorption, described procedures for determining bioavailability of drug products, set forth requirements for submission of in vivo bioavailability data, and provided general guidelines for the conduct of in vivo bioavailability studies. Subpart C set forth requirements for marketing a drug product subject to a bioequivalence requirement. ANDAs were generally still restricted to duplicates of drug products approved prior to October 10, 1962 and determined to be effective for at least one indication in a DESI notice. A duplicate drug product had to meet bioequivalence requirements if well-controlled trials showed that it was either not therapeutically equivalent or bioequivalent to other pharmaceutically equivalent products. Narrow therapeutic index (NTI) drugs also had to meet bioequivalence requirements, as did drugs with low aqueous solubility, poorly absorbed drugs, drugs with nonlinear pharmacokinetics, drugs that underwent extensive first-pass metabolism, drugs which were unstable in the GI tract, and drugs for which absorption was limited to a specific portion of the GI tract. Finally, a duplicate drug product had to meet bioequivalence requirements if competent medical determination concluded that a lack of bioequivalence would have a serious adverse effect in the treatment or prevention of a serious disease or condition.

An important feature of the 1977 regulations was the provision for waiver of in vivo bioequivalence study requirements (biowaivers) under certain circumstances. Applicants could file waiver requests for parenteral solutions, topically applied preparations, oral dosage forms not intended to be absorbed, gases or vapors administered by the inhalation route, and oral solubilized dosage forms. Waivers could be granted for duplicate

DESI-effective parenteral drug products (suspensions excluded) and duplicate DESI-effective immediate-release oral drug products which were not on the list of FDA pharmacological classes and drugs for which in vivo bioequivalence testing was required. Biowaivers could also be granted for drug products in the same dosage form, but a different strength, and proportionally similar in active and inactive ingredients to a drug product from the same manufacturer for which in vivo bioavailability had been demonstrated. Both drug products were required to meet an appropriate in vitro test (generally dissolution) approved by the FDA.

The FDA did allow some duplicate drug versions of post-1962 drug products to be marketed under a "paper NDA" policy (14). Under this policy, in lieu of conducting their own tests, manufacturers of such duplicate drug products could submit safety and effectiveness information derived primarily from published reports of well-controlled studies. However, such reports of adequate and well-controlled studies in the literature were limited, and the FDA staff effort involved in reviewing paper NDA's became a substantial and often inefficient use of resources.

In 1984, the Drug Price Competition and Patent Term Restoration Act (the Hatch–Waxman Amendments) amended the Federal Food, Drug, and Cosmetic Act (15) by creating Section 505(j) of the Act (21 USC 355 (j)), which established the present ANDA approval process. Section 505(j) extended the ANDA process to duplicate versions of post-1962 drugs, but also required that an ANDA for any new generic drug product shall contain information to show that the generic product is bioequivalent to the reference listed drug product. Evidence of bioequivalence was now required for all dosage forms: tablets, capsules, suspensions, solutions, topical ointments and creams, transdermal patches, ophthalmics, injectables, and so on. The new law stated that a drug shall be considered to be bioequivalent to a listed drug if "the rate and extent of absorption of the drug do not show a significant difference from the rate and extent of absorption of the listed drug when administered at the same molar dose and of the therapeutic ingredient under similar experimental conditions in either a single dose or multiple doses . . ."

In 1992, the FDA revised the *Bioavailability and Bioequivalence Requirements* of 21 CFR Part 320 to implement the Hatch–Waxman Amendments (14). In its present form, 21 CFR Part 320 consists of Subpart A, *General Provisions*, and Subpart B, *Procedures for Determining the Bioavailability and Bioequivalence of Drug Products*. Subpart A describes general provisions including definitions of bioavailability and bioequivalence. Subpart B states the basis for demonstrating in vivo bioavailability or bioequivalence and lists types of evidence to establish bioavailability or bioequivalence, in descending order of accuracy, sensitivity, and reproducibility. Subpart B also provides guidelines for the conduct and design of an in vivo bioavailability study and lists criteria for waiving evidence of in vivo bioequivalence. The present biowaiver regulations now apply to solutions of all parental preparations, including intraocular, intravenous, subcutaneous, intramuscular, intraarterial, intrathecal, intrasternal, and interperitoneal, but no longer permit automatic biowaivers for all topical and nonsystemically absorbed oral dosage products (16). Waivers of in vivo testing can now be granted for ophthalmic, otic, and topical solutions. A DESI-effective immediate-release oral drug product can be granted a waiver of in vivo testing, provided it is not listed in the FDA's *Approved Drug Products with Therapeutic and Equivalence Evaluations* as having a known or potential bioequivalence problem (17). Other aspects of the present regulations governing biowaivers are similar to the 1977 regulations.

4. STATISTICAL EVALUATION OF BIOEQUIVALENCE DATA

Statistical evaluation of most bioequivalence studies is based on analysis of drug blood or plasma/serum concentration data. The area under the plasma concentration vs. time curve (AUC) is used as an index of the extent of drug absorption. Generally, both AUC determined until the last blood sampling time (AUC_{0-t}) and AUC extrapolated to infinity (AUC_∞) are evaluated. Drug peak plasma concentration (C_{max}) is used as an index of the rate of drug absorption.

Criteria for approval of generic drugs have evolved since the 1970s (18). In the early 1970s, approval was based on mean data. Mean AUC and C_{max} values for the generic product had to be within $\pm 20\%$ of those of the brandname product. In addition, plasma concentration–time profiles for immediate-release products had to be reasonably superimposable. Beginning in the late 1970s, the 75/75 (or 75/75-125) rule was added to the criteria. According to the 75/75 rule, the test/reference ratios of AUC and C_{max} had to be within 0.75–1.25 for at least 75% of the subjects. This was an attempt to consider individual variability in rate and extent of absorption. In the early 1980s, the power approach was applied to AUC and C_{max} parameters in conjunction with the 75/75 rule. The power approach consisted of two statistical tests: (1) a test of the null hypothesis of no difference between formulations using the F test; and (2) the evaluation of the power to a test to detect a 20% mean difference in treatments.

Statistically, the power approach and the 75/75 rule have poor performance, and the FDA discontinued the use of these methods in 1986. Since 1986, the FDA has used the two one-sided tests statistical procedure, also referred to as the 90% confidence interval approach. The two one-sided tests procedure encompasses two questions (19). Stated simply, the first test asks if the test product is significantly less bioavailable than the reference product. The second question asks if the reference product is significantly less bioavailable than the test product. A significant difference is defined as 20% at the alpha equals 0.05 level. Based on these statistical criteria, the mean test/reference ratio of the data is usually close to one. The criteria above may be re-stated to illustrate the rationale for the 0.80–1.25 (or 80–125%) confidence interval criteria. In the first case illustrated above, test/reference = 0.80 and in the second case (or bioequivalence limit) reference/test = 0.80 (expressed by convention as test/reference = 1.25, i.e., the reciprocal of 0.80). This may be stated in clinical terms as follows: if a patient is currently receiving a brand-name reference product and is switched to a generic product, the generic product should not deliver significantly less drug to the patient than the brand-name product, conversely, if a patient is currently receiving the generic product and is switched to the brand-name reference product the brand-name product should not deliver significantly less drug to the patient than the generic product.

The two one-sided tests procedure is the statistical procedure used to evaluate bioequivalence rather than the hypothesis testing procedure, which is the statistical procedure usually used to evaluate whether one treatment produces a result significantly different from another treatment (20). This is because, in evaluating bioequivalence studies, we want to establish whether the difference between the generic and brand-name formulation is acceptable. Thus, the evaluation of bioequivalence data is based on the 90% confidence interval approach rather than hypothesis testing (20,21). As described above: (1) the 90% confidence interval encompasses the two one-tailed tests, each carried out at the alpha = 0.05 (5%) level; and, (2) the FDA specifies that the bioavailability of the generic formulation relative to the brand-name should be within 0.80–1.25 and must be known with a 90% confidence. The analysis of variance (ANOVA) is applied to bioequivalence study data to determine the 90% confidence limits of the differences.

Until 1992, for bioequivalence statistical analysis, the FDA generally recommended that applicants perform ANOVA on untransformed AUC and C_{max} data to determine the 90% confidence limits of the differences. Following a 1991 meeting of the Generic Drugs Advisory Committee which focused on statistical analysis of bioequivalence data, the FDA began to recommend that applicants perform ANOVA on log-transformed data. Since AUC and C_{max} values are log-normally distributed, the Advisory Committee and FDA statisticians concluded that log-transformed data better satisfy the assumptions underlying the ANOVA than untransformed data. Since 1992, the FDA has formally recommended that applicants perform ANOVA on log-transformed data and determine the 90% confidence interval for the ratios of the test/reference least squares geometric means in performing average bioequivalence analysis (22).

5. CURRENT METHODS AND CRITERIA FOR DOCUMENTING BIOEQUIVALENCE

A new FDA guidance for industry posted in 2003 updates recommendations for documentation of bioavailability and bioequivalence in regulatory submissions. *Bioavailability and Bioequivalence Studies for Orally Administered Drug Products—General Considerations* provides recommendations to sponsors planning to include bioavailability and bioequivalence information for orally administered drug products in regulatory submissions (23). The guidance addresses how to meet the *Bioavailability/Bioequivalence Requirements* set forth in 21 CFR Part 320 as they apply to oral dosage forms. The guidance also applies to nonorally administered drug products where reliance on systemic exposure measures is suitable to document bioavailability/bioequivalence (e.g., transdermal systems, certain rectal and nasal drug products).

There are several types of studies commonly used for demonstration of bioequivalence. The preferred study for most orally administered dosage forms is a two-way crossover, two-period, two-sequence single-dose study, under fasting conditions performed in volunteers. In this design, each study subject receives each treatment, test and reference, in random order. Plasma or blood samples are collected for approximately three pharmacokinetic half-lives for determination of the rate and extent of drug release from the dosage form and absorption by each subject. A washout period is scheduled between the two periods to allow the subjects to completely eliminate the drug absorbed from the first dose before administration of the second dose. Although this design is carried out for most orally absorbed drug products, it may become impractical for drugs with long pharmacokinetic half-lives, i.e., longer than 30 h (e.g., amiodarone, clomiphene, mefloquine). In this case a single-dose parallel design may be used instead (24). For drugs with very long half-lives, concentration sampling may be carried out for a period of time corresponding to two times the median T_{max} (time to C_{max}) for the product. For drugs that demonstrate low intrasubject variability in distribution and clearance, an AUC truncated at 72 h may be used in place of AUC_{0-t} or AUC_∞ (23). An alternative study design that may be useful for highly variable drug products is a replicate design (23). In this design, each treatment is repeated in the same subject on two separate occasions. This is performed as either a partial (three-way) or full (four-way) replication of treatments. The replicate design (22) has the advantage that fewer subjects can be used.

Because food can influence the bioequivalence between test and reference products, the FDA recommends that applicants conduct bioequivalence studies under fasting as well as under fed conditions for most orally administered immediate-release drug products (25). Fed bioequivalence studies are particularly recommended for immediate-release oral dosage forms whenever the innovator's label makes statements about the effect of food on absorption or administration. However, if the label states that the product should be taken only on an empty stomach, fed bioequivalence studies are not recommended. Fed bioequivalence studies are generally conducted using meal conditions expected to provide the greatest effects on formulation performance and gastrointestinal physiology such that systemic drug bioavailability may be maximally effected. Typically, the drug is administered to subjects within 30 min of consuming a high-fat, high-calorie meal. Fed bioequivalence studies should be conducted for all modified-release oral dosage forms because the bioavailability of these products is likely to be altered by co-administration with meals. The FDA recommends that these studies use a randomized, balanced, single-dose, two-treatment (fed vs. fasting), two-period, two sequence crossover design (25). For a few drug products, bioequivalence is evaluated only under fed conditions because there are safety concerns associated with administration of the product on an empty stomach.

The FDA recommends that in vivo bioequivalence studies be conducted in individuals representative of the general population, taking into account age, sex, and race factors (23). For example, if a drug product is to be used in both sexes, the sponsor should attempt to include similar proportions of males and females in the study; if the drug product is to be used predominantly in the elderly, the applicant should attempt to include as many subjects of 60 years of age or greater as possible. Restrictions on admission into the study should generally be based solely on safety considerations.

Bioequivalence studies should be conducted in the intended patient population when there are significant safety concerns associated with use in healthy subjects. For example, bioequivalence of an antineoplastic drug intended for short-term therapy, such as etoposide, can be evaluated following a single dose either in cancer patients in remission or in patients under active treatment by sampling on the first day of a treatment cycle (24). For a medication such as clozapine, on which normal subjects may experience serious orthostatic hypotension with the first dose, the most appropriate study design is a steady-state (multiple dose) crossover bioequivalence study in patients (24,26). These studies can be conducted either in naive patients, or in patients who are already stabilized on the medication of interest.

6. TYPES OF EVIDENCE TO ESTABLISH BIOAVAILABILITY AND BIOEQUIVALENCE

Subpart B of the *Bioavailability and Bioequivalence Requirements* in 21 CFR Part 320 lists the following in vivo and in vitro approaches to determining bioequivalence in descending order of accuracy, sensitivity, and reproducibility (27):

- in vivo measurement of active moiety or moieties in biologic fluid;
- in vivo pharmacodynamic comparison;
- in vivo limited clinical comparison;
- in vitro comparison;
- any other approach deemed appropriate by FDA.

Figure 1 illustrates, for a model of oral dosage form performance, why the most sensitive approach is to measure the drug in biological fluids, such as blood, plasma, or serum. The active ingredient leaves the solid dosage

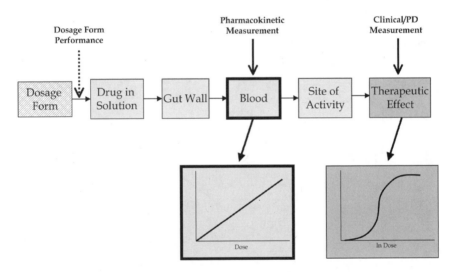

FIGURE 1 The most sensitive approach in evaluating bioequivalence of two formulations is to measure drug concentration in biological fluids, as illustrated in this diagram showing the relationship between dosage form performance and therapeutic response. Following oral dosing, the active ingredient leaves the solid dosage form, dissolves in the gastrointestinal tract, and, following absorption through the gut wall, appears in the systemic circulation. Formulation performance is the major factor determining the critical steps of dosage form disintegration and drug substance dissolution prior to absorption. All other steps following in vivo drug substance dissolution are patient- or subject-determined processes not directly related to formulation performance. The variability of the measured endpoint increases with each additional step in the process, such that variability of clinical measures is quite high compared to that of blood concentration measures. As a result, a pharmacodynamic or clinical approach is not as accurate, sensitive, and reproducible as an approach based on plasma concentrations.

form and dissolves in the gastrointestinal tract, and following absorption through the gut wall, appears in the systemic circulation. The step involving dissolution of the drug substance prior to absorption is the critical step that is determined by the formulation. Other steps illustrated in the diagram are patient- or subject-determined processes not directly related to formulation performance. Variability of the measured endpoint increases with each additional step in the process. Therefore, variability of clinical measures is quite high compared to blood concentration measures. Figure 2 shows that the blood concentration of a drug directly reflects the amount of drug delivered from the dosage form.

In situations where a drug cannot be reliably measured in blood, it may be appropriate to base bioequivalence evaluation on an in vivo test in humans in which an acute pharmacologic (pharmacodynamic) effect is

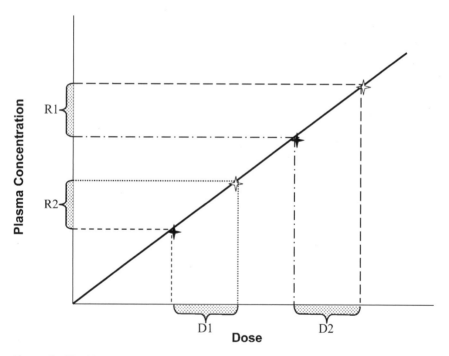

FIGURE 2   The blood concentration of a drug directly reflects the amount of drug delivered from the dosage form. The corresponding responses over a wide range of doses will be of adequate sensitivity to detect differences in bioavailability between two formulations. This is illustrated for two widely different doses, D_1 and D_2. Any differences in dosage form performance are reflected directly by changes in blood concentration (R_1 and R_2).

measured as a function of time. Generally, the pharmacodynamic response plotted against the logarithm of dose appears as a sigmoidal curve, as shown in Figure 3. It is assumed that, after absorption from the site of delivery, the drug or active metabolite is delivered to the site of activity and, through binding to a receptor or some other mechanism, elicits a quantifiable pharmacodynamic response. Since additional steps contribute to the observed pharmacodynamic response, a pharmacodynamic assay is not as sensitive to drug formulation performance as blood drug concentrations. In developing a pharmacodynamic assay for bioequivalence evaluation, it is critical to validate the assay by selecting the correct dose. The dose should be in the range that produces a change in response, as shown in the midportion of the curve. In other words, the pharmacodynamic assay should be sensitive to

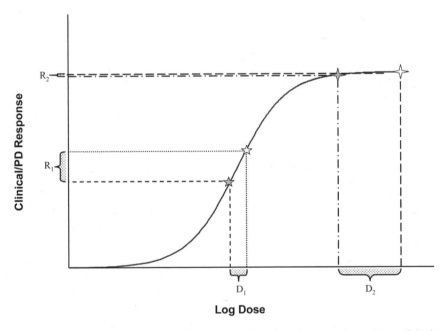

FIGURE 3 In evaluating bioequivalence in a study with pharmacodynamic or clinical endpoints, it is critical to select a dose that falls on the middle ascending portion of the sigmoidal dose–response curve. The most appropriate dose for a study based on pharmacodynamic or clinical endpoints should be in the range that produces a change in response (R_1), as shown in the midportion of the curve (D_1). A dose that is too high will produce a minimal response at the plateau phase of the dose–response curve, such that even large differences in dose (D_2) will show little or no change in pharmacodynamic or clinical effect (R_2). Thus, two formulations that are quite different may appear to be bioequivalent.

small changes in dose. A dose that is too high will produce a minimal response at the plateau phase of the dose–response curve, such that even large differences in dose will show little or no change in pharmacodynamic effect. A pharmacodynamic study can be conducted in healthy subjects. The pharmacodynamic response selected should directly reflect dosage form performance but may not necessarily reflect therapeutic efficacy.

If it is not possible to develop reliable bioanalytical or pharmacodynamic assays, then it may be necessary to evaluate bioequivalence in a well-controlled trial with clinical endpoints. This type of bioequivalence study is conducted in patients and is based on evaluation of a therapeutic, i.e., clinical, response. The clinical response follows a similar dose–response pattern to the pharmacodynamic response, as shown in Figure 3. Thus, in designing bioequivalence studies with clinical endpoints, the same considerations for dose selection apply as for bioequivalence studies with pharmacodynamic endpoints. As with a pharmacodynamic study, the appropriate dose for a bioequivalence study with clinical endpoints should be on the linear rising portion of the dose–response curve, since a response in this range will be the most sensitive to changes in formulation performance. Due to high variability and the subjective nature of clinical evaluations, the clinical response is often not as sensitive to differences in drug formulation performance as a pharmacodynamic response. For these reasons, the clinical approach is the least accurate, sensitive, and reproducible of the in vivo approaches to determining bioequivalence.

Most bioequivalence studies submitted to the FDA are based on measuring drug concentrations in plasma. In certain cases, whole blood or serum may be more appropriate for analysis. Measurement of only the parent drug released from the dosage form, rather than a metabolite, is generally recommended because the concentration–time profile of the parent drug is more sensitive to formulation performance than a metabolite, which is more reflective of metabolite formation, distribution, and elimination (23). Measurement of a metabolite may be preferred when parent drug concentrations are too low to permit reliable measurement. In this case, the metabolite data are subject to a confidence interval approach for bioequivalence demonstration. Both the parent and metabolite are measured in cases where the metabolite is formed by presystemic or first-pass metabolism and contributes meaningfully to safety and efficacy. In this case, only the parent drug data are analyzed using the confidence interval approach. The metabolite data are not subjected to confidence interval analysis but rather is used to provide supportive evidence of comparable therapeutic outcome.

Urine measurements are not as sensitive as plasma measurements, but are necessary for some drugs such as orally administered potassium chloride (28), because serum concentrations are too low to allow for accurate measurement of drug absorbed from the dosage form. Both cumulative amount of drug excreted (A_e) and maximum rate of urinary excretion (R_{max}) are evaluated statistically in bioequivalence studies which rely on urine concentrations.

The FDA accepts pharmacodynamic effect methodology to approve generic topical corticosteroid drug products (29). This approach is based on the ability of corticosteroids to produce blanching or vasoconstriction in the microvasculature of the skin.

Bioequivalence study designs with clinical endpoints are used for some oral drug products that are not systemically absorbed, such as sucralfate tablets. Bioequivalence studies with clinical endpoints generally employ a randomized, blinded, balanced, parallel design. Studies compare the efficacy of the test product, innovator product, and placebo to determine if the two products containing active ingredient are bioequivalent. The placebo is included to assure that the two active treatments in the clinical trial actually are being studied at a dose which effects the therapeutic response(s). Failure to assure that the treatments are clinically active in the trial would show that the trial has no sensitivity to differences in formulation, i.e., the response is on the flat bottom of the dose–response curve (Figure 3). A generic equivalent of the innovator product should be able to demonstrate bioequivalence for selected clinical endpoint(s) that adequately reflect drug appearance at the site(s) of activity and therefore formulation performance. For example, for sucralfate tablets, the clinical endpoint is duodenal ulcer healing at 4 weeks (24). The test and reference clinical responses are considered bioequivalent if the 90% confidence interval for the differences in proportions between test and reference treatment is contained within -0.20 to 0.20.

With suitable justification, bioavailability and bioequivalence may be established by in vitro studies alone. This approach is also suitable for some types of locally acting products, such as cholestyramine resins (30), which form nonabsorbable complexes with bile acids in the intestine. For cholestyramine resins, the in vitro measures of bioequivalence are based on the rates of binding to bile acid salts. The 90% confidence of the test/reference ratios of the equilibrium binding constants should fall within the limits of 0.80–1.25.

As described above, most studies determining bioequivalence between generic products and the corresponding brand-name products are based on evaluation of blood concentration data in healthy subjects. It is true that drug pharmacokinetic profiles may differ between healthy subjects and particular types of patients. This is because some disease states affect different aspects of drug substance absorption, distribution, metabolism, and elimination. However, the effects of disease on relative formulation performance, i.e., release of the drug substance from the drug product, are rare.

Bioequivalence studies are designed to measure and compare formulation performance between two drug products within the same individuals. It is expected that any difference between in vivo drug release from the two formulations will be the same whether the two formulations are tested in patients or normal subjects. Thus, generic and brand-name products which are bioequivalent can be substituted in patients because they will produce the same effect(s). This is illustrated by findings from a recent observational cohort study comparing effectiveness and safety in patients switched from brand-name warfarin sodium tablets to generic warfarin sodium tablets (31). The generic product was approved based on standard bioequivalence studies in normal volunteers. The observational cohort study showed that the two products had no difference in clinical outcome measures.

7. WAIVERS OF IN VIVO BIOEQUIVALENCE BASED ON IN VITRO DISSOLUTION TESTING

Under certain circumstances, product quality bioavailability and bioequivalence can be documented using in vitro approaches (27). In vitro dissolution testing to document bioequivalence for nonbioproblem DESI drugs remains acceptable. In vitro dissolution characterization is encouraged for all product formulations investigated, including prototype formulations, particularly if in vivo absorption characteristics are being defined for the different product formulations. Such efforts may enable the establishment of an in vitro–in vivo correlation. When an in vitro–in vivo correlation is available (16), the in vitro test can serve as an indicator of how the product will perform in vivo.

For immediate-release products, an in vivo bioequivalence demonstration of one or more lower strengths can be waived based on acceptable dissolution testing and an in vivo study on the highest strength (23). All strengths should be proportionally similar in active and inactive ingredients. For reasons of safety of study subjects, it is sometimes appropriate to conduct the in vivo study on a strength that is not the highest. In these cases, the FDA will consider a biowaiver request for a higher strength if elimination kinetics are linear over the dose range, if the strengths are proportionally similar, and if comparative dissolution testing on all strengths is acceptable. Examples of drug products for which an in vivo study is not recommended on the highest strength due to safety include mirtazapine tablets (17) and terazosin hydrochloride capsules and tablets (24).

For modified-release oral drug products, application of dissolution waivers varies depending on whether the product is formulated as a beaded capsule or tablet. For capsules in which the strength differs only in the number of identical beads containing the active moiety, in vivo testing can be waived based on acceptable dissolution testing and an acceptable in vivo study on the highest strength. For tablets, a biowaiver may be considered when the drug product is in the same dosage form but in a different strength, is proportionally similar in its active and inactive ingredients, and has the same drug release mechanism. All strengths should exhibit similar dissolution profiles in at least three media (e.g., pH 1.2, 4.5, and 6.8) (23).

Applicants can request biowaivers for immediate-release products based on an approach termed the biopharmaceutics classification system (BCS) (32). The BCS is a framework for classifying drug substances based on solubility and intestinal permeability. With product dissolution, these are the three major factors governing rate and extent of absorption from immediate-release products. The BCS classifies drug substances as:

Class 1: high solubility, high permeability;
Class 2: low solubility, high permeability;
Class 3: high solubility, low permeability;
Class 4: low solubility, low permeability.

The FDA believes that demonstration of in vivo bioequivalence may not be necessary for immediate-release products containing BCS Class 1 drug substances, as long as the inactive ingredients do not significantly affect absorption of the active ingredient(s). This is because, when a drug dissolves rapidly from the dosage form (in relation to gastric emptying) and has high intestinal permeability, the rate and extent of its absorption are unlikely to depend on dissolution and/or gastrointestinal transit time.

The CDER Guidance for Industry: *Waiver of In Vivo Bioavailability and Bioequivalence Studies for Immediate Release Solid Oral Dosage Forms Based on a Biopharmaceutics Classification System* (32), recommends methods for determining drug solubility and permeability for applicants who wish to request biowaivers based on BCS. The drug solubility class boundary is based on the highest dose strength of the product that is the subject of the biowaiver request. The permeability class can be determined in vivo (mass balance, absolute bioavailability, or intestinal perfusion approaches) or in vitro (permeation studies using excised tissues or a monolayer of cultured epithelial cells). Dissolution testing should be conducted in three media: 0.1 N HCl or simulated gastric fluid without enzymes; pH 4.5 buffer, and pH 6.8 buffer or simulated intestinal fluid without enzymes and the f_2 test applied (23).

8. COMPLEX DRUG SUBSTANCES

There are many drug substances that may fit into the category of "Complex Drug Substances". These include many proteins, peptides, botanicals, synthetic hormones, biotechnology products, and complex mixtures. For most of these drugs, the most difficult problem is to demonstrate pharmaceutical equivalence. In many cases, current technology is not sufficient to unequivocally characterize the drug substance in two different manufacturer's products or after a single manufacturer wishes to make pre- or post-approval changes in manufacturing procedures. These deficiencies in drug substance characterization methods currently may stand in the way of the approval of generic products for many of these products containing complex drug substances.

9. NARROW THERAPEUTIC INDEX DRUGS

There are no additional approval requirements for generic versions of NTI drugs vs. non-NTI drugs. The FDA does not set specific standards based on therapeutic index (23,33). The bioequivalence criteria, using the 90% confidence interval approach, are quite strict; there is no need to apply stricter criteria for NTI drugs. The current FDA position is that any generic product may be switched with its corresponding reference listed drug.

10. FAILED BIOEQUIVALENCE STUDIES

There are several reasons why bioequivalence studies fail. Figure 4 shows various scenarios of bioequivalence results for several hypothetical formulations (labeled F1–F7). For simplicity, the width of the 90% confidence interval is shown as a bar, although it is important to remember that the results are truly not an even distribution but a normal or log-normal distribution. The log-transformed test/reference ratios from a bioequivalence study are distributed as a bell-shaped curve, with most of the subjects' ratios centered around the center or mean, and fewer subjects' ratios falling at the edges. The top bar in Figure 4 (F1) represents a study with a 90% confidence interval of the test to reference ratio falling between the limits of 0.80–1.25 and the test/reference ratios centered around 1.00. This is what most applicants would like to achieve with the to-be-marketed formulation for a given product. The second bar (F2) also represents a 90% confidence interval of test/reference ratios falling within 0.8–1.25. Although the mean test/reference ratio is less than 1.00, the variability is very low with the result that this product also meets the 90% confidence interval criteria. The remaining bars in Figure 4 show various scenarios of failure to demonstrate bioequivalence. The third bar (F3) from the top depicts a situation where the test/reference ratios are still centered around 1.00, but because of high variability and probably inadequate sample size, the 90% confidence interval is very wide. This example illustrates how highly variable drugs often need

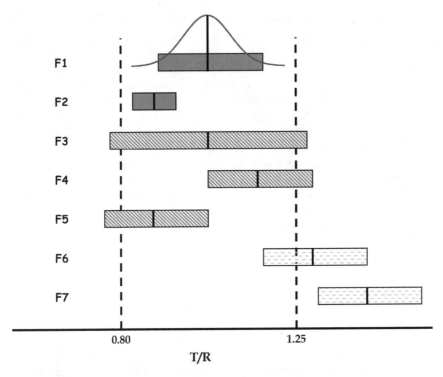

FIGURE 4 Hypothetical bioequivalence study results for formulations F1–F7 illustrate various scenarios of passing and failing bioequivalence criteria. The width of each 90% confidence interval (CI) is shown as a bar, although in actuality, the log-transformed test/reference (T/R) ratios are distributed as a bell-shaped curve. F1 and F2 represent results of studies in which the 90% CIs of the test/reference ratios (T/R) fall between 0.80 and 1.25 (pass bioequivalence criteria). For F1, the ratio of T/R means (point estimate) is near 1.00. For F2, the point estimate is less than 1.00, but because of low variability, the 90% CI of T/R ratios still falls within acceptable limits. F3–F7 show ways in which studies fail to pass CI criteria. With F3, the point estimate is near 1.00, but because of high variability, the 90% CI is very wide and the drug does not pass bioequivalence criteria. F3 may pass CI criteria if the number of study subjects is increased. By contrast, F4–F7 have variability comparable to F1. F4 represents a failure on the low side (T is less bioavailable than R), and F5 represents a failure on the high side (R is less bioavailable than T). Since the point estimates for F3 and F4 are still within the 0.8–1.25 range, these formulations may also meet CI criteria if a greater number of subjects are dosed. F6 does not meet the upper bound of the 90% CI, and the point estimate exceeds 1.25. For F7, the entire CI is outside the acceptance criteria (bioinequivalence). Formulations F6 and F7 are so different from the reference that both will still fail CI criteria even if the number of subjects is increased.

more subjects to attain sufficient statistical power to pass bioequivalence criteria. It is very likely that a new study on the same formulation would pass if more subjects were enrolled, thereby increasing the power of the study and decreasing the resulting width of the 90% confidence interval. The next two bars (F4 and F5) show results of studies which fail to meet bioequivalence criteria, one a failure on the low side (test product has lower bioavailability than reference product), the other a failure on the high side (reference product has lower bioavailability than test product). These two formulations have comparable variability to the formulation that passed (F1), but fail because there is a difference between the test and reference formulations. Because the ratio of means, or point estimate, is still within the 0.80–1.25 limits in each of these two cases, it is also possible that these two formulations may pass another study if many more subjects were enrolled. The product represented by the bar that is second from the bottom (F6) not only does not meet the upper bound of the 90% confidence interval, but the point estimate exceeds 1.25. It is likely that this product will not pass even if the power of the study is increased by enrolling more subjects. The bottom bar (F7) represents a very extreme case in which the entire confidence interval is outside the acceptance criteria. In this extreme case, the two products are bioinequivalent. The two products are so different that it is highly improbable that repeat studies would ever demonstrate bioequivalence.

In bioequivalence studies of generic products, the most common reason for failure is that the study was underpowered with respect to the number of subjects in the data set. The width of the confidence interval is controlled by the number of subjects and by the variability of the pharmacokinetic measures. Studies may be underpowered for various reasons. The applicant may have failed to enroll an adequate number of subjects. There may be an excessive number of withdrawals, or there may be missing data because of lost samples. Sometimes a study may fail because of outliers. For example, noncompliant subjects may cause the study to fail. The FDA discourages deletion of outlier values, particularly for nonreplicated study designs (22).

Until recently, applicants did not include failed bioequivalence study data in ANDA submissions. Although applicants submitting NDAs are required to submit data from all clinical studies to the FDA, this is not the case for ANDAs. The Food Drug and Cosmetic Act Section 505(b)(1)(A) states that, for NDAs, all human investigations made to show whether or not a drug is safe for use and whether such drug is effective must be submitted. Similar language was not included in Section 505(j), the section covering the submission of ANDAs. Therefore, generic firms for many years interpreted this language to mean that failed bioequivalence studies did not have to be submitted in their ANDAs. In November of 2000, the Advisory Committee for Pharmaceutical Science recommended that generic applicants submit to the FDA results of all bioequivalence studies on the to-be-marketed formulations (34). The Committee expressed the opinion that applicants should submit the results of failed bioequivalence studies as complete summaries, further suggesting that the FDA should do a brief, but careful examination to identify potential problems worthy of requesting additional information. In 2003, the FDA posted a proposed rule relating to failed bioequivalence studies in the Federal Register for notice and comment (35). The proposed rule would amend the Bioavailability/ Bioequivalence Regulations to require an ANDA applicant to submit data from all bioequivalence studies that an applicant conducts on a drug product formulation submitted for approval. The proposed rule is consistent with the recommendations of the Advisory Committee, in that it will require applicants to submit summary data for all bioequivalence studies other than those upon which the applicant relies for approval.

11. BIOEQUIVALENCE EVALUATION OF GENERIC DRUG PRODUCTS IN OTHER COUNTRIES

11.1. Canada

In Canada, applicants can seek approval of generic drug products by submitting abbreviated drug submissions (ANDS) to Health Canada's Therapeutic Products Directorate (36). A subsequent entry (generic) product is eligible for an ANDS against a Canadian reference product if it is given by the same route of administration, is shown to be pharmaceutically equivalent and bioequivalent to the Canadian reference product, and if it falls within the same condition(s) of use as the Canadian reference product. Applicants may also seek approval of subsequent entry products compared to a foreign reference product if the foreign reference meets a number of specific requirements (37).

The applicant may request that the results of a single comparative bioavailability study be extrapolated for all strengths in a product series provided that the proportions of the medicinal and nonmedicinal ingredients fall within specified limits and exhibit the same dissolution profiles. The Therapeutic Products Directorate screens ANDS upon receipt, and if judged to be acceptable for review they are subjected to in-depth evaluation. The Therapeutic Products Directorate has issued a number of guidances related to comparative bioavailability studies and bioequivalence studies. Three of particular relevance provide guidance on the general format of ANDS (38) and the conduct and analysis of bioavailability/bioequivalence studies of solid oral dosage forms intended for systemic effects in immediate-release (38) and modified-release (39) dosage forms. In general, single-dose fasting and single-dose fed bioequivalence studies may be designed as either two single-dose, randomized, two-period, two-treatment crossover studies or as one single-dose, randomized, four-period, four-treatment crossover study. Multiple-dose bioequivalence studies are also to be conducted for modified-release products that are used at a dose likely to lead to accumulation. Bioequivalence studies generally enroll healthy adult male subjects. Studies in patients may be required if the use of healthy volunteers is precluded for reasons of safety. Normally data for only the parent compound or active ingredient is required if it can be accurately measured, e.g., measurement of the active component may be appropriate if the parent compound is a prodrug. An Expert Advisory Committee on Bioavailability also recommended more stringent requirements be considered for drugs which exhibit "complicated" pharmacokinetics, e.g., drugs with a narrow therapeutic range, highly toxic drugs, drugs that exhibit nonlinear kinetics, etc (40). The Therapeutic Products Directorate is developing guidances related to such drugs (41,42). In general, for a drug that demonstrates "uncomplicated pharmacokinetics" in an immediate-release dosage form, the standards for bioequivalence are that the 90% confidence interval of the relative mean AUC_{0-t} of the test to reference product should be within 0.8–1.25 and for C_{max} only the relative mean of the test to reference product should be between 0.8 and 1.25 (i.e., point ratio only for C_{max} must fall within the limits of 80–125% and no 90% confidence interval requirement). These standards are to be met, normally in the fasted state, on log-transformed parameters calculated from the measured data and also data corrected for measured drug content (percent potency of label claim). For drugs that exhibit "complicated" pharmacokinetics the standards for bioequivalence are more stringent (40). For example, for a drug that exhibits a narrow therapeutic range the 95% confidence interval of the relative mean AUC_{0-t} and C_{max} of the test to reference product should be within 0.8–1.25 in single-dose studies conducted under both fasted and fed conditions. Again, these standards must be met on log-transformed parameters calculated from the measured data and also from data corrected for measured drug content (41). For drugs with nonlinear kinetics resulting in greater than proportional increases in AUC with increasing dose, the bioequivalence standards for "uncomplicated" drugs apply, i.e., 90% confidence limits, but bioequivalence studies are to be conducted under fasted and fed conditions on at least the highest strength. Similarly, for drugs with nonlinear kinetics resulting in less than proportional increases in AUC with increasing dose, bioequivalence studies are conducted on at least the lowest strength (42).

11.2. Japan

In Japan, the Organization for Pharmaceutical Safety and Research (OPSR) reviews data in applications for approval of generic medications to verify equivalency between the proposed generic and the medicine which has already been approved. These reviews are conducted under commission from the Japanese Ministry of Health, Labor, and Welfare (MHLW). The Japanese National Institute of Health Sciences (NIHS) has responsibility for preparation of guidelines and has issued a guideline for bioequivalence studies of generic products (43). In general, applicants conduct single-dose crossover studies using healthy adult subjects. Multiple-dose studies are conducted for drugs that are repeatedly issued to patients. For modified-release products, single-dose fasted and postprandial bioequivalence studies are conducted. A high-fat diet is administered for a postprandial bioequivalence study. If a high incidence of severe adverse events is indicated after dosing in the fasted state, a fasting study is replaced with a postprandial dose study that uses a low fat meal. If the test and reference products show a significant difference in dissolution at about pH 6.8, subjects with low gastric acidity (achlorohydric subjects) are used unless the application of the drug is limited to a special population. If adverse events preclude administration to healthy subjects, then patients are used. Bioequivalence analysis is generally based on drug concentrations in blood. Urine samples are used if there is a rationale. The parent drug is generally measured but major active metabolites may be measured instead of the parent drug, if there is a rationale. The acceptable range of bioequivalence is generally 0.8–1.25 as the ratios of average AUC and C_{max} of the test product to reference product, when the parameters are logarithmically distributed. For drugs with pharmacologically mild actions, a wider range can be acceptable. The acceptable ranges for other parameters, such as T_{max}, are determined for each drug. If two products do not meet the 90% confidence interval criteria, they can still be considered bioequivalent if three additional conditions are satisfied: (1) the total sample size of the initial bioequivalence study is at least 20 or the pooled sample size of initial and add-on subject studies is at least 30; (2) the differences in average values of log-transformed AUC and C_{max} between two products are between $\log(0.9) - \log(1.11)$; and (3) dissolution rates of test and reference products are evaluated to be equivalent under all dissolution testing conditions. Pharmacodynamic studies can be conducted for products which do not produce measurable blood or urine concentrations. In studies based on pharmacodynamic endpoints, efficacy–time profiles are compared and acceptance criteria are established by considering the drug's pharmacologic activity. If bioequivalence and pharmacodynamic studies are impossible or inappropriate, a clinical study can be conducted.

The acceptance criteria in a clinical study are established by considering the drug's pharmacologic characteristics and activity.

11.3. European Union

The European Agency for the Evaluation of Medicinal Products (EMEA) is in charge of supervising medicinal products for human use throughout the European Union (EU). The EU is an international organization of Member States that have set up common institutions to which they delegate some of their sovereignty so that decisions on specific matters of joint interest can be made at the European level (44). The marketing of medicinal products throughout the EU is authorized by the European Commission, which bases its decision on recommendations made by the EMEA.

Applicants submit to the EMEA an abridged application for marketing approval of a generic drug product that claims essential similarity to a reference product by demonstrating bioequivalence (45). The reference product is an innovator product that has been approved on the basis of a full dossier, including chemical, biological, pharmaceutical, pharmacological–toxicological and clinical data. An approved essentially similar product can be substituted for the innovator product. The EU defines essential similarity as follows: "A medicinal product is essentially similar to an original product where it satisfies the criteria of having the same qualitative and quantitative composition in terms of active substances, of having the same pharmaceutical form, and of being bioequivalent unless it is apparent in the light of scientific knowledge that it differs from the original product as regards safety and efficacy." A generic firm can submit to numerous EU Member States an abridged application claiming essential similarity to a reference product based on bioequivalence with a reference product from one Member State.

The EMEA has posted a guidance, *Note for Guidance on the Investigation of Bioavailability and Bioequivalence*, to provide recommendations for study design, statistical analysis, and requirements for biowaiver requests (45). In general, applicants conduct single-dose crossover studies in healthy male and nonpregnant female adult subjects. Steady-state studies are conducted in the case of dose- or time-dependent pharmacokinetics, for some modified-release products. Steady-state studies may also be conducted if drug concentrations in plasma cannot be reliably measured following a single dose, or if high intra-individual pharmacokinetic variability precludes the possibility of demonstrating bioequivalence in a reasonably sized single-dose study and this variability is reduced at steady state. In most cases bioequivalence evaluation is based on measured concentrations of the parent compound. A metabolite can be used if concentrations of the parent drug are too low to be accurately measured. If a metabolite contributes significantly to activity and the pharmacokinetic system is nonlinear, parent and metabolite are evaluated separately. For acceptance criteria, the 90% confidence interval for AUC and C_{max} ratios (test/reference) should fall within 0.8–1.25. The acceptance interval may be tightened for narrow therapeutic range drugs. In certain cases, a wider acceptance range is used with sound clinical justification. Statistical evaluation of T_{max} is conducted when there is a clinically relevant claim for rapid release or action or signs related to adverse events. In this case, the nonparametric 90% confidence interval for T_{max} should lie within a clinically determined range. Applicants can request exemption from in vivo bioequivalence studies based on BCS Class 1 classification, if the drug has linear pharmacokinetics, does not show evidence of bioinequivalence, and does not require monitoring for critical plasma concentrations. A bioequivalence study based on only one strength of a product series is acceptable, provided that the choice of strength used for the in vivo study is justified, the drug has linear pharmacokinetics, the different strengths are proportionally similar, and dissolution profiles are acceptable. Pharmacodynamic or comparative clinical studies are conducted for products intended for local use (after oral, nasal, inhalation, ocular, dermal, rectal, vaginal, etc. administration) intended to act without systemic absorption. If there is a risk of systemic toxicity resulting from a locally applied, locally acting medicinal product, then systemic exposure is measured.

12. SUMMARY

Current bioequivalence methods in the US and other countries are designed to provide assurance of therapeutic equivalence of all generic drug products with their innovator counterparts. The sole objective of bioequivalence testing is to measure and compare formulation performance between two or more pharmaceutically equivalent drug products. For generic drugs to be approved in the US and most other countries, they must be pharmaceutically equivalent and bioequivalent to be considered therapeutically equivalent and therefore approvable. In the US, a mechanism for submitting ANDA's for generic products was initiated in 1962 and expanded by the Hatch–Waxman amendment of 1984. The requirement that ANDA submissions contain information showing that a generic drug product is bioequivalent to the innovator product is mandated by law, under Section 505(j) of the US Federal Food, Drug, and Cosmetic Act. Additional Federal laws, published under Title 21 of the Code of Federal Regulations, implement Section 505(j). Part 320 of 21 CFR, the *Bioavailability and Bioequivalence Requirements*, states the basis for demonstrating in vivo bioequivalence, lists the types of evidence to establish bioequivalence (in descending order of accuracy, sensitivity, and reproducibility), and provides guidelines for the conduct and design of an in vivo bioavailability study. Through the years, the US FDA has published Guidances for Industry which address how to meet the *Bioavailability and Bioequivalence Requirements* set forth in 21 CFR Part 320. The FDA makes every attempt to update these Guidances as the need arises to ensure that they reflect state-of-the art scientific thinking regarding the most accurate and sensitive methods available to demonstrate bioequivalence between two products. Consulting with panels of experts such as Advisory Committees, participating in meetings and workshops with Academia and Industry (both in the US and abroad), and inviting public comment on draft guidances are among the mechanisms that the FDA employs to keep Guidance development current.

Current statistical criteria for determining acceptability of bioequivalence studies in the US and in other countries assure that the test product is not significantly less bioavailable than the reference (usually the innovator) product, and that the reference product is not significantly less bioavailable than the test product. The difference for each of these two tests is 20%, with the result that the test/reference ratios of the bioequivalence measures must fall within the limits of 0.80–1.25. A generic product that does not meet these criteria is not approved. The FDA and regulatory agencies in other countries agree that the most accurate, sensitive, and reproducible method for determining bioequivalence is to measure drug concentrations in blood/plasma/serum in a single-dose study using human subjects. If it is not possible to accurately and reproducibly measure drug concentrations in such biological fluids, other approaches may be used, such as measuring active metabolite or measuring drug in urine. For locally active drug products with little systemic availability, bioequivalence may be evaluated by pharmacodynamic, clinical-endpoint, or highly specialized in vitro studies. Because of the strictness of the therapeutic equivalence criteria, there is not yet a mechanism for approving generic versions of many complex drug substances such as proteins, botanicals, and complex mixtures. Recently, the FDA considered requesting that applicants submit results of all in vivo studies on the to-be-marketed formulation, whether these studies pass or fail the 90% confidence interval criteria to identify potential problems worthy of seeking additional information.

Biowaivers are granted in some circumstances. Conditions under which waivers may be granted are also stipulated in 21 CFR Part 320. For those drug products which are systemically available and have demonstrated acceptable in vivo bioequivalence, the requirement for an in vivo study may be waived for lower strengths only if the strengths are proportionally similar and show acceptable in vitro dissolution by a method approved by the FDA. Biowaivers may also be granted if an applicant satisfactorily demonstrates that a drug dissolves rapidly from the dosage form and has high intestinal permeability (BCS Class 1).

It should be clear that regulatory bioequivalence evaluation of generic drug products is quite rigorous. In approving a generic product, the FDA and the regulatory agencies of other countries make a judgement that it is therapeutically equivalent to the corresponding reference product. A health-care provider can substitute an approved generic product for the brand product with assurance that the two products will produce an equivalent therapeutic effect in each patient.

ACKNOWLEDGMENTS

The authors would like to acknowledge the assistance of Mr. Donald Hare, Ms. Rita Hassall, Dr. Henry Malinowski, Dr. Conrad Pereira, Dr. Norman Pound, and Dr. Lizzie Sanchez in the preparation of this manuscript.

REFERENCES

1. Kefauver-Harris Amendments. Public Law (PL) 87-781, 87th Congress, Oct. 10, 1962.
2. Drug Efficacy Study: A Report to the Commissioner of Food and Drugs, National Academy of Sciences, National Research Council, Washington, DC, 1969.
3. 34 Fed Regist 2673, Feb. 27, 1969.
4. 35 Fed Regist 6574, Apr. 24, 1970.
5. 35 Fed Regist 11273, Jul. 14, 1970.
6. Glazko AJ, Kinkel AW, Alegnani WC, Holmes EL. An evaluation of the absorption characteristics of different chloramphenicol preparations in normal human subjects. Clin Pharmacol Ther 1968; 9:472–483.
7. Barr WH, Gerbracht LM, Letchen K, Plaut M, Strahl N. Assessment of the biologic availability of tetracycline products in man. Clin Pharmacol Ther 1972; 13:97–108.
8. Chiou WL. Determination of physiological availability of commercial phenylbutazone preparations. Clin Pharmacol Ther 1972; 12:296–299.
9. Blair DC, Barnes RW, Wildner EL, Murray WJ. Biologic availability of oxytetracycline HCl capsules: a comparison of all manufacturing sources supplying the United States market. JAMA 1971; 215:251–254.
10. Lindenbaum J. et al. Variations in biological availability of digoxin from four preparations. N Eng J Med 1971; 285:1344.
11. Office of Technology Assessment. Drug Bioequivalence. A Report of the Office of Technology Assessment Drug Bioequivalence Study Panel, US Government Printing Office, Washington, DC, 1974.
12. Office of Technology Assessment. Scientific commentary: Drug bioequivalence. J Pharmacokinet Biopharm 1974; 2:433–466.

13. 42 Fed Regist 1648, Jan. 7, 1977.
14. 57 Fed Regist 17950, Apr. 28, 1992.
15. Drug Price Competition and Patent Term Restoration Act of 1984, Public Law
     98-417, 98 Stat 1585-1605, Sept. 24, 1984.
16. 57 Fed Regist 17998, Apr. 28, 1992.
17. Food and Drug Administration, Center for Drug Evaluation and Research.
     Approved Drug Products with Therapeutic Equivalence Evaluations. 24th ed.
     Superintendent of Documents. Washington, DC: US Government Printing
     Office, 2004.
18. Dighe SV, Adams WP. Bioequivalence: a United States regulatory perspective.
     In: Welling PG, Tse FLS, Dighe SV, eds. Pharmaceutical Bioequivalence. New
     York: Marcel Dekker, Inc, 1991:347–380.
19. Schuirmann DJ. A comparison of the two one-sided tests procedure and
     the power approach for assessing the equivalence of average bioavailability.
     J Pharmacokinet Biopharm 1987; 15:657–680.
20. Gibaldi M, Perrier D. Absorption kinetics and bioavailability. In: Pharmacoki-
     netics. 2nd New York: Marcel Dekker, 1982:145–198.
21. Hauck WW, Anderson S. A new statistical procedure for testing equivalence in
     two-group comparative bioavailability studies. J Pharmacokinet Biopharm
     1984; 12:83–91.
22. US Dept of Health and Human Services, Food and Drug Administration,
     Center for Drug Evaluation and Research. Guidance for Industry: Statistical
     Approaches to Establishing Bioequivalence. Jan. 2001.
23. US Dept of Health and Human Services, Food and Drug Administration, Center
     for Drug Evaluation and Research. Guidance for Industry: Bioavailability and
     Bioequivalence Studies for Orally Administered Drug Products—General
     Considerations. Mar. 19, 2003.
24. Freedom of Information Staff, Food and Drug Administration, Center for Drug
     Evaluation and Research, Rockville, MD. Summary Basis of Approval.
25. US Dept of Health and Human Services, Food and Drug Administration, Center
     for Drug Evaluation and Research. Draft Guidance for Industry: Food-Effect
     Bioavailability and Bioequivalence Studies. Dec. 2002.
26. US Dept of Health and Human Services, Food and Drug Administration, Cen-
     ter for Drug Evaluation and Research. Draft Guidance for Industry: Clozapine
     Tablets In Vivo Bioequivalence and In Vitro Dissolution Testing. Feb. 29, 2003.
27. 57 Fed Regist 29354, Jul. 1, 1992.
28. US Dept of Health and Human Services, Food and Drug Administration, Cen-
     ter for Drug Evaluation and Research. Draft Guidance for Industry: Potassium
     Chloride (slow-release tablets and capsules) In Vivo Bioequivalence and
     In Vitro Dissolution Testing. Aug. 6, 2002.
29. US Dept of Health and Human Services, Food and Drug Administration, Center
     for Drug Evaluation and Research. Guidance for Industry: Topical Dermato-
     logic Corticosteroids: In Vivo Bioequivalence. Mar. 6, 1998.
30. US Dept of Health and Human Services, Food and Drug Administration, Center
     for Drug Evaluation and Research. Interim Guidance for Industry: Cholestyra-
     mine Powder In Vitro Bioequivalence. Jul. 15, 1993.

31. Swenson CN, Fundak G. Observational cohort study of switching warfarin sodium products in a managed care organization. Amer J Health Syst Pharm 2000; 57:452–455.
32. US Dept of Health and Human Services, Food and Drug Administration, Center for Drug Evaluation and Research. Guidance for Industry: Waiver of In Vivo Bioavailability and Bioequivalence Studies for Immediate-Release Solid Oral Dosage Forms Based on a Biopharmaceutics Classification System. Aug. 31, 2000.
33. Nightingale S. From the Food and Drug Administration. JAMA 1998; 279:645.
34. Advisors and Consultants Staff, Food and Drug Administration, Center for Drug Evaluation and Research, Rockville, MD. Meeting of the Advisory Committee for Pharmaceutical Science. Nov. 16, 2000.
35. 68 Fed Regist 61640, October 29, 2003.
36. Health Canada. Therapeutic Products Directorate Guideline: Preparation of Drug Submissions: Comparative Bioavailability Studies. 1997.
37. Canadian Reference product: Policy Issue from the Drugs Directorate. Use of a non-Canadian Reference Product, Section C.08.002.1 (c) of then Food and Drug Regulations, December 5, 1995.
38. Health Canada. Therapeutic Products Directorate Guideline: Conduct and Analysis of Bioavailability and Bioequivalence Studies—Part A: Oral Dosage Formulations Used for Systemic Effects. 1992.
39. Health Canada. Therapeutic Products Directorate Guideline: Conduct and Analysis of Bioavailability and Bioequivalence Studies—Part B: Oral Modified Release Formulations. 1996.
40. Health Canada. Report C. Expert Advisory Committee on Bioavailability, Report on Bioavailability of Oral Dosage Formulations, not in Modified Release Form, of Drugs Used for Systemic Effects, Having Complicated or Variable Pharmacokinetics. 1992.
41. Health Canada. Therapeutic Products Directorate Draft Guideline: Standards for Comparative Bioavailability Studies Involving Drugs with a Narrow Therapeutic Range. 1997.
42. Health Canada. Therapeutic Products Directorate Draft Guideline: Bioequivalence Requirements (Draft): Drugs Exhibiting Non-Linear Pharmacokinetics. 1997.
43. National Institute of Health Sciences, Japan. Guideline for Bioequivalence Studies of Generic Products. 1997.
44. http://www.eurunion.org/states/home.htm.
45. The European Agency for the Evaluation of Medicinal Products. Note for Guidance on the Investigation of Bioavailability and Bioequivalence. Jul. 26, 2001.

11

Statistical Considerations for Establishing Bioequivalence

Sanford Bolton
University of Arizona, Tucson, Arizona, U.S.A.

1. INTRODUCTION

The assessment of "Bioequivalence" (BE) refers to a procedure that compares the bioavailability of a drug from different formulations. Bioavailability is defined as the rate and extent to which the active ingredient or active moiety is absorbed from a drug product and becomes available at the site of action. For drug products that are not intended to be absorbed into the bloodstream, bioavailability may be assessed by measurements intended to reflect the rate and extent to which the active ingredient or active moiety becomes available at the site of action. In this chapter, we will not present methods for drugs that are not absorbed into the bloodstream (or absorbed so little as to be unmeasurable), but may act locally. However, statistical methodology, in general, will be approached in a manner consistent with methods presented for drugs that are absorbed.

Thus, we are concerned with measures of the release of drug from a formulation and its availability to the body. Bioequivalence can be simply defined by the relative bioavailability of two or more formulations of the same drug entity. According to 21 CFR 320.1 (1), BE is defined as "...the absence of a significant difference in the rate and extent to which the active ingredient or active moiety ... becomes available at the site of drug action when administered ... in an appropriately designed study."

Bioequivalence is an important part of an NDA in which formulation changes have been made during and after pivitol clinical trials. Bioequivalence studies as part of ANDA submissions, in which a generic product is compared to a marketed, reference product, are critical parts of the submission. Bioequivalence studies may also be necessary when formulations for approved marketed products are modified.

In general, most BE studies depend on accumulation of pharmacokinetic (PK) data which provide levels of drug in the bloodstream at specified time points following administration of the drug. These studies are typically performed, using oral dosage forms, on volunteers who are incarcerated (housed) during the study to ensure compliance with regard to dosing schedule as well as other protocol requirements. This does not mean that BE studies are limited to oral dosage forms. Any drug formulation that results in measurable blood levels after administration can be treated and analyzed in a manner similar to drugs taken orally. For drugs that act locally and are not appreciably absorbed, either a surrogate endpoint may be utilized in place of blood levels (e.g., a pharmacodynamic response) or a clinical study using a therapeutic outcome may be necessary. Also, in some cases where assay methodology in blood is limited, or for other relevant reasons, measurements of drug in the urine over time may be used to assess equivalence.

To measure rate and extent of absorption for oral products, PK measures are used. In particular, model independent measures used are (a) area under the blood level vs. time curve (AUC) and the maximum concentration (C_{max}), which are measures of the amount of drug absorbed and the rate of absorption, respectively. The time at which the maximum concentration occurs (T_{max}) is a more direct measure of absorption rate, but is a very variable estimate.

In this chapter, we will discuss single dose studies, where blood levels are measured following ingestion of a single dose. Multiple dose, steady state studies have been required for certain kinds of drugs and formulations, but recently the FDA has discouraged the use of multiple dose studies. One objection to the use of such studies is that they are less sensitive to formulation differences than single dose studies. On the other hand, multiple dose studies are closer to reality for drugs taken on a chronic basis. This is a controversial area.

2. TWO-TREATMENT–TWO-PERIOD (TTTP) DESIGNS— ANALYSIS OF AVERAGE BIOEQUIVALENCE

Two-treatment, two-period, two-sequence (TTTP) crossover designs are used to compare the average BE of two products. The statistical model for this design can be expressed as follows (2):

$$Y_{ijk} = \mu + G_i + S_{ik} + P_j + T_{t(ij)} + \varepsilon_{ijk} \tag{1}$$

where μ is the overall mean, G_i, the effect of sequence group ($i = 1,2$), S_{ik} the Effect of subject k in sequence i ($k = 1,2,3,\ldots,N$), $T_{t(ij)}$ the treatment effect t ($t = 1,2$) in sequence i and period j and ε_{ijk} the residual error.

Average BE addresses the comparison of average results derived from the TTTP BE study, and does not consider differences in within subject variance and interactions in the evaluation. The design and analysis of two-period crossover designs are relatively straightforward. The design consists of randomly assigning subjects to two sequences. In one sequence, Product A is administered in the first period, followed by a suitable wash-out period, followed by administration of Product B. In the second sequence, the order of administration of the products is reversed. Product B is administered in the first period, followed by a suitable wash-out period, followed by administration of Product A (see Figure 1). Typically, the wash-out period should be at least 5–6 drug elimination half-lives. The design aims to have an equal number of subjects in each sequence. Although this is optimal, it is not necessary. For example, drop-outs may result in unequal number of subjects in each sequence. Immediately prior to dosing and at specified intervals after dosing, blood samples are taken for analysis of drug. This results in a typical "pharmacokinetic" profile of drug blood levels over time (Figure 2).

The analysis of the data consists of determining the maximum blood level (C_{max}) and the area under the blood level vs. time curve (AUC) for each subject, for each product. AUC is determined using the trapezoidal rule. The area between adjacent time points may be estimated as a trapezoid (Figure 2). The area of each trapezoid, up to and including the final time point, where a measurable concentration is observed, is computed, and the sum of these areas is the AUC, designated as AUC(t). The area of a trapezoid is $1/2$(base) (sum of two sides). For example in Figure 2, the area of the trapezoid shown in the blood level vs. time curve is 4. In this figure, C_{max} is 5 ng/mL and T_{max}, the time at which C_{max} occurs is 2 h.

	Period 1		Period 2
Sequence 1:	Product A →	(Wash-out) →	Product B
Sequence 2:	Product B →	(Wash-out) →	Product A

FIGURE 1 TTTP design.

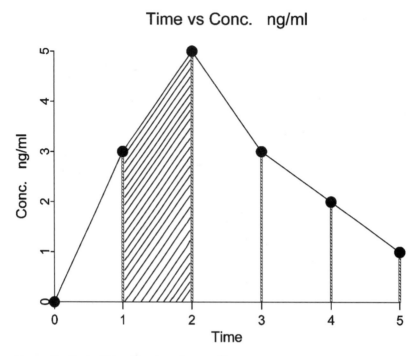

FIGURE 2 Typical blood level vs. time profile.

Having performed this calculation for each subject and product, the AUC and C_{max} values are transformed to their respective logarithms. Either natural logs (ln) or logs to the base 10 (log) may be used. Typically, one uses the natural log, or ln. The details of the analysis are described later in this chapter.

The analysis of AUC and C_{max} was not always performed on the logs of these values. Several years ago, the actual, observed (non-transformed) values of these derived parameters were used in the analysis. (This history will be discussed in more detail below.) However, examination of the theoretical derivations and mathematical expression of AUC and C_{max}, as well as the statistical properties has led to the use of the logarithmic transformation. In particular, data appear to show that these values follow a log-normal distribution more closely than they do a normal distribution. The form of expression for AUC suggests a multiplicative model

$$\text{AUC} = FD/VK_e$$

where F is the fraction of drug absorbed, D the dose, V the volume of distribution and K_e the elimination rate constant.

The distribution of AUC is complex because of the non-linearity; it is a ratio. Ln(AUC) is equal to $\ln(F) + \ln(D) - \ln(V) - \ln(K_e)$. This is linear, and the statistical properties are more manageable. A similar argument can be made for C_{max}.

2.1. Statistical Analysis

For purposes of illustrating the statistical analyses, data from Table 1 will be used. Analysis of variance (ANOVA) tables for average BE based on these data are shown in Table 2, A, B; ANOVA on the log-transformed C_{max} (A) for periods 1 and 2 and on the original C_{max} data for periods 1 and 2 (B). In these analyses, the residual error term is used in statistical computations, e.g., to construct confidence intervals (CI). The between subject mean square is the error term for testing sequence differences.

As previously noted, in BE studies, we compute parameters derived from the blood level vs. time curve obtained from the individual blood levels at various collection times. In particular, three derived parameters are estimated for each individual and product. These are AUC(t), AUC(inf), and C_{max}. AUC(inf) is computed as AUC(t), AUC up to the last analyzed time point, plus $C(\text{final})/K_e$ where $C(\text{final})$ is the final measurable blood concentration, and K_e is the drug elimination rate constant (0.693/half-life). Each of these parameters is analyzed separately. The discussion below applies to each of the analyses, AUC(t), AUC(inf), and C_{max}. T_{max} and half-life are also computed, but these are not crucial to product approval unless these results are inconsistent and/or troublesome, which is rarely a problem.

This design is described above (Figure 1), and is a variation of a Latin square. In Latin squares, certain effects are confounded and cannot be directly estimated. Confounding of effects means that a variance estimate in the ANOVA is a combination of two or more effects, and one cannot be sure how much of each effect contributes to the observed variance. In designed experiments, we try to confound effects in a way such that one effect predominates in the confounded estimate (2). Although we can never be sure which effect predominates, we can make educated guesses. For example, a main effect (e.g., product difference) will usually be more prominent than an interaction. (e.g., product × period interaction). In the TTTP design, for example, the estimate of a differential carryover effect is confounded with a group effect (2). A carryover (CO) effect may be described as an effect of a preceeding observation on a subsequent observation. In the TTTP design, if the treatment in the first period affects the blood levels in the second period, this would result in an CO effect. A differential CO effect is one in which the CO effect when Treatment A is given first is different from the CO effect when Treatment B is given first. A group, or sequence effect as it is often called,

TABLE 1 Results of a Four-Period, Two-Sequence, Two-Treatment, Replicate Design (C_{max})

Subject	Product	Sequence	Period	C_{max}	Ln (C_{max})
1	Test	1	1	14	2.639
2	Test	1	1	16.7	2.815
3	Test	1	1	12.95	2.561
4	Test	2	2	13.9	2.632
5	Test	1	1	15.6	2.747
6	Test	2	2	12.65	2.538
7	Test	2	2	13.45	2.599
8	Test	2	2	13.85	2.628
9	Test	1	1	13.05	2.569
10	Test	2	2	17.55	2.865
11	Test	1	1	13.25	2.584
12	Test	2	2	19.8	2.986
13	Test	1	1	10.45	2.347
14	Test	2	2	19.55	2.973
15	Test	2	2	22.1	3.096
16	Test	1	1	22.1	3.096
17	Test	2	2	14.15	2.650
1	Test	1	3	14.35	2.664
2	Test	1	3	22.8	3.127
3	Test	1	3	13.25	2.584
4	Test	2	4	14.55	2.678
5	Test	1	3	13.7	2.617
6	Test	2	4	13.9	2.632
7	Test	2	4	13.75	2.621
8	Test	2	4	13.25	2.584
9	Test	1	3	13.95	2.635
10	Test	2	4	15.15	2.718
11	Test	1	3	13.15	2.576
12	Test	2	4	21	3.045
13	Test	1	3	8.75	2.169
14	Test	2	4	17.35	2.854
15	Test	2	4	18.25	2.904
16	Test	1	3	19.05	2.947
17	Test	2	4	15.1	2.715
1	Reference	1	2	13.5	2.603
2	Reference	1	2	15.45	2.738
3	Reference	1	2	11.85	2.472
4	Reference	2	1	13.3	2.588
5	Reference	1	2	13.55	2.606
6	Reference	2	1	14.15	2.650

(*Continued*)

TABLE 1 (Continued)

Subject	Product	Sequence	Period	C_{max}	Ln (C_{max})
7	Reference	2	1	10.45	2.347
8	Reference	2	1	11.5	2.442
9	Reference	1	2	13.5	2.603
10	Reference	2	1	15.25	2.725
11	Reference	1	2	11.75	2.464
12	Reference	2	1	23.2	3.144
13	Reference	1	2	7.95	2.073
14	Reference	2	1	17.45	2.859
15	Reference	2	1	15.5	2.741
16	Reference	1	2	20.2	3.006
17	Reference	2	1	12.95	2.561
1	Reference	1	4	13.5	2.603
2	Reference	1	4	15.45	2.738
3	Reference	1	4	11.85	2.472
4	Reference	2	3	13.3	2.588
5	Reference	1	4	13.55	2.606
6	Reference	2	3	14.15	2.650
7	Reference	2	3	10.45	2.347
8	Reference	2	3	11.5	2.442
9	Reference	1	4	13.5	2.603
10	Reference	2	3	15.25	2.725
11	Reference	1	4	11.75	2.464
12	Reference	2	3	23.2	3.144
13	Reference	1	4	7.95	2.073
14	Reference	2	3	17.45	2.859
15	Reference	2	3	15.5	2.741
16	Reference	1	4	20.2	3.006
17	Reference	2	3	12.95	2.561

is the difference in the average results for those subjects given the sequence Treatment A followed by B (AB) and the average results for those subjects given the sequence Treatment B followed by A (BA). In TTTP designs, the subjects are assigned to sequence groups in a random manner. In TTTP designs, the differential CO effect cannot be measured directly. However, we can estimate the group (or sequence) effect. If this is significant, we may suspect a differential CO effect is responsible, because the two sequence groups should not be different except by chance; the sequence groups are chosen in a random manner. At one time the FDA considered a significant sequence effect to be a serious problem because of the implications of

TABLE 2 ANOVA for Data from First Two Periods of Table 1
(A) LN TRANSFORMATION
General linear models procedure
Dependent variable: LN C_{MAX}

Source	DF	Sum of squares	Mean square	F value	Pr > F
Model	18	1.65791040	0.09210613	10.34	0.0001
Error	15	0.13359312	0.00890621		
Corrected total	33	1.79150352			

Mean	R-Square	CV	Root MSE	
2.67483698	0.925430	3.528167	0.09437271	LN C_{MAX}

Source	DF	Type I SS	Mean square	F value	Pr > F
SEQ	1	0.09042411	0.09042411	10.15	0.0061
SUBJ(SEQ)	15	1.48220203	0.09881347	11.09	0.000
PER	1	0.00039571	0.00039571	0.04	0.8359
TRT	1	0.08488855	0.08488855	9.53	0.0075

General linear models procedure
Least squares means

TRT	LN C_{MAX} LSMEAN
Reference	2.62174427
test	2.72185203

		T for H0:		
Parameter	Estimate	Parameter = 0	Pr > |T|	Std error of estimate
T vs. R	0.10010777	3.09	0.0075	0.03242572

(B)
General linear models procedure
Dependent variable: C_{MAX}

Source	DF	Sum of squares	Mean square	F value	Pr > F
Model	18	381.26362847	21.18131269	9.07	0.0001
Error	15	35.01637153	2.33442477		
Corrected total	33	416.28000000			

Mean	R-square	CV	Root MSE	C_{MAX}
0.915883	10.25424	1.52788245	14.90000000	

(*Continued*)

TABLE 2 (*Continued*)

Source	DF	Type I SS	Mean square	F value	Pr > F
SEQ	1	18.59404514	18.59404514	7.97	0.0129
SUBJ(SEQ)	15	346.22095486	23.08139699	9.89	0.0001
PER	1	0.24735294	0.24735294	0.11	0.7493
TRT	1	16.20127553	16.20127553	6.94	0.0188

Least Squares Means

TRT	C_{MAX} LSMEAN
Reference	14.1649306
Test	15.5479167

Dependent variable: C_{MAX}

Parameter estimate	Estimate	T for H0: Parameter = 0	Pr > |T|	Std error of estimate
T VS. R	1.38298611	2.63	0.0188	0.52496839

differential CO. A significance test was applied to the sequence effect, and if significant at the 10% level, most such studies were deemed to be a failure. There was a serious problem with this evaluation. This approach would result in rejecting 10% of otherwise good studies submitted, because of a chance significance of the sequence effect. Also, differential CO is extremely unlikely in TTTP design where a suitable wash-out period is applied, and blood levels of drug are absent at time 0 in the second period. At the time of this writing, significant sequence effects are usually not a cause for failure of a BE study.

Other effects that are confounded include a sequence × period interaction and the treatment effect (difference between treatments). A sequence × period interaction means that the difference between the results in periods I and II is different for the two sequences. Suppose that the following average results occurred in an TTTP designed experiment.

	Period I	Period II
Sequence I	10	20
Sequence II	20	10

These results could indicate a significant sequence × period interaction. The interaction can be defined as $1/2$; $[(20-10) - (10-20)] = 10$. Suppose that Sequence I was Treatment A followed by Treatment B, and Sequence II was B followed by A. The results could then be expressed as:

	Treatment A	Treatment B
Sequence I	10	20
Sequence II	10	20

The treatment effect is $\frac{1}{2}[(20-10) + (20-10)] = 10$. Examination of these estimates of the sequence × period interaction and the treatment effect shows that the results will always be identical. In this example, a difference between treatments is more likely than the sequence × period interaction, and we would not attribute a difference between treatments to be due to the interaction. Even so, such an interaction would be quite disturbing, and does not make much sense.

2.1.1. Analysis of Variance

An ANOVA is computed for each parameter based on the model. The ANOVA table is not meant for the performance of statistical hypothesis tests, except perhaps to test the sequence effect, which uses the between subject within sequences mean square as the error term. Rather, the analysis removes some effects from the total variance to obtain a more "efficient" or pure estimate of the error term. It is the error term, or estimate of the within subject variability (assumed to be equal for both products in this analysis) that is used to assess the equivalence of the parameter being analyzed.

In the analysis of the TTTP design, we estimate the effects that have meaning. Interactions are considered to be small or absent (except possibly a differential CO effect in unusual situations). The ANOVA separates the variance due to the effects specified in the model (Eq. (1)).

The effects that are modeled in the ANOVA are:

difference between subjects;
difference between treatments;
difference between periods;
difference between sequences.

At the time of this writing, the great majority of BE studies are analyzed using the TTTP design, with a log transform of C_{max} and AUC, and a 90% CI that must lie between 80% and 125% in order to be acceptable. If the sponsor feels that a log transform is not appropriate, FDA will consider this, if sufficient justification is given prior to completion of the study and availability of study data. The TTTP designs are used to assess average BE.

Some history may be of interest with regard to the analysis recommended in the most recent FDA Guidance (3). In the early evolution of BE analysis, a hypothesis test was used at the 5% level of significance. The raw data were used in the analysis; i.e., a logarithmic transformation was not recommended. The null hypothesis was simply that the products were equal, as opposed to the null hypothesis that the products were different. This had the obvious problem with regard to the power of the test. Products that showed nearly the same average results, but with very small variance, could show a significant difference, and be rejected. Alternatively, products that showed large differences with large variance could show a non-significant difference, and be deemed equivalent. Similarly, products could be shown to be equivalent if a small sample size was used in the BE study.

Because of these problems, an additional caveat was added to the requirements. If the products showed a difference of less than 20%, and the power of the study to detect a difference of 20% exceeded 80%, the products would be considered to be equivalent. This helped to avoid undersized studies and prevent products with observed large differences from passing the BE study. The following examples illustrate this problem.

Example 1. In a BE two period, crossover study, with eight subjects, the test product showed an average AUC of 100, and the reference product showed an average AUC of 85. The observed difference between the products is $(100 - 85)/85$, or 17.6%. The error term from the ANOVA (see below for description of the analysis) is 900, s.d. $= 30$. The test of significance (a t test with 6 d.f.) is

$$[100 - 85]/[900(1/8 + 1/8)]^{1/2} = 1.00$$

This is not statistically significant at the 5% level (a t value of 2.45 for 6 d.f. is needed for significance). Therefore, the products may be deemed equivalent.

However, this test is under-powered based on the need for 80% power to show a 20% difference. A 20% difference from the reference is $0.2 \times 85 = 17$. The approximate power (2) is:

$$Z = [17/42.43][6]^{1/2} - 1.96 = -0.98$$

Referring to a Table of the Cumulative Standard Normal Distribution (2), the approximate power is 16%. Although the test of significance did not reject the null hypothesis, the power of the test to detect a 20% difference is weak. Therefore, this product would not pass the BE requirements.

Example 2. In an BE two period, crossover study, with 36 subjects, the test product showed an average AUC of 100, and the reference product showed an average AUC of 95. The products differ by approximately only 5%. The error term from the ANOVA is 100, s.d. $= 10$. The test of significance (a t test with 34 d.f.) is

$$[100 - 95]/[10(1/36 + 1/36)]^{1/2} = 6.7$$

This is statistically significant at the 5% level (a t value of 2.03 for 34 d.f. is needed for significance). Therefore, the products may be deemed non-equivalent.

However, this test passes the criterion based on the need for 80% power to show a 20% difference. A 20% difference from the reference is $0.2 \times 95 = 19$. The approximate power is (2):

$$Z = [19/14.14][34]^{1/2} - 1.96 = 5.88$$

The approximate power is almost 100%. Although the test of significance rejected the null hypothesis, the power of the test to detect a 20% difference is extremely high. Therefore, this product would pass the BE requirements.

Other requirements at that time included the 75/75 rule (4). This rule stated that 75% of the subjects in the study should have ratios of test/reference between 75% and 125%. This was an attempt to control the variability of the study. Unfortunately, this criterion has little statistical basis, and would almost always fail with highly variable drugs. In fact if a highly variable drug (CV greater than 30–40%) is tested against itself, it would most likely fail this test. Eventually, this requirement was correctly phased out.

Soon after this phase in the evolution of BE regulations, the hypothesis test approach was replaced by the two-one-sided t test or, equivalently, the 90% CI, or two-one-sided t test approach (5). This approach resolved the problems of hypothesis testing, and assumed that products that are within 20% of each other with regard to the major parameters, AUC and C_{max}, are therapeutically equivalent. For several years, this method was used without a logarithmic transformation. However, if the study data conformed better to a log-normal distribution than a normal distribution, a log transformation was allowed. An appropriate statistical test was applied to test the conformity of the data to these distributions.

To illustrate some of the concepts and statistical analyses, the reader is referred to Tables 1 and 2(A,B). The ANOVA (2) for the data in the first two periods from Table 1 is shown in Table 2. The analysis is performed on the log-transformed data as well as the original non-transformed values of C_{max}.

The form of the statistical procedure to determine the confidence limits for the derived parameters (C_{max} and AUC) prior to the implementation of the log transformation was as follows:

$$1 + \{|\text{average (test)} - \text{average (reference)}| \\ \pm t(\text{variance}(2/N))^{1/2}\}/\text{average reference}$$

This interval must lie between 0.8 and 1.2 for approval of equivalence.

The value of t is for a 90% CI with d.f. based on the variance estimate (residual mean square) in the ANOVA. N is the sample size for the two-period design. This test is not exact. For example, the denominator (the average value of the reference) is considered fixed in this calculation, when, indeed, it is a variable measurement. Also, the decision rule is not symmetric with regard to the average results for the test and reference. That is, if the reference is 20% greater than the test, the ratio test/reference is not 0.8 but is $1/1.2 = 0.83$. Conversely, if the test is 20% greater than the reference, the ratio will be 1.2. Nevertheless, this approximate calculation was considered satisfactory for the purposes of assessing BE. Note that the usual concept of power does not play a part in the approval process. It behooves the sponsor of the BE study to recruit sufficient number of subjects to help ensure approval based on this criterion. If the products are truly equivalent (the ratio of test/reference is truly between 0.8 and 1.2), the more subjects recruited, the greater the probability of passing the test. Note again that in this scenario the more subjects, the better the chance of passing. In practice, one chooses a sample size sufficiently large to make the probability of passing reasonably high. This probability may be defined as power in the context of proving equivalence. Sample size determination for various assumed differences between the test and reference products for various values of power (probability of passing the CI criterion) has been published by Dilletti et al. (6).

The computation (prior to the use of the log transformation) is illustrated using the results for the analysis for periods 1 and 2 of the data of Table 1 as shown in Table 2(B).

$$1 + \{|\text{average (test)} - \text{average reference}| \\ \pm t(\text{variance}(2/N))^{1/2}\}/\text{average reference} \\ = 1 + (1.383 \pm 1.75(2.3344 \times 2/34)^{1/2}/14.165) \\ = (1.383 \pm 0.648)/14.165 = 1.14, 1.05$$

Since these limits are within 0.8–1.2, this would pass the FDA criterion at that time.

This is very close to the CI using log-transformed data (see below). When the variance is small, both methods will give very similar results.

2.1.2. Analysis Using the Log Transformation

Examination of BE submissions, in addition to theoretical evaluations, resulted in the conclusion that the BE parameters conformed more to a log-normal distribution than a normal distribution (see discussion above). Therefore, the FDA currently requires that the AUC and C_{max} parameters be transformed to logarithms prior to statistical analysis. The log transformation simplifies the calculations used previously and leads to a more direct interpretation of the experiment as the ratio of the parameters, rather than the difference of the parameters. One only has to place a 90% CI on the difference of the average of the logs for the two products. Note that the difference of the two logs is equivalent to the log of their ratio. Also, the analysis makes the reference and test products symmetric. That is, we reach the same conclusion whether we look at reference/test or test/reference, which was not necessarily the case in the previously recommended analysis.

Consider the following example from Table 2(A) where the difference in the averages of the log-transformed values is 0.1001 and the error variance is 0.00890621.

The CI takes the following form:

$$[\ln(\text{test}) - \ln(\text{reference})] \pm t_{0.05}(\text{error} \times 2/N)^{1/2}$$

where t is from a t table with appropriate degrees of freedom.

$$= (0.1001 \pm 1.74(0.00890621 \times 2/17)^{1/2}$$
$$= (0.1001 \pm 0.05632) = 0.0438, 0.1564$$

We then take the antilog of these limits to put them into more understandable terms.

The back-transformed limits are 1.17–1.04.

Note that if we placed an CI on ln (test) – ln (reference), the limits would be −0.0156 to 0.0438. The antilogs are 0.86, 0.96, which are the reciprocals of the above limits.

The antilog of the mean of the treatment mean of the log-transformed values is the geometric mean.

The residual or remaining variance in the ANOVA is considered to be error. Error in this ANOVA is assumed to the within subject variability, an average of the variability for each treatment or product. We cannot directly estimate the variability of each product separately, a deficiency that is considered to be of importance by some persons (see Individual Bioequivalence below).

2.1.3. Test for Differential Carryover

Another criterion that was imposed during these years was a test for differential CO as discussed above. This was a test of the group or sequence effect at the 10% level. This test and a test for equality of T_{max} are not enforced on a regular basis at the present time.

We cannot directly estimate differential CO or product × subject interaction. To estimate these effects, a replicate design would be necessary. As previously noted, differential CO is now considered to be an unlikely event, and has taken a position of lesser importance in the analysis of BE studies. The test for sequence effects uses the between subject (within sequences) mean square as the error term. The test for sequence would be an F test. Using the ANOVA for the analysis of ln C_{max} in Table 2(A), a test for the sequence or carryover effect is $F_{1,15} = 90/0.99 = 0.91$, which is not significant.

For the data from Table 2 (B), non-transformed C_{max}, $F_{1,15} = 18.6/23.1 = 0.8$, which is not statistically significant.

All of the criteria for BE must pass the CI test, 0.8–1.25. This would include AUC(inf), AUC(t), and C_{max} for all moieties tested, including metabolites if applicable. In addition, some products need testing under both fed and fasted conditions, and/or need multiple dose, steady state, studies. As noted previously, at the present time, in general, the use of multiple dose studies is not recommended.

3. REPLICATE STUDY DESIGNS

Replicate studies in the present context are studies in which individuals are administered one or both products on more than one occasion. For purposes of BE, either three or four period designs are recommended. The 4-period design will be further discussed in the discussion of Individual Bioequivalence (IB), for which it is recommended. The FDA (1) gives sponsors the option of using replicate design studies for all BE studies. However, the agency recommends use of replicate studies for modified-release dosage forms and highly variable drugs, those with within subject CV > 30%. The purpose of these studies is to provide more information about the drug products than can be obtained from the typical, non-replicated, two-period design. The FDA is interested in obtaining information from these studies to aid them in evaluation of the need for IB. In particular, replicate studies provide information on within subject variance of each product separately, as well as potential product × subject interactions.

The FDA recommends that submissions of studies with replicate designs be analyzed for average BE (1). The analysis of IB will be the

TABLE 3 Analysis of Data From Table 1 for Average Bioequivalence

---

Analysis for Ln-transformed C_{MAX}
The MIXED procedure

Class level information

Class	Levels	Values
SEQ	2	1 2
SUBJ	17	1 2 3 4 5 6 7 8 9 10 11 12 13 14 15 16 17
PER	4	1 2 3 4
TRT	2	1 2

Covariance parameter estimates (REML)

Cov Parm	Subject	Group	Estimate
FA(1,1)	SUBJ		0.20078553
FA(2,1)	SUBJ		0.22257742
FA(2,2)	SUBJ		-0.00000000
DIAG	SUBJ	TRT 1	0.00702204
DIAG	SUBJ	TRT 2	0.00982420

Tests of fixed effects

Source	NDF	DDF	Type III F	Pr $> F$
SEQ	1	13.9	1.02	0.3294
PER	3	48.2	0.30	0.8277
TRT	1	51.1	18.12	0.0001

Estimate statement results

Parameter T vs. R Alpha $= 0.1$	Estimate	Std error	DF	t	Pr $> \lvert t \rvert$	
	0.09755781	0.02291789	51.1	4.26	0.0001	
			Lower	0.0592	Upper	0.1360

Least squares means

Effect	TRT	LSMEAN	Std error	DF	t	Pr $> \lvert t \rvert$
TRT	1	2.71465972	0.05086200	15	53.37	0.0001
TRT	2	2.61710191	0.05669416	15.3	46.16	0.0001

responsibility of the FDA, but will be only for internal use, not for evaluating BE for regulatory purposes. The following is an example of the analysis of a two-treatment-4 period replicate design to assess average BE. The design has each of two products, balanced in two sequences, ABAB and BABA, over four periods. Table 1 shows the results for C_{max} for a replicate study. Eighteen subjects were recruited for the study and 17 completed the study. An analysis using the usual approach for the TTTP design, as discussed above, is not recommended. The FDA (1) recommends use of a mixed model approach as in SAS PROC MIXED (7). The recommended code is:

```
PROC MIXED;
CLASSES SEQ SUBJ PER TRT;
MODEL LNCMAX=SEQ PER TRT/DDFM=SATTERTH;
RANDOM TRT/TYPE=FA0 (2) SUB=SUBj G;
REPEATED/GRP=TRT SUB=SUBJ;
LSMEANS TRT;
ESTIMATE 'T VS. R' TRT 1-1/CL ALPHA=0.1;
RUN;
```

The abbreviated output is shown in Table 3.

Note that the CI using the complete design (0.0592–0.1360) is not much different from that observed from the analysis of the first two periods (above), 0.0438, 0.1564. This should be expected because of the small variability exhibited by this product.

4. INDIVIDUAL BIOEQUIVALENCE[*]

Individual bioequivalence (IB) is an assessment that accounts for product differences in the variability of the PK parameters, as well as differences in their averages. The IB evaluation is based on the statistical evaluation of a metric, which represents a "distance" between the products. In average BE, this distance can be considered the square of the difference in average results. In IB, in addition to the difference in averages, the difference between the within subject variances for the two products, and the formulation × subject interaction (FS) are evaluated. In this section, we will not discuss the evaluation of population BE. The interested reader may refer to the FDA guidance (1).

Although analysis of data using IB criteria is not recommended at the present time, the FDA will consider IB analysis if, a priori, the sponsor requests this analysis.

---

[*] Recently, the FDA has indicated that BE data should only be analyzed using average bioequivalence, unless there is a compelling reason to use an alternative analysis.

The design and analysis of replicate studies for IB can be very complex and ambiguous. The practitioner is encouraged to follow FDA guidelines when designing such studies.

The metric to be evaluated for IB is

$$\theta = [\delta^2 + \sigma_I^2 + (\sigma_T^2 - \sigma_R^2)]/\sigma_R^2 \tag{2}$$

where δ to the difference between means of test and reference, σ_I^2 the subject $\times$ treatment interaction variance, σ_T^2 the within subject test variance and σ_R^2 the within subject reference variance.

The evaluation of IB is based on a 95% upper confidence limit on the metric, where the upper limit for approval, theta (θ), is defined as 2.4948. Note that we only look at the upper limit because the test is one-sided, i.e., we are only interested in evaluating the upper value of the confidence limit, upon which a decision of passing or failing depends. A large value of the metric results in a decision of inequivalence. Referring to Eq. (2), a decision of inequivalence results when the numerator is large and the denominator is small in value. Large differences in the average results, combined with a large subject $\times$ formulation interaction, a large within subject variance for the test product and a small within subject variance for the reference product, will increase the value of theta (and vice versa).

Using the within subject variance of the reference product in the denominator as a scaling device, allows for a less stringent decision for BE in cases of large reference variances. That is, if the reference and test products appear to be very different based on average results, they still may be deemed equivalent if the reference within subject variance is large. This can be a problem in the interpretation of BE, because if the within subject variance of the test product is sufficiently smaller than the reference, an unreasonably large difference between their averages could still result in BE (see Eq. (2)). This could be described as a compensation feature or trade-off, i.e, a small within subject variance for the test product can compensate for a large difference in averages. To ensure that such apparently unreasonable conclusions will not be decisive, the FDA guidance has a provision that the observed T/R ratio must be not more than 1.25 or less than 0.8.

4.1. Constant Scaling

The FDA Guidance (1) also allows for a constant scaling factor in the denominator of Eq. (2). If the variance of the reference is very small, the IB metric may appear very large, even though the products are reasonably close. If the within subject variance for the reference product is less than 0.15, a value of 0.15 may be used in the denominator, rather than the observed variance. This prevents an artificial inflation of the metric for cases of a small within subject reference variance. This case will not be discussed further, but is a simple extension of the following discussion. The reader may refer to the FDA Guidance for further discussion of this topic (1).

4.2. Statistical Analysis for Individual Bioequivalence

For average BE, the distribution of the difference in average results (log transformed) is known based on the assumption of a log-normal distribution of the parameters. One of the problems with the definition of BE based on the metric, Eq. (2), is that the distribution of the metric is complex, and cannot be easily evaluated. At an earlier evolution in the analysis of the metric, a bootstrap technique, a kind of simulation, was applied to the data in order to estimate its distribution. The nature of the distribution is needed in order to construct a CI so that a decision rule of acceptance or rejection can be determined. This bootstrap approach was time consuming, and not exactly reproducible. At the present time, an approximate "parametric" approach is recommended (8), which results in a hypothesis test that determines the acceptance rule. We refer to this aproach as the "Hyslop" evaluation. This will be presented in more detail below.

To illustrate the use of the Hyslop approach, the data of Table 4 will be used. This data set has been studied by several authors during the development of methods to evaluate IB (9).

The details of the derivation and assumptions can be found in the FDA guidance (1) and a paper by Hyslop et al. (8).

I will make an effort to describe the calculations as simply as possible. First, let us define some terms that are used in the calculations. The various estimates are obtained from the data of Table 4, using SAS (6), with the following code:

```
proc mixed data = lasix;
    class seq subj per trt;
    model ln = seq per trt;
    random int subject /subject = trt;
repeated/grp = trt sub = subj;
    estimate 't vs. r' trt 1 −1/cl alpha = 0.1;
run;
```

Table 5 shows the estimates of the variance components and average results for each product from the data of Table 4.

Basically, the Hyslop procedure obtains an approximate upper CI on the sum of independent terms (variables) in the IB metric equation (Eq. (2)). However, the statistical approach is expressed as a test of a

TABLE 4 Data From a Two-Treatment, Two-Sequence, Four Period Replicated Design (9)

Subject	Sequence	Period	Product	Ln C_{max}
1.00	1.00	1.00	1	5.105339
1.00	1.00	3.00	1	5.090062
2.00	1.00	1.00	1	5.59434
2.00	1.00	3.00	1	5.45916
3.00	2.00	2.00	1	4.991792
3.00	2.00	4.00	1	4.693181
4.00	1.00	1.00	1	4.553877
4.00	1.00	3.00	1	4.682131
5.00	2.00	2.00	1	5.168778
5.00	2.00	4.00	1	5.213304
6.00	2.00	2.00	1	5.081404
6.00	2.00	4.00	1	5.333202
7.00	2.00	2.00	1	5.128715
7.00	2.00	4.00	1	5.488524
8.00	1.00	1.00	1	4.131961
8.00	1.00	3.00	1	4.849684
1.00	1.00	2.00	2	4.922168
1.00	1.00	4.00	2	4.708629
2.00	1.00	2.00	2	5.116196
2.00	1.00	4.00	2	5.344246
3.00	2.00	1.00	2	5.216565
3.00	2.00	3.00	2	4.513055
4.00	1.00	2.00	2	4.680278
4.00	1.00	4.00	2	5.155601
5.00	2.00	1.00	2	5.156178
5.00	2.00	3.00	2	4.987025
6.00	2.00	1.00	2	5.27146
6.00	2.00	3.00	2	5.035003
7.00	2.00	1.00	2	5.019265
7.00	2.00	3.00	2	5.246498
8.00	1.00	2.00	2	5.249127
8.00	1.00	4.00	2	5.245971

hypothesis. If the upper limit of the CI is less than 0, the products are deemed equivalent, and vice versa. The following discussion relates to the scaled metric, where the observed reference within subject variance is used in the denominator. An analogous approach is used for the case where the reference variance is small and the denominator is fixed at 0.15 (see Ref. 1).

The IB criterion is expressed as

$$\theta = [\delta^2 + \sigma_d^2 + (\sigma_T^2 - \sigma_R^2)]/\sigma_R^2 \tag{2}$$

It can be shown that

$$\sigma_1^2 = \sigma_d^2 + 0.5(\sigma_T^2 - \sigma_R^2) \tag{3}$$

where σ_d^2 is the pure estimate of the subject $\times$ formulation interaction component.

We can express this in the form of a hypothesis test, where the IB metric is linearized as follows.

Substituting Eq. (3) into Eq. (2), and linearizing:

$$\text{Let} \quad \eta = (\delta)^2 + \sigma_i^2 + 0.5\sigma_T^2 - \sigma_R^2(-1.5 - \theta) \tag{4}$$

We then form a hypothesis test with the hypotheses:

$$\text{Ho}: \eta > 0 \qquad \text{HA}: \eta < 0$$

Howe's method (Hyslop) effectively forms a CI for η by first finding an upper or lower limit for each component in η. Then, a simple computation allows us to accept or reject the null hypothesis at the 5% level (one-sided test). This is equivalent to seeing if an upper CI is less than the FDA specified criterion, θ. Using Hyslop's method, if the upper confidence limit is less than θ, the test will show a value less than 0, and the products are considered to be equivalent.

The computation for the method is detailed below.

We substitute the observed values for the theoretical values in Eq. 4. The observed values are shown in Table 5.

The next step is to compute the upper 95% confidence limits for the components in Eq. (4). Note that δ is normal with mean, true delta,

TABLE 5 Parameter Estimates from Analysis of Data of Table 4 With Some Definitions

μ = mean of test; estimate = 5.0353
μ = mean of reference; estimate = 5.0542
δ = difference between observed mean of test and reference = -0.0189
σ_I^2 = interaction variance; estimate = MI = 0.1325
σ_T^2 = within subject variance for the test product; estimate = MT = 0.0568
σ_R^2 = within subject variance for the reference product; estimate = MR = 0.0584
n = degrees of freedom
s = number of sequences

TABLE 6 Computations for Evaluation of Individual Bioequivalence

$H_q = (1 -\text{alpha})$ level upper confidence limit	$E_q = $ point estimate	$U_q = (H_q - E_q)^2$
$H_D = [\,\|\delta\| + t\,(1 - \alpha, n - s)$ $(1/s^2 \, \Sigma n_i^{-1} \, M_i)^{\frac{1}{2}}]^2$	$E_D = \delta^2$	U_d
$H_I = ((n - s)\, M_I)/\chi^2(\alpha, n - s)$	$E_I = M_I$	U_i
$H_T = (0.5(n - s)\, M_T)/\chi^2(\alpha, n - s)$	$E_T = 0.5\, M_T$	U_t
$H_R{}^* = (-(1.5 + \theta_I)\,(n - s)\,M_R)/$ $\chi^2(1 - \alpha, n - s)$	$E_R = -(1.5 + \theta_I)\, M_R$	U_r

*Note that we use the $1 - \alpha$ percentile here because of the negative nature of this expression.
$n = \Sigma n_i$, $s = $ number of sequences and n_i are the number of subjects in sequence i.

and variance $2\sigma_d{}^2/N$. The variances are distributed as $(\sigma^2)\,\chi^2(n)/n$, (where $n = $ d.f.) For example, $M_T \sim \sigma_T{}^2\,(n)\,\chi^2(n)/n$.

The equations for calculations are given in Table 6 (4).

Table 7 shows the results of these calculations.

Examples of calculations:

$$H_D = [\|0.0189\| + 1.94((1/4)0.1325/2)^{1/2}))]^2 = 0.07213,$$
$$H_I = ((6)0.1325)/1.635 = 0.486,$$
$$H_T = (0.5(6)0.0568)/1.635 = 0.104,$$
$$H_R = (-(1.5 + 2.4948)(6)0.0584)/12.59 = -0.1112.$$

If the upper CI exceeds theta, the hypothesis is rejected, and the products are bio-inequivalent. This takes the form of a one-sided test of hypothesis at the 5% level.

Since this value exceeds 0, the products are considered to be inequivalent.

TABLE 7 Results of Calculations for Data of Table 6

$H_i = $ confidence limit	$E_i = $ point estimate	$U_i = (H - E)^2$
$H_d = 0.07213$	$E_d = 0.000361$	0.0052
$H_i = 0.486$	$E_i = 0.1325$	0.1251
$H_t = 0.104$	$E_t = 0.0284$	0.0057
$H_r = -0.1112$	$E_r = 0.2333$	0.0149
Sum	-0.0720	0.1509

$H = \Sigma(Ei) + \Sigma(Ui)^{0.5} = -0.0720 + .0.3885 = 0.3165$

5. THE FUTURE

At the present time, the design and analysis of BE studies use TTTP designs with a log transformation of the estimated parameters. The 90% CI of the back-transformed difference of the average results for the comparative products must lie between 0.8 and 1.25 for the products to be deemed equivalent. Four period replicate designs are recommended for controlled release products and, in some cases, very variable products. However, FDA recommends that these designs be analyzed for average BE. The results of these studies will be analyzed for IB by the FDA in order to assess the need for IB, i.e., is there a problem with formulation X subject interactions and differences between within subject variance for the two products? If the result of this venture shows that replicate designs are not needed, i.e., the data does not show significant interaction or within subject variance differences, it is likely that IB will be reserved for occasions where these designs will be advantageous in terms of cost and time. For example, IB analysis may be optimal for very variable drugs, requiring less subjects than would be required using an TTTP design for average BE. On the other hand, if IB analysis shows the existence of problems with interaction and within subject variances, it is likely that the four period replicate design and IB analysis will be required for at least some subset of drugs or drug products that exhibit problems.

Based on experience at this time, it does seem likely that we will see more of IB as time progresses. This may be accompanied with new ways of assessing and analyzing these complex problems and designs.

REFERENCES

1. Guidance for Industry, Bioavailability and Bioequivalence Studies for Orally Administered Drug Products, General Considerations. FDA, CDER, October, 2000.
2. Bolton S. Pharmaceutical Statistics. 3rd ed. New York, NY: Marcel Dekker, 1997.
3. Statistical Approaches to Establishing Bioequivalence. US Department of Health and Human Services FDA CDER, January 2001.
4. Haynes JD. J Pharm Sci 1981; 70:673.
5. Schuirmann DJ, Pharmacokinet J. Biopharm 1987; 15:656–680.
6. Dilletti E, Hauschke D, Steinjens VW. Int J Clin Pharm Toxical 1991; 29:1.
7. The SAS System for Windows, Release 6.12, Cary, NC, 27513.
8. Hyslop T, Hsuan F, Hesney M. Stat Med 2000; 19:2885–2897.
9. Eckbohm, Melander H. Biometrics 1989; 45:1249–1254.

12

Scale-up, Post-approval Changes, and Post-marketing Surveillance

**Sadie M. Ciganek, Aruna J. Mehta,
Frank J. Mellina, and Leon Shargel**

1. INTRODUCTION

Approval of an Abbreviated New Drug Application (ANDA) is only the beginning of a generic drug product's history. Frequently, changes are made to the chemistry and manufacturing controls of an ANDA following approval and continue throughout the life of the product. A pharmaceutical manufacturer may make changes in the drug formulation, batch size, process, equipment, or manufacturing site, which affects the identity, strength, quality, purity, and potency of the finished product. Therefore, any change must be fully evaluated prior to implementation to determine its impact on the finished product as they may relate to safety or effectiveness.

Changes to an approved ANDA can be initiated for a number of reasons, i.e., revised market forecast affecting batch size requirements, qualification of a new active pharmaceutical ingredient source, optimization of the manufacturing process, upgrade of the container/closure system, or enhancement of the analytical test methods and specifications to name a line.

A change within a given parameter can have varied adverse effects depending on the type or dosage form of the product. For example, a change in the container/closure system of a solid oral dosage form will have less impact on the drug product than it would for a semisolid or oral liquid dosage form where the primary packaging component becomes critical for the shelf life of the finished product. To illustrate further, a small change in the concentration ratio of an inactive ingredient may have less impact on an immediate release drug product than it would for a modified release product, where that same ingredient may adversely affect the release rate, thereby impacting bioequivalence. Under such circumstances, the reporting requirements for one will differ from those for the other depending on the dosage form and route of administration.

Single or multiple changes within the same ANDA over time can have an impact and must be considered in the overall life of the drug product as well. Numerous changes to the manufacturing parameters occurring over time may render the drug product approved in the original ANDA substantially different than the one on the market. Therefore, data submitted in an application to support most changes should include a comparison to the original exhibit batch or bio-batch wherever possible.

Pharmaceutical manufacturers are also required to file periodic Post-Market Reports for an approved ANDA to FDA through the *Post-Marketing Surveillance System,* which will be described in greater detail in this chapter.

2. HISTORY AND BACKGROUND

2.1. FDAMA

On November 21, 1997, the Food and Drug Administration Modernization Act (FDAMA) was signed into law. The FDAMA initiative was directed at providing more definite language to the current Food, Drug, and Cosmetic (FD&C) Act and further defining the statutory requirements for marketing approved drugs in the United States. FDAMA added section 506A (21U.S.C. 356a) to the FD&C Act, which provided specific language for manufacturing changes to an approved application, and reporting requirements for those changes. Following FDAMA, and further decodifying the statutory requirements for post-approval changes, the FDA issued a *Guidance for Industry: Changes to an Approved NDA or ANDA* in November 1999 (1). This guidance is the current standard used in the pharmaceutical industry to assess and report manufacturing changes.

FDAMA was effectively a rewrite for Title 21 Code of Federal Regulation (CFR) part 314.70, which had previously defined post-approval changes, but not to the extent that FDAMA considered. FDAMA also relaxed certain requirements for changes that were determined to have little or no impact on the finished products. This was intended to lessen the regulatory burden for FDA and industry alike. In addition to relaxing certain change requirements, FDAMA also provided a new reporting category known as *Supplement—Changes Being Effected in 0 Day* (CBE 0 day). The CBE 0 day enabled sponsors to implement changes immediately after first notifying FDA without a waiting period. In effect, the current CBE 30 days reporting category already provided for in (CFR) part 314.70 was expanded to include another level of notification less stringent than what existed.

In summary, FDAMA provided for four reporting categories as follows:

1. *Prior Approval Supplement*: Major changes that require FDA approval before implementation
2. *Supplement—Changes Being Effected (30 Days)*: Moderate changes that require 30 days' notice before implementation
3. *Supplement—Changes Being Effected (0 Day)*: Moderate changes that can be implemented immediately
4. *Annual Report:* Minor changes that can be implemented immediately and filed in the next Periodic Report

2.2. SUPAC

Prior to FDAMA, the basis for revision of the FD&C Act was the *Guidance for Industry: Immediate Release Solid Dosage Forms—Scale-Up and Post-Approval Changes (SUPAC)* (2). This guidance was a first attempt beyond the Case of Federal Regulation (CFR) to provide industry with clear and definitive language regarding the regulatory notification process and requirements for post-approval changes. It also attempted to reduce the regulatory burden for industry. SUPAC classified changes according to "levels" and provided requirements to support each level. The reporting category for the change was determined by the "level" classification, which will be described in greater detail below. When SUPAC was first introduced, it became a milestone for the pharmaceutical industry. The criteria for the different level changes and the documentation required to support the change were based on three independent studies: (a) research conducted by the University of Maryland in Association with the FDA, (b) results from a workshop between the American Association Pharmaceutical Scientists (AAPS), US Pharmaceutical Convention, and FDA, and (c) research conducted at the University of Michigan and the University of Uppsala.

In summary, the SUPAC guidance expanded 21 CFR part 314.70 and defined in much greater detail the types of changes and reporting category required. The guidance describe the following areas where change is likely:

- Components and composition of the drug product
- Manufacturing site change
- Scale-up of the drug product

- Manufacturing equipment
- Packaging

The SUPAC guidance describes three levels of change and the recommended chemistry, manufacturing and controls tests, in vitro dissolution tests, and bioequivalence tests for each level. It also describes the documents required to support the change. The three level changes as described by FDA are provided below.

Level	Definition
1	Changes that are unlikely to have any detectable impact on formulation quality and performance
2	Changes that could have a significant impact on formulation quality and performance
3	Changes that are likely to have a significant impact on formulation quality and performance

A level 1 change such as a small change in the excipient amount (e.g., starch, lactose) is unlikely to alter the quality or performance of the drug product, whereas a level 3 change where the qualitative or quantitative change in the excipients is outside an allowable range, particularly for drug products with a narrow therapeutic range, may require an in vivo bioequivalence study to demonstrate that the drug quality and performance were not altered by the change.

A manufacturing change must be assessed for its effect on the identity, strength, quality, purity, and potency of the product, as these factors may relate to the safety or effectiveness of the product (506A(b)). The assessment of the effect of a change should include a determination that the drug substance, in-process materials, and/or drug product affected by the change conforms to *specifications*, which are provided in the *approved application*. Moreover, the manufacturer must confirm the quality of drug substance, drug product, and in-process materials. If a specification needs to be revised as a result of the change, this is considered a multiple change. Additional testing such as chemical and physical behavior, microbiological, biological, bioavailability, and/or stability may also be required in order to ensure that the identity, strength, quality, purity, or potency of the product is not changed. The type of additional testing that an applicant should perform depends on the type of manufacturing changes, the type of drug substance and/or drug product, and the effect of the change on the quality of the product, e.g.,

- Evaluation of changes in the purity or degradant profile
- Toxicology tests to qualify a new impurity or degradant or to qualify an impurity that is above a previously qualified level
- Evaluation of the hardness or friability of a tablet
- Assessment of the effect of a change on bioequivalence, which may include multipoint and/or multimedia dissolution profiling and/or an in vivo bioequivalence study
- Evaluation of extractables from new packaging components or moisture permeability of a new container/closure system

If an assessment concludes that a change has adversely affected the identity, strength, quality, purity, or potency of the drug product, the change should be filed in a Prior Approval Supplement, regardless of the reporting category of the change.

Following the publication of the SUPAC-IR, FDA issued numerous other SUPAC guidances specific for modified release drug products, active pharmaceutical ingredients, analytical equipment, etc. The same principles of assessment of changes, i.e., level 1, 2, or 3, are used in these guidances. This discussion will focus mainly on the original SUPAC Immediate Release Drug Products guidance.

3. CURRENT REQUIREMENTS FOR POST-APPROVAL CHANGES

3.1. Components/Composition

In general, changes to the qualitative/quantitative composition of the formulation are considered major changes. Therefore, these changes must be considered carefully before implementation. Such changes require a Prior Approval Supplement unless otherwise exempted by regulation or guidance documents. The current guidance for industry, *Changes to an Approved ANDA or NDA,* does not address components/composition in detail; therefore, the SUPAC guidance remains in effect for defining components and composition changes and the reporting category thereof.

The addition or deletion of an ingredient can have an adverse effect on the dissolution profile of the finished product and on the in vivo bioequivalence to the reference listed drug. In general, any addition or deletion of an ingredient must be filed as a Prior Approval Supplement. The exception to this applies to colors, which can be removed or reduced from the formulation and filed in an annual report. Only in certain circumstances can changes to the components/composition be made with a less stringent reporting category. These instances are defined in SUPAC and summarized in Table 1.

TABLE 1 Components/Composition Change

Level	Definition	Category and example	Test documentation	Filing documentation
1 (Minor changes)	Changes unlikely to have any detectable impact on formulation quality and performance	i. Deletion/partial deletion of color or flavor or change in the ingredient of the printing ink ii. Changes in excipient (% w/w) of total for mulation not greater than 5%	i. *Chemistry*: Compendial release and stability testing **Stability**: Long-term stability testing on one batch in annual report ii. *Dissolution*: None beyond application/compendial requirement iii. *In vivo BE*: None	Annual Report (all information including long-term stability data)
2 (Moderate changes)	Changes could have significant impact on formulation quality and performance as a result of change in therapeutic range, solubility, and permeability (low or high)	Changes in technical grade of an excipient or changes in excipient amount greater than expressed in level 1, but total additive effect of all excipients should not be greater than 10%	i. *Chemistry*: Compendial release, batch record **Stability**: one batch with 3 months' accelerated stability data in supplement and one batch on long-term stability ii. *Dissolution*: Using case A, B, and C as described in the guidance iii. *In Vivo BE*: None if situation does not meet above dissolution description	Changes Being Effected (CBE) Supplement with long-term stability data

| 3 (Major changes) | Changes likely to have a significant impact on formulation quality and performance as a result of change in therapeutic range, solubility, and permeability (low or high) | i. Qualitative and quantitative changes to a narrow therapeutic drug beyond the ranges of excipients noted in level 1

ii. High solubility and permeability drug, low permeability and high solubility drug and high permeability and low solubility drugs not meeting the dissolution criteria as stipulated in the guidance

iii. Changes in the excipient ranges of low solubility, low permeability drugs listed under level 1 | i. *Chemistry*: Compendial release and batch records
Stability: (**a**) 3 months' accelerated stability testing on one batch in supplement and long-term stability data on one batch in Annual Report if significant body of information is available; (**b**) 3 months' accelerated (supplement) and long-term stability (Annual Report) on up to three batches

ii. *Dissolution*: Multi-point dissolution profile in compendial medium at 15, 30, 45, 60, and 120 min or until asymptote is reached

iii. *In Vivo BE*: Full BE study except for the cases when in vitro/ in vivo correlation is established | Prior Approval Supplement on all information including accelerated stability and long-term stability in Annual Report |

3.2. Site Changes

The sponsor of an ANDA must include in its application the site of manufacture, where the drug product will be produced, tested, packaged, and/or labeled. A change in any of these sites can adversely affect the identity, strength, quality, purity, or potency of the finished product. Therefore, any site change under SUPAC-IR calls for the new site to be in compliance with good manufacturing practice (cGMP) regulations. A stand-alone packaging operation site change, utilizing container(s)/closure(s) in the approved application, may be submitted as a Change Being Effected Supplement. The facility should also have a current and satisfactory cGMP compliance profile with FDA for the type of packaging operation in question before submission of the supplement. If the facility has not received a satisfactory cGMP inspection within the previous two years for the type of packaging operation involved, a Prior Approval Supplement with the same commitment for stability is recommended. The supplement should also contain a commitment to place the first production batch of the product on long-term stability studies using the approved protocol in the application and to submit the resulting data in annual reports. Likewise, a stand-alone analytical testing laboratory site change may also be submitted as a Change Being Effected Supplement if the new facility has a current and satisfactory cGMP compliance profile with the FDA for the type of testing operation in question.

Different levels and the regulatory requirements for site changes are discussed in Table 2.

3.3. Change in Batch Size

Change in batch size from pivotal/pilot scale bio-batch to larger or smaller production batches tends to change the operating parameters. Therefore, all the parameters, such as mixing time, speed, etc., are adjusted according to the equipment (large or small) used in the process. This requires proper validation of the batches before submission of additional information in the application. Any change in the production batch for which the operating parameter falls within the range established for the ANDA batch and validation batches will be regarded as a level 1 change. If it falls outside the validation ranges, the change would be permitted under SUPAC-IR as a level 2 change. Regardless, SUPAC-IR does not address scale-down below 100,000 units. Changes in batch size are characterized in two levels as cited in Table 3.

3.4. Manufacturing

This includes any change made in equipment and the process used in manufacturing a drug product.

TABLE 2 Site Change

Level	Definition	Test documentation	Filing documentation
1 (Minor changes)	Site change within facility and using same equipment, SOPs, environment conditions (temperature and humidity), and controls, no changes made in manufacturing batch records	i. *Chemistry*: Compendial release ii. *Dissolution*: Compendial release iii. *In-vivo BE*: None	Annual Report
2 (Moderate changes)	Site change within a contiguous campus or between facilities in adjacent city blocks using same equipment, SOPs, environment conditions (temperature and humidity), and controls, no changes made to manufacturing batch records	i. *Chemistry*: Updated batch records, compendial release, Stability: Long-term stability on one batch reported in Annual Report ii. *Dissolution*: Compendial release iii. *In Vivo BE*: None	Changes Being Effected (CBE) Supplement, Annual Report
3 (Major changes)	Changes in manufacturing site to a different campus. Same equipment, SOPs, environment conditions and controls should be used at the new site. No changes in the manufacturing batch records	i. *Chemistry*: Updated batch records, compendial release, Stability: 3 months' accelerated stability data reported in supplement, long-term stability data on up to three batches in Annual Report ii. *Dissolution*: Case B of the guidance, multipoint profile in compendial medium at 15, 30, 45, 60, and 120 min or until an asymptote is reached. Dissolution profile should be similar at both current and proposed site iii. *In Vivo BE*: None	Changes Being Effected (CBE) Supplement, Annual Report

TABLE 3 Batch Size Change

Level	Definition	Test documentation	Filing documentation
1 (Minor changes)	Change in batch size by 10 times the pilot/bio-batch using equipment having the same design and operating principles as that used to produce the test batch. The batch should be manufactured under full compliance with cGMPs and SOPs using the same formulation and manufacturing procedures	i. *Chemistry:* Compendial release, notification of changes, and updated batch records in annual report, Stability: Long-term stability on one batch ii. *Dissolution:* Compendial release iii. *In vivo BE:* None	Annual Report including long-term stability data
2 (Moderate changes)	Change in batch size beyond a factor of 10 times the size of the pilot / bio-batch using equipment having the same design and principles. The batch should be manufactured under full compliance with cGMPs and SOPs using the same formulation and manufacturing procedures	i. *Chemistry:* Compendial release, notification of change, and updated batch records, Stability: 3 month' accelerated stability and long-term stability on one batch ii. *Dissolution:* Case B of the guidance, multiple point profile in compendial medium at 15, 30, 45, 60, and 120 min or until an asymptote is reached iii. *In vivo BE:* None	Changes Being Effected Supplement, Annual Report including long-term stability data

3.4.1. Equipment Change

Any change in manufacturing equipment other than that used in the approved application requires appropriate validation studies to demonstrate that the new equipment is similar to the original equipment. Equipment within the same class and subclass would be considered to have the same design and operating principal under SUPAC-IR. For example, a change in V-blender from one manufacturer to another manufacturer would not represent a change in operating principle, and hence be considered to be the same under SUPAC-IR, whereas a change in equipment from one class (V-blender) to a different class (ribbon blender) would be considered a change in design and operating principle and would be considered different under SUPAC-IR. A guidance for industry, *SUPAC-IR/MR: Immediate Release and Modified Solid Oral Dosage Forms—Manufacturing Equipment Addendum, 1999* (3), explains in detail about various changes in equipment and the regulatory requirements.

The two different levels of change and regulatory requirements on change in equipment are summarized in Table 4.

3.4.2. Process Change

Change in manufacturing process or technology from that currently used by the applicant may have the potential for adverse effects on the identity, strength, quality, purity, or potency of a drug product. The safety or effectiveness of the product depends on the type of the manufacturing process and the changes being instituted for the drug substance or drug product. Any fundamental change in the manufacturing process, e.g., dry to wet granulation or change from one type of drying process to another (e.g., oven tray, fluid-bed) is considered a major change, whereas change in mixing time, operating speed, etc., within an approved range is considered a minor change. The guidance defines three levels of in-process change, as indicated in Table 5.

3.5. Specifications

Specifications are the standards a drug product must meet to ensure conformance to predetermined criteria for consistency, reproducibility, and quality. Such changes generally require a Prior Approval Supplement unless the specification is tightening or otherwise exempted by regulation guidance documents.

Prior approval is required on the following *major changes* in specification except as provided in the SUPAC-IR guidance:

- Relaxing an acceptance criterion

TABLE 4 Equipment Change

Level	Definition	Test documentation	Filing documentation
1	a. Changes from nonautomated to automated equipment to move ingredients b. Changes to alternative equipment of the same design and operating principles (same or different capacity)	i. *Chemistry*: Notification of change, compendial release, and Updated batch records Stability: Long-term stability on one batch ii. *Dissolution*: Compendial release iii. *In vivo BE*: None	Annual Report including long-term stability data
2	Changes in equipment to a different design and Different operating principles.	i. *Chemistry*: Compendial release, notification of change, updated batch records Stability: (a) Significant body of data available, which includes 3 months' accelerated stability data in supplement and long-term stability on one batch reported in Annual Report; (b) significant body of data not available, Which includes 3 months' accelerated stability on up to three batches in supplement and long-term stability on up to three batches reported in annual report ii. *Dissolution*: Case C dissolution profile of the guidance, which is multipoint dissolution, provides in water, 0.1 N HCl, and USP buffer media at pH 4.5, 6.5, and 7.5 for the proposed and currently accepted formulation iii. *In vivo BE*: None	Prior Approval Supplement with justification for change, Annual Report including long-term stability data

TABLE 5 Process Change

Level	Definition	Test documentation	Filing documentation
1	Changes such as mixing times and operating speeds within application/validation changes	i. *Chemistry*: Compendial release ii. *Dissolution*: Compendial release. iii. *In vivo BE*: None	Annual Report
2	Any changes outside of application/validation ranges (mixing time, operating speed)	i. *Chemistry*: Compendial release, notification of change, updated batch records Stability: Long-term stability on one batch ii. *Dissolution*: Case B dissolution profile of the guidance, multipoint dissolution in the application/compendial medium at 15, 30, 45, 60, and 120 min or until an asymptote is reached iii. *In vivo BE*: None	Changes Being Effected (CBE) Supplement, Annual Report including long-term stability data
3	Any change in process such as wet-granulation to direct compression	i. *Chemistry*: Compendial release, notification of change, updated batch records Stability: (a) Significant body of data available, which is 3 months' accelerated stability on one batch in supplement and long-term stability on one batch reported in Annual Report; and (b) significant body of data not available 3 this includes 3 months' accelerated stability on up to three batches in supplement and long-term stability on up to three batches reported in Annual Report. ii. *Dissolution*: Case B dissolution profile of the guidance, multipoint dissolution profile in the application/compendial medium at 15, 30, 45, 60, and 120 min or until an asymptote is reached iii. *In Vivo BE*: Full BE study. BE study may be waived if *IVIVC* is established	Prior Approval Supplement with justification, Annual Report including long-term stability data

- Deleting any part of a specification
- Changing or establishing a new regulatory analytical procedure that does not provide the same or increased assurance of the identity, strength, quality, purity, or potency of the material being tested as the analytical procedure described in the approved application

A 30 days' Changes Being Effected Supplement needs to be filed in case of *moderate changes* in specifications, e.g.,

- Change in regulatory analytical procedures other than editorial or identified as major
- A change in analytical procedure or deletion of a test for raw materials used in drug substance manufacturing or in-process materials prior to the final intermediate

The following include changes in specifications that are considered to have minimal potential for an adverse effect on the identity, strength, quality, purity, or potency of a product as they may relate to the safety or effectiveness of the product, and therefore can be submitted in an annual report:

- Change in specification made to comply with an official compendium
- Change in analytical procedure for testing raw material, drug substance or drug product that provides the same or increased assurance of identity, strength, purity, or potency of the material being tested as the analytical procedure described in the approved application
- Tightening of acceptance criteria

3.6. Packaging

A container/closure system for a solid oral dosage form tends to be low risk and will have little impact on the shelf life of the finished product. Therefore, under the new guidance for industry, and the stability guidance, the requirements for packaging changes have been relaxed significantly.

4. COMPARABILITY PROTOCOLS

A *comparability protocol* is a plan for anticipated future CMC changes. FDA recently published a draft guidance, *Comparability Protocols—Chemistry, Manufacturing, and Controls Information,* to provide recommendations on preparing and using comparability protocols for post-approval changes in the CMC section of an NDA or ANDA (4). Although applications for protein products are not included in the guidance, well-characterized synthetic peptides are included within the scope of this guidance.

According to the guidance, "A comparability protocol is a well defined, detailed, written plan for assessing the effect of specific CMC changes in the identity, strength, quality, purity, and potency of a specific drug product as these factors relate to the safety and effectiveness of the product. A comparability protocol describes the changes that are covered under the protocol and specifies the tests and studies that will be performed, including analytical procedures that will be used, and acceptance criteria that will be achieved to demonstrate that specified CMC changes do not adversely affect the product."

A comparability protocol may be submitted with an ANDA or NDA application or as a Prior Approval Supplement (post-approval). The benefit of the comparability protocol is that an FDA request for additional information to support a change is less likely when the change is covered under an approved protocol. Thus, the sponsor could implement a CMC post-approval change as described in the comparability protocol. This would allow the sponsor to place the product in distribution sooner.

5. POST-MARKETING SURVEILLANCE

Once the FDA approves a generic drug product, manufacturers are responsible for conducting post-marketing surveillance. Post-marketing reporting requirements for an approved ANDA are set forth in the US Federal Code of Regulations, 21 CFR 314.80 (5) and 314.98. The main component of this requirement is the reporting of adverse drug experiences(ADEs). According to 21 CFR 314.80(a), an *adverse drug experience* is defined as "any adverse event associated with the use of a drug in humans, whether or not considered drug related" (6). The definition continues by stating that adverse events include those that occur in the course of the use of a drug product in professional practice, occur from drug overdose (accidental or intentional), abuse, or withdrawal, or involve failure of expected pharmacological action. According to the definition, it is irrelevant whether or not an event is considered drug related. A known or proven cause and effect relationship between the drug and the event is not required. The fact that an adverse event occurred while a person was using a drug product is reason enough to consider it an adverse drug experience.

It is important to examine who is involved in the process of ADE reporting. Generally, there are three members that take part in this process: a reporter, a manufacturer, and the FDA. Essentially anyone can report an ADE. The *reporter* can be a patient, doctor, pharmacist, nurse, or anyone else aware of such an event. This person can report it to either the manufacturer of the drug product or directly to the FDA. If the manufacturer receives the report first, the manufacturer is responsible for investigating the ADE and reporting it to the FDA. If the FDA is notified directly by the reporter, the agency informs the manufacturer so that the ADE can be investigated. Part of investigating an ADE may include, but is not limited to, contacting the patient's physician, the prescriber (if different from the physician), and the pharmacy that filled the prescription. Other investigations include performing all required testing of the retain sample from the lot of the product that was used by the patient. Of course, there are many times when the lot number is not known and therefore, this testing cannot be conducted. Once an investigation is complete, the manufacturer is responsible for submitting the information in a report to the FDA.

There is certain information that must be known, though, before a report is submitted to the FDA. Among this information are four elements: an identifiable patient, an identifiable reporter, a suspect drug/biological product, and an adverse event or fatal outcome. If any of these basic elements remain unknown after being actively sought by the applicant/ manufacturer, a report on the incident should not be submitted to the FDA, because reports without this information make interpretation of their significance difficult, if not impossible. In these cases, the applicant/manufacturershould track the steps taken to acquire the additional information in their safety files for the product. To facilitate the reporting process, FDA created the *MedWatch* program (7). MedWatch is the FDA Medical Products Reporting Program. It was originally designed to emphasize the responsibility of healthcare providers to identify and report ADEs. Through the MedWatch program, healthcare professionals can report ADEs with the use of FDA Form 3500 (6) (MedWatch Form). However, this reporting is done on a voluntary basis. Currently, there are no regulations that require healthcare professionals to report adverse drug experiences to the FDA or the manufacturer. In contrast, a manufacturer aware of an ADE is required by law to report it to the FDA (provided the four elements noted earlier are known). The FDA/ MedWatch Form 3500A is used for mandatory reporting by manufacturers. It is interesting to point out that on the bottom portion of both MedWatch forms there is a note that reads: "Submission of report does not constitute an admission that the product caused or contributed to the event." This is a reiteration of what was stated earlier in the CFR definition of an ADE.

After an adverse event is reported to a manufacturer, two classifications must be made. First, the adverse event must be categorized as either serious or nonserious. Second, it must be determined whether the ADE is expected or unexpected. Again, these terms are defined in 21 CFR 314.80. A serious adverse drug experience is "any ADE occurring at any dose that results in any of the following outcomes: death, a life-threatening adverse drug experience, inpatient hospitalization or prolongation of existing hospitalization, a persistent or significant disability/incapacity, or a congenital anomaly/birth defect." In addition, the regulations include an "important medical event" that may endanger the patient and may require medical involvement to prevent one of the outcomes listed above. A nonserious ADE is one that does not result in any outcome listed in the definition of a serious ADE.

In regards to the expected and unexpected designation, the labeling of the product is used to determine the type of ADE. If the product labeling lists a particular adverse event, it is considered expected. If not, it is considered unexpected. This classification of ADEs is not always clear. Unexpected ADEs also include events that may be symptomatically and pathophysiologically related to an event listed in the labeling, but differ from the event because of greater severity or specificity. For example, if a report is received that a patient experienced complete loss of vision while using a marketed product and the labeling of the product lists visual disturbances in the adverse effects section, the manufacturer may consider this an expected event. However, since complete loss of vision is more severe than the description in the labeling, this ADE would be classified as unexpected rather than expected. The key here is that manufacturers should not give the FDA the impression that reports or details of reports are being hidden or glossed over. It is important to note that by submitting an ADE report to the FDA, manufacturers are simply notifying FDA. As discussed earlier, it is not an admission of guilt or even agreement that the product caused the event.

It is important to correctly classify an ADE as either serious or nonserious and either expected or unexpected. The classification of the ADE will determine the type of report that is submitted to the FDA. ADEs that are considered both serious and unexpected must be submitted to the FDA in an expedited manner and are known as *15-Day Alert Reports*. Manufacturers must submit these reports to the FDA as soon as possible, but in no case later than 15 calendar days of the initial receipt of the information. All other ADEs (those that are serious and expected, nonserious and expected, or nonserious and unexpected) should be reported to the FDA as Periodic Reports. Periodic Reports must be submitted at quarterly intervals for three years from the date of FDA approval of the product, and then annually. Any follow-up information received after the initial submission to the FDA should be submitted to the FDA and should follow the same rules depending on whether the original ADE report was classified as a 15-Day Alert Report or Periodic Report.

During the investigation and submission of the ADE report to the FDA, patient privacy should be maintained. The manufacturer should not identify patients by name or address in the reports. Instead, the manufacturer should assign a unique code (e.g., patient's initials or a tracking number) to each report. In addition, names of patients, healthcare professionals, hospitals, and geographical identifiers in adverse drug experience reports are not releasable to the public under FDA's public information regulations.

Although there is some complexity at times, the ADE reporting system is efficient and straightforward. The main goal of the requirement is to identify new or previously unrecognized adverse events that are caused by drug products. This often results in the addition of safety information to a product's labeling, but can also lead to more severe actions like product recalls or withdrawals. In any case, the objective is to expand the information available to the medical community and the public regarding a product's adverse event profile and therefore increase public safety.

REFERENCES

1. Guidance for Industry. Changes to an Approved NDA or ANDA. US Department of Health and Human Services, Food and Drug Administration, Center for Drug Evaluation and Research (CDER), November 1999, CMC.
2. *Guidance for Industry.* Immediate Release Solid Oral Dosage Forms—Scale-Up and Postapproval Changes: Chemistry, Manufacturing, and Controls, In Vitro Dissolution Testing, and In Vivo Bioequivalence Documentation. Center for Drug and Research (CDER), November 1995, CMC 5.
3. Guidance for Industry. SUPAC-IR/MR: Immediate Release and Modified Release Solid Oral Dosage Forms—Manufacturing Equipment Addendum. US Department of Health and Human Services, Food and Drug Administration, Center for Drug Evaluation and Research (CDER), January 1999, CMC9 (Revision 1).
4. Guidance for Industry. Comparability Protocols—Chemistry, Manufacturing, and Controls Information. FDA, Center for Drug Evaluation and Research (CDER), February 2003, http://www.fda.gov/cder/guidance/5427dft.pdf.
5. Office of the Federal Register. 21 CFR 314.80. Revised as of April 1, 2002: 119–122.
6. Guidance for Industry. Postmarketing Adverse Experience Reporting for Human Drug and Licensed Biological Products: Clarification of What to Report. Food and Drug Administration, August 1997.
7. Food and Drug Administration. MedWatch FDA Form 3500/3500A. http://www.fda.gov/cder/guidance/5427dft.pdf, June 1993.

13

Outsourcing Bioavailability and Bioequivalence Studies to Contract Research Organizations

Patrick K. Noonan

PK Noonan & Associates, LLC, Richmond, Virginia, U.S.A.

1. WHY OUTSOURCE?

1.1. What is the Goal/Reason for Outsourcing?

Contract Research Organizations (CROs) provide a much needed service to the pharmaceutical sector. Full service CROs offer a comprehensive selection of capabilities, while smaller "niche" CROs may focus on a narrow segment of services (e.g., clinical or analytical only). All of these organizations fulfill a need in that they provide the services necessary for the approval of new clinical entities or generic drug products. A sampling of these services is included in Table 1.

Many of the larger pharmaceutical companies have in-house capabilities for most, if not all, of these services. For example, many often have their own clinical and bioanalytical units that provide full support for Phase I studies. However, even these internal resources can become saturated due to the drive to develop more compounds in shorter time intervals.

Unlike their larger counterparts, the smaller companies, virtual firms and generic companies do not have the luxury of their own dedicated clinical unit or full in-house capabilities and are required to outsource their clinical

TABLE 1 Check Sheet Providing Typical Services Outsourced for BA/BE Studies

Service	Sponsor (✓)	CRO (✓)
Bioanalytical Analysis		
Bioanalytical Site Selection and Qualification		
Clinical Study Design		
Clinical Protocol Development		
Clinical Site Selection and Qualification		
Clinical Conduct		
Clinical Monitoring		
Data Management		
Pharmacokinetic Analyses		
Statistical Analyses		
Pharmacokinetic Report Writing		
Integrated ICH Report Writing		
Project Management		
FDA/Regulatory Consultation		

trials, including bioavailability (BA) and bioequivalence (BE) studies. Although generic companies have internal resources for product development, manufacturing and release testing, they do not have clinical and bioanalytical capabilities.

It is critical that the CRO and client realize the importance of close collaboration and seamless communication between their organizations. This collaboration is necessary to achieve study success in a timely manner. Key elements necessary for success include:

- *Communication* at all levels between the CRO and the pharmaceutical company.
- *Sensitivity* to both the project specific requirements and timelines.
- *Flexibility* to recognize and adjust to unexpected events throughout the project timeline.

As the number of outsourced services may vary with each client, it is important that the CROs demonstrate a flexible attitude and responsive approach that will enable a better partnership with the pharmaceutical company.

1.2. Outsourcing Relationship: Vendor vs. Partnership

Prior to selecting a CRO, a company needs to evaluate their goal for outsourcing and assess the relationship they wish to have with the CRO. The most common relationships include the CRO as a vendor, a preferred provider or a development partner.

1.2.1. Vendor

Some projects may require only a "one-off" type of relationship; that is, the outsourced project is a one-time event and there is no need for a long-term relationship with the CRO. Some questions that need to be resolved include:

- Is the project a one-time event?
- What is most critical to the company: timing or cost?
- Will the deliverable be a commodity that is awarded to the CRO with the lowest price?
- Will the study be awarded to the CRO with the earliest dosing date and fastest timelines?
- Does the firm require a single service CRO (e.g., bioanalytical services)?

Outsourcing managers are cautioned to avoid the "commodity" mindset. Many CRO services are considered to be or are evaluated as if the service was a commodity. Commodities are purchased based on price; quality and value are all considered to be equal (between brands, or CROs). Unfortunately (for the accountants), this mindset is not generally successful in the drug development arena and the phrase "you get what you pay for" is applicable. In the long run, it is important to also focus on quality, timelines, and service level when considering contracting a single service.

1.2.2. Preferred Provider

A preferred provider or vendor relationship/agreement works in two directions. It is assumed that the company or sponsor prefers to give work to those companies with which it has developed this relationship. In return, the CRO is expected to provide better than average timelines and prices. Often these agreements provide for a tiered discount (that is, the more studies that a client places with the CRO, the greater the discount on the pricing).

1.2.3. Partner

As mentioned above, an effective CRO/client relationship requires close collaboration and seamless communication to achieve study success in a timely manner. The best outsourcing results are obtained when pharmaceutical firms develop a long-term partner relationship with a quality CRO (or at least assume a partner "mentality" or perspective).

Partners work towards a common goal and benefit. It is important to realize that CROs are made up of individuals who value their work. To them, their work is more than just a commodity. Partnering with these individuals results in a feeling of ownership; this type of relationship will motivate individuals to go beyond the minimum requirements and will result in a higher quality end product.

As a full development partner, a CRO will help to develop the entire program. As a partner, the CRO has a vested interest in the success of the program and will run with it as if it were its own drug product. Virtual pharmaceutical companies, that do not have the in-house expertise for full development, must rely on consultants or a full service CRO to assist with the successful development and execution of their program. Although most CROs do not provide the capabilities for full partnership, a few have demonstrated that they can successfully develop a drug product from inception to clinical proof-of-concept.

1.3. Timing/Cost Considerations

Outsourcing becomes attractive, even to those companies who have in-house resources, when these resources are committed to different projects. Timing and costs are two major considerations that come into play when a pharmaceutical company decides to outsource.

Timing is a major consideration for many projects. Although most Phase I studies are not a critical path to an NDA submission, there are times that bioavailability data are necessary to design a Phase II or III study. Occasionally, a bioequivalence study, comparing the Phase III formulation with the final marketed product, becomes rate limiting for an NDA submission. At these times, outsourcing is necessary and cost effective since approval (and marketing) delays can be quite costly when compared to lost revenue.

Generic BE studies are often on very tight timelines since the company's objective is to file an ANDA within 3–4 months of manufacturing the clinical lot. The goal of most Generics is to be the first to market because the first generic approval provides that manufacturer with a higher profit margin. Each additional approval increases competition and decreases prices (eroding margins). Timing is even more critical when a generic manufacturer intends to file an ANDA with a paragraph IV patent certification. The first generic to file (as a paragraph IV) is entitled to 6 months of exclusivity (i.e., no generic competition). Six months of exclusivity (for branded or generic products) provide a substantial financial incentive to the pharmaceutical firm. Therefore, since it is critical that the bioequivalence trial be completed expeditiously, these companies approach CROs to provide dedicated resources that can meet the company's timeline.

For those studies where timing is not critical, many companies evaluate cost as a basis for outsourcing. These companies will send an RFP (request for proposal) to a number of CROs. The CROs, in turn, will provide study quotations that detail the price for the services. Interestingly, many companies will compare internal costs vs. the cost to outsource. However, this comparison often includes only "out-of-pocket" costs (internal salaries) and does not include overhead expenses (benefits, offices, computers, training, etc.).

It is important to compare "apples to apples" when comparing costs/ prices (both internal and external). Companies comparing internal costs should utilize all costs (not just salaries). When comparing bids from multiple CROs, it is also important to assess both the prices and deliverables from each CRO. An RFP that is not clearly written may yield a number of proposals with a wide range of prices. It is important for each CRO to identify the assumptions and deliverables behind each proposal. Firms may be disappointed with the end-results if they select a CRO based on price alone.

2. IDENTIFICATION OF APPROPRIATE CROS

It is important that your CRO has validated corporate procedures for all segments of clinical study conduct. These procedures are used to ensure that all aspects of a study, including but not limited to clinical conduct, laboratory analysis, data management, biostatistics, pharmacokinetics, and medical writing, are performed in compliance with Good Clinical Practices (GCP), Good Laboratory Practices (GLP), and other applicable regulatory practices and guidelines. These procedures, in short, guarantee the credibility of the data and protect the rights and integrity of the study subjects.

2.1. Assessment of Capabilities and Experience

Before "shopping" for a CRO or vendor, a company needs to first identify specific services to be outsourced. If the pharmaceutical company has project management resources available, then it may be able to work with multiple vendors to complete a single study. For example, the company could separately contract with a clinical facility (a university clinic, a commercial standalone clinic or a CRO with clinical capabilities), an analytical unit and a pharmacokineticist to write the report. Note that the company could also contract the project management duties to one of these three vendors. Alternatively, the company could contract with a CRO that provides clinical, bioanalytical, pharmacokinetic, statistical and report writing services. This "one stop shopping" generally facilitates the conduct of these studies, assuming that the CRO can provide the experience and meet the company's timeline and pricing expectations.

In order to identify the CRO that will conduct a potential study, it is necessary to first develop a list of potential CROs. The list will be made up of those CROs that provide all services and those that provide clinic only or analytical only services. The list is often comprised of those CROs with which the company (or individuals) have worked with in the past. Although there are many CROs that advertise in the trade publications, most of these will not have the necessary BA/BE expertise or capabilities that are required for the study. Thus, the company will need to evaluate all CROs and will need to make the initial "cut". Evaluating the experience and capabilities of the CRO and their ability to meet the company's timeline are the first two screening criteria. For the purpose of this discussion, it is assumed that the pharmaceutical firm will use a single CRO for all services. For those companies who prefer to subcontract the clinical, bioanalytical, and pharmacokinetic resources, the mechanism to identify the most appropriate vendor is the same, but must be repeated for each vendor.

2.2. Clinical Capabilities

The first step to CRO qualification is the assessment of their capabilities and experience. The ability of a CRO to recruit a particular patient or volunteer population is a primary requirement. The CRO should be able to recruit the entire study population at a single center, preferably as a single group. Healthy volunteer populations are the easiest to recruit; however, some studies may require large numbers of subjects or replicate designs. In these cases, the ability of the CRO to recruit this large population as a single group should be assessed. When conducting replicate design studies, the dropout rate is often higher than a simple two period crossover design. As always, the CRO clinic should be capable of recruiting an adequate number of subjects to account for dropouts. Some drug products also require special populations. For example, estrogens are generally dosed to postmenopausal females. Other drugs may be targeted to an elderly population. It is essential that the CRO be assessed for its ability to recruit these special populations.

2.3. Bioanalytical Capabilities

Just as the clinical capabilities must be assessed, the bioanalytical capabilities are equally important. Validation lists (lists of analytical methods that are currently available and validated) are available from most CROs. It is critical that the bioanalytical facility be experienced in analyzing the drug (and metabolite, as appropriate) and should be able to provide a written validation report. The validation should be assessed prior to awarding the study, or at least prior to dosing. In addition to having an appropriately validated method, the facility should follow cGLPs and have a clean FDA inspection history.

2.4. Pharmacokinetic Capabilities

Most companies focus primarily on the clinical and bioanalytical capabilities for CRO selection. However, the pharmacokinetic capabilities should also be critically assessed. The CRO should have validated pharmacokinetic and statistical programs in place and should be compliant with 21 CFR Part 11 (especially in regard to change control).

2.5. Timeline Assessment

The list of CROs that meet the company's clinical, bioanalytical, and pharmacokinetic criteria must be assessed for their ability to meet the company's timeline. The CRO must be able to meet the timelines as established by the company management team. In the rare instance that no CRO can meet the timeline, then the company may need to reassess their strategy and internal submission timelines.

Often the large list of commercial CROs and/or laboratories can be whittled down to between one and three candidates at this point. Once the list has been narrowed, the candidate CRO sites should be evaluated "in person". If, however, too many sites are viable candidates, the sites can be "interviewed" via telephone to evaluate their qualifications. However, the final candidate should be qualified with an on-site inspection.

3. CRO QUALIFICATION

3.1. Due Diligence

If the pharmaceutical firm has used the CRO in the past, they should objectively evaluate their past experience with this CRO. If the experience was good, the firm should identify those components that were successful and insure that they are used for their new study. However, caution should be exercised and due diligence pursued if the new study requires a different subject population or analytical technique. For example, a CRO may specialize in recruiting healthy male and female volunteers, but may have difficulty in the recruitment of postmenopausal females. Similarly, a successful bioanalytical project using LC does not guarantee success with more complex methods such as LC/MS. On the other hand, if the firm had a negative experience with a particular CRO, the firm should objectively assess the cause of that experience.

All CRO evaluations should begin with an assessment of information in the public domain. The firm should obtain copies of past FDA inspection reports (483s and Establishment Inspection Reports {EIRs}) through the Freedom of Information (FOI). Also, the firm should request any FDA warning letters that may have been issued to the CRO.

The CRO should provide the client with a written and signed statement that neither the CRO nor any of its employees or any subcontractors has been debarred by the Food and Drug Administration (under the provisions of the United States Generic Drug Enforcement Act of 1992). The CRO should also provide performance metrics used for tracking timelines and financial metrics. The company should request "references"; these references should include those companies which outsourced studies that resulted in successful ANDA or NDA approvals.

The firm should carefully evaluate any external providers (subcontractors) that the CRO proposes to employ (for example, clinical labs, medical specialists, specialized assay laboratories). The success of the clinical program (in this case a BA or BE study) is dependent on the weakest link.

Another important aspect (but one that is difficult to objectively assess) is the support that will be provided by the study program manager. This individual is responsible for overseeing the various functions within the CRO and often functions as the "program champion", and must be capable of managing a multi-disciplinary development team. The program manager also manages timelines and serves as communication facilitator within the CRO team and between team and sponsor. This individual has a focus on overall objectives with eye on the final deliverable and timelines.

The larger CROs have expertise in a number of therapeutic areas and can provide consulting capabilities if needed. Although some CROs provide some limited *gratis* consulting, the real expertise is usually available on an hourly billing rate. The consulting that is available in the larger CROs covers regulatory, medical, clinical, biopharmaceutics, pharmacokinetic, and statistical issues. Availability of this consulting is key when the "unexpected" happens during the study conduct. The unexpected can include analytical failure or unanticipated adverse events, abnormal pharmacokinetic behavior or inability to prove bioequivalence.

After evaluating the credentials and performance metrics of each CRO, the sponsor should physically visit and audit the clinical, bioanalytical, and pharmacokinetic capabilities of the CRO.

3.2. Clinical Site Qualification/Audit

The sponsor should conduct a site qualification visit. In addition to a cGCP site audit, this evaluation should include an assessment of the areas in Table 2.

3.3. Bioanalytical Site Qualification

Candidate CROs for bioanalytical laboratory work (for drug, metabolite and/or biomarker assays) should also be assessed. The personnel, their

TABLE 2   List of Those Areas to be Included in the Clinical Site Assessment

	Check (✓) when complete
Clinical site evaluation	
Assess the volunteer (or patient) population pool	
Evaluate CRO procedures for handling an unexpected	
and serious adverse event (AE) investigation	
Assess training records for the clinical team	
Evaluate CRO's ability to coordinate plasma/urine	
shipments to different bioanalytical facilities	
Assess ability to coordinate functional handoffs (e.g.,	
timely delivery of protocol to clinic, samples to lab,	
bioanalytical data to the pharmacokineticist)	
Assess clinical project management capabilities	
Clinical data management	
Assess the validation of the data collection system	
Evaluate query generation, SOPs, CRF and database	
correction, change control	
Evaluate clinical deliverables	
CRFs (CRO or sponsor format)	
Data Base (when applicable)	
Blood/plasma/urine collection procedures/SOPs and	
transport procedures to bioanalytical unit	
Content of the written clinical report (i.e., CRO	
clinical report to be incorporated into the final study	
report)	

qualifications, and analytical method, and validation should be assessed prior to awarding the study. The company audit should also include cGLP compliance and an assessment of the laboratory's inspection history. Copies of the inspection history with all FDA 483s and EIRs should be reviewed. Laboratory project management should be assessed for their ability to coordinate all processes with the client, clinic, and pharmacokineticist.

Finally, the CRO should provide written documentation as to the content of the final analytical report that should contain additional project specific validation data (e.g., frozen matrix stability determined for the length of sample storage—i.e., from time of first clinical sample collection to the time that the last sample is analyzed) to support the BA/BE study. The FDA requires that full validation be performed to support bioavailability and bioequivalence studies in new drug applications (NDA) and abbreviated new drug applications (ANDA) (1,2).

3.4. Pharmacokinetic Site Qualification

The pharmaceutical firm should also qualify the CRO site (or department) that is responsible for PK and statistical analyses and completion of the final integrated report (and possibly the EVA). The group should have all programs fully validated according to FDA programming guidelines. During the pharmacokinetic site audit, the following areas should be carefully assessed:

- Qualifications of pharmacokinetic and statistical personnel.
- Validation of pharmacokinetic and statistical programs (usually SAS).
- Compliance with 21CFR Part 11. At the time of this publication, full and complete compliance with Part 11 was not being enforced. However, the CRO should have a written plan and timeline for bringing all postlaboratory functions into compliance.
- Evaluate format and completeness of pharmacokinetic tables and graphs, statistical output (listings) and a mock final report.

3.5. Culture

Although culture can not be quantitatively assessed, it is important to consider the following key areas:

- Is the culture of the CRO compatible with that of the pharmaceutical company?
- Does the firm expect the CRO to make all decisions with regard to minor protocol deviations?
- Does the firm wish to manage all communications and decisions?

4. COMPETITIVE BIDS/DEFINING THE DELIVERABLES

In an effort to quickly place a clinical study, the development of the RFP (request for proposal) may be rushed and result in a document that is subject to various degrees of interpretation. In light of this, it is important for companies to carefully evaluate competitive bids to assure that each CRO has made the same set of assumptions.

4.1. Final Report Content and Format

Ideally, the development of an effective RFP and proposal should begin with the outcomes in mind. That is, the focus on the proposal should begin with the objective of a final deliverable (the report) and should include a description of the content and format of the final report.

4.1.1. Final Written Report

CROs work with a large number of different clients; each client often has their own report format preferences. Therefore, if the RFP does not specifically address the report format, the CRO often will make an assumption regarding the report format. This assumption may or may not be explicitly stated in the resulting proposal. This assumption can make or break a proposal since the report format assumes a number of other important deliverables.

A full ICH-formatted report requires a substantial amount of data analysis of all data in the CRFs (Case Report Forms). Thus, the CRO statisticians will provide additional statistical tables, analysis listings, and graphs. This additional work increases the cost of the study due to the additional statistical and medical writing man-hours needed. Although these data may be required for an NDA BA study, they are not required for a generic BE study.

Many CROs have developed their own "standardized" format for bioequivalence studies which, although quite abbreviated, is adequate for submission to OGD (the FDA Office of Generic Drugs). These reports include a relatively short summary of the clinical and analytical conduct and the pharmacokinetic and statistical results. The clinical report, analytical report, CRFs, and statistical output are merely attached to the report as supportive documentation. This report format requires fewer man-hours and is substantially less expensive that its ICH counterpart.

If the client requires a report that may also be submitted (at a later date) to the European Authorities, then they may expect a report suitably formatted for ICH. However, if the CRO assumes a report formatted for OGD, then the client will not be satisfied with the final product (i.e., report). On the other hand, if the CRO assumes that an ICH format and content are necessary, but the client requires only the more abbreviated OGD report, then the price of the study will be much higher than needed. The CRO will appear to be noncompetitive with other CROs that assumed an OGD format.

4.1.2. Electronic BE Study Reports (EVA) (6)

The FDA Office of Generic Drugs currently recommends that all BE studies be submitted electronically within 30 days of submission of the "paper" application. The EVA (Entry Validation Application) is not a requirement, and not all companies submit an EVA. If a sponsor company anticipates that they will be submitting an EVA, then this fact should be included in the RFP. In order to meet the 30-day timeline, the CRO needs to work on the EVA in parallel (at the same time) as the paper report.

Once a sponsor decides that the EVA will be included as part of the deliverables, then a number of additional considerations must be addressed.

The EVA and "companion document" contain all data needed for an FDA Biopharm review. This includes a number of CMC-related items (for all product strengths within the ANDA) that are not normally provided to CROs. For example, qualitative and quantitative composition, dissolution profiles, batch sizes, and manufacturing dates are required fields that should be entered into the EVA database.

The FDA provides a degree of latitude for these data; that is, a sponsor (or the CRO) does not have to enter these data but can reference the paper application. However, if these data are going to be included in the EVA, then the sponsor must decide (early in the process) as to whether the CRO or the sponsor will enter these data into the database. If the CRO provides the data entry, then these data must be provided in a timely manner. However, many sponsors consider these CMC data to be highly confidential and may insist that their own regulatory affairs department enters these data. In this case, the CRO must have both the report and the EVA prepared one to two weeks before the deadline in order to allow sufficient time for the client to enter and review these data.

4.2. Clinical

4.2.1. Protocol Development

Prior to 1999, the FDA Office of Generic Drugs published a large number of drug-specific guidances that provided the basic information needed to conduct a generic BE trial. However, FDA determined that they could not support the development and maintenance of these guidances and provide timely reviews of abbreviated drug applications. With the publication of general BA/BE Guidance, the Agency "withdrew" the drug-specific guidances. Although the FDA now expects the Pharmaceutical Industry (and CROs) to determine the optimal protocol design and criteria necessary to establish bioequivalence (or bioavailability), they will review protocols on a case-by-case basis. However, at the time of this publication, these protocol reviews were placed in the review queue at FDA and this review often took between three and six months.

Since these drug product specific guidances are no longer available (3), it is important that an RFP specifies the expectations for protocol development. Three possible options exist, each with a different cost structure:

Level 1: Client provides final clinical protocol.

Level 2: Client provides protocol "outline" including design and all specifications; CRO provides final protocol.

Level 3: Client provides objective; CRO provides design and protocol.

Unless the sponsor provides the final clinical protocol (as in Level 1), the following items must be addressed in the RFP in order to obtain an accurately priced study.

4.2.2. Protocol Format

Some pharmaceutical firms are quite strict when it comes to formatting requirements. If the firm requires the CRO to follow a specific format (developed by the company) then this information (and the format) should be provided within the RFP. On the other hand, many companies do not have a preference for protocol format. They are only concerned that all of the relevant parameters are included in the protocol. For these companies, CROs can often provide a standardized (and shorter) format for less money. Another advantage to using this standardized approach is that the CRO clinical personnel are often more familiar with the CRO format which will result in fewer questions back to the client.

4.2.3. Clinical Study Population

Many, if not most, BA/BE studies are conducted in healthy volunteers. In the past, apparently in order to reduce variability and liability, most sponsors chose to perform most BA/BE studies in healthy, young, male volunteers. However, the most recent FDA guidance for BA/BE studies (3) states as follows:

> Unless otherwise indicated by a specific guidance, subjects recruited for in vivo BE studies should be 18 years of age or older and capable of giving informed consent. This guidance recommends that in vivo BE studies be conducted in individuals representative of the general population, taking into account age, sex, and race factors. If the drug product is intended for use in both sexes, the sponsor should attempt to include similar proportions of males and females in the study.

The FDA guidance provides leeway for the clinical study population. However, the RFP needs to specifically address the expected composition of the volunteer population. In order to expedite recruitment, it is best to use males and females without specifying a specific ratio of males to females. The study population is also defined by the drug product; for example, an oral contraceptive BE study would be conducted only in females while that for a hormone replacement product should be conducted in postmenopausal females. Given the difficulties in recruiting some of these special populations, it is important that the sponsor define (up-front) the maximum number of dosing groups that may be allowed.

4.2.4. Inclusion/Exclusion Criteria

The protocol inclusion/exclusion criteria such as acceptable ranges for age and weight, race restrictions and whether smokers will be allowed to participate can affect the clinic's ability to recruit and can have a significant effect on the cost of the clinical trial. The FDA BA/BE guidance (3) continues as follows:

> If the drug product is to be used predominantly in the elderly, the sponsor should attempt to include as many subjects of 60 years of age or older as possible. The total number of subjects in the study should provide adequate power for BE demonstration, but it is not expected that there will be sufficient power to draw conclusions for each subgroup. Statistical analysis of subgroups is not recommended. Restrictions on admission into the study should generally be based solely on safety considerations. In some instances, it may be useful to admit patients into BE studies for whom a drug product is intended. In this situation, sponsors and/or applicants should attempt to enter patients whose disease process is stable for the duration of the BE study. In accordance with 21 CFR 320.31, for some products that will be submitted in ANDAs, an IND may be required for BE studies to ensure patient safety.

Since a BA/BE study for any given drug product may or may not require special inclusion criteria, it is best that any expectations be documented in the RFP. These criteria will affect recruitment and the study cost; when comparing proposals between different CROs, it is best to evaluate any additional assumptions that the CRO made with regard to these criteria.

4.2.5. Lab Chemistries/Special Tests/Physicals

The number of lab chemistries, physical examinations (by a physician), and special tests (such as ECGs, x-rays, blood glucose monitoring, special biomarkers, etc.) will have a significant effect on the cost of the study. Although the protocol may be very specific regarding the timing and numbers of tests, this information must be present in the RFP in order to provide an accurate proposal.

4.2.6. Dose and Safety Considerations

For most drug products, the RLD (reference listed drug) and strength(s) to be used in the BE study are provided in the FDA "Orange Book" (4). Generally the dose of the RLD is safe to administer to healthy volunteers. However, for some drug products, that dose may cause adverse events and the clinical trial will require additional safety considerations. For example, prazosin has a significant first dose effect that is exhibited by marked postural hypotension; prazosin studies usually require that volunteers stay in a reclined position for several hours after dosing and that blood pressure be routinely monitored. Diltiazem and other calcium channel blockers can cause significant AV block; studies with this drug should include serial lead II ECGs in order to monitor for cardiac adverse events.

Since it is in the best interest (and required by the IRB) for both the CRO and the pharmaceutical company to ensure subject safety, any known adverse events should be communicated early in the RFP process so that safety procedures can be included in the study budget. If this information is left out of the RFP, then competitive bids may or may not include safety considerations (depending on each CRO's experience with the drug) that could result in two proposals with very different prices.

4.2.7. Clinical Conduct

Clinical bids are based on the version of the study outline or protocol submitted with the RFP. A number of factors affect the price of clinical studies. Some of these are shown below:

- Population (volunteers vs. patients, males vs. males and females, postmenopausal females).
- Number of volunteers or patients.
- Inclusion/exclusion criteria.
- Volunteer stipend.
- Number of lab chemistries and special tests (ECGs, blood glucose monitoring, etc.).
- Dose (with regard to safety and adverse events).
- Washout period.
- Number of blood draws and urine collections and times of sampling.

Protocol revisions or amendments that change or add services, including but not limited to labs, samples, procedures, personnel or clinical summary report writing, will usually require a revised or amended cost quotation.

4.2.8. Clinical Database

A clinical database (which contains all of the information on the case report forms) is not necessary for BE submissions to the Office of Generic Drugs. Also, it is rare that such a database would be required by FDA for a single dose BE or BA study (in volunteers) to support an NDA submission. However, some companies require all CRF data to be entered into a database so that these data can be included in the overall safety database for the NDA. It should be apparent that inclusion of such a database will increase the cost of the study. Companies should carefully review proposals from CROs to determine if such a database has been included.

4.3. Bioanalytical

Any bioanalytical method used for a human BA/BE study should conform to current FDA guidance (2) on analytical validation and should be conducted according to FDA cGLP (current good laboratory practices).

4.3.1. Bioanalytical Method/Technology Requirements

Generally the technology used for bioanalysis is dependent on the requirements for sensitivity, specificity, accuracy and precision, and throughput. It is not necessary to use a mass spectrometry (MS) assay when these needed criteria can be met using HPLC or GC methods. In fact, most CROs charge more for assays that are based on MS as compared to those using HPLC.

Ideally, any CRO should have a validated analytical method in place prior to dosing the clinical trial. On occasion, a pharmaceutical company may need to contract the method development and validation to a CRO. Since the method ruggedness is dependent on the development and validation processes, these processes should be closely evaluated prior to committing a BA or BE study to any CRO.

4.3.2. Project Timelines and Turnaround Times

Project timelines are highly method-specific. Sample analysis timing and throughput should be discussed, understood, and agreed upon before project agreement. Most CROs have standard turnaround times that will apply unless they are otherwise negotiated. It is also important to negotiate the timeline for the final written analytical report otherwise standard CRO timelines will be assumed. These standard timelines may be acceptable; however, it is important to get all timelines committed in writing.

4.3.3. Analytical Report and Data Format

If a client-specific bioanalytical report format, template, or file is to be used to record data, the format, template, or file, along with any instructions, must be provided to the laboratory before or with the shipment of samples. Sponsors should be aware that implementation of client-specific formats may result in additional charges.

4.3.4. Assay of Samples from Placebo-treated Subjects

Generally, samples from placebo-treated subjects are not an issue with BE studies. However, some BA studies may include placebo treatments so that safety can be more appropriately evaluated. For these studies, it is essential to communicate with the CRO regarding the handling and analysis of these samples. All CROs will charge for each sample that is assayed; some CROs will assay all samples, whether or not they were generated in a placebo-treated subject. If the firm does not require placebo-treated samples to be analyzed (since they generally would not provide any meaningful pharmaco-kinetic data), it is important to provide the randomization schedule to the laboratory before analysis.

4.3.5. SOPs

There must be prior agreement and upfront expectations with regard to SOPs. Some firms require that the CROs follow the firm's SOPs while other companies permit the CRO to operate under their own SOPs. Since the scope of work is affected by the standard operating procedures, this specifi-cation must be defined during the RFP process and in the CROs proposal.

4.3.6. Bioanalytical Sample Handling, Shipping, and Storage

Samples originating in HIV-exposed, or other infectious subject populations may involve liabilities to clients, clinics, couriers, and laboratories. These samples will require special documentation, shipping, and handling. The clinic, shipping service, regulatory agencies, customs authorities, and the bioanalytical laboratory must be formally notified of all special handling requirements before shipment to the laboratory. Thorough documentation of potentially infectious samples must be included with each shipment container.

Incomplete, illegible, or conflicting information in the sample inven-tory documentation may delay analytical timelines. Most CROs will accept electronic sample inventory information files; these should be received with the samples provided to the CRO with the electronic information that will be used to support the final analytical report.

Sample storage conditions must be described in the protocol and are usually dependent on the conditions used for the analytical validation. The samples should be stored using conditions consistent with the validation. Long-term storage charges should be negotiated with each CRO.

4.3.7. Quality Assurance

All bioanalytical data should be reviewed by and released from the labora-tory's Quality Assurance Unit. Although the laboratory may provide data that are reviewed via a quality control process, these data should not be considered final until after the QA audit and release. Note that QA approved data are especially important for GLP studies. The timelines for the final QA-approved data and bioanalytical report should be part of the negotiations with each CRO.

4.3.8. Miscellaneous Bioanalytical Billing Practices

As mentioned earlier, most CROs charge on a per-sample pricing basis (based on the number of samples assayed). However, it is important to point out that the sample count may change without the laboratory's knowledge. For example, the study protocol may be altered to dose fewer (or more) subjects or subjects may drop out of the study due to adverse events. Thus the final analytical price (based on the number of samples received and assayed) may differ from that in the proposal. Also, some CROs charge for additional sample analyses when sample concentrations exceed the calibration range; in these cases, the samples must be diluted and reassayed. Additionally, some CROs may charge for client-requested repeat analyses (e.g., for reanalyzing samples that appear to be pharmacokinetic outliers or fall outside of the calibration range). Although FDA discourages this practice, many pharmaceutical clients still require aberrant samples to be repeated. In these cases, it is important that the company consider the CRO policy for reassays prior to awarding a study to any particular CRO.

4.4. Pharmacokinetic and Statistical Analyses

4.4.1. Pharmacokinetic Analyses and Statistical Assessment
of PK Data

The costs of providing pharmacokinetic services are dependent on a number of variables. Table 3 provides the requirements that should either be available in the protocol or be explicitly stated in the RFP.

4.4.2. Statistical Assessments

The costs of providing statistical services are also dependent on a number of variables. This information must be explicitly stated in the RFP or must be available to be extracted from the protocol:

- Since the statistical analysis plan (SAP) is a long and comprehensive document, the number of review cycles that the client company expects can have significant effect on the cost of this document.
- Expedited timelines for production of statistical tables, listings and graphs can affect the cost of this deliverable.
- Requirements for client-specific table, listing, and graph formats can affect the cost of these services. Most CROs offer standard formats (which are ready for ICH-recommended NDA appendices). These standard formats should be considered if cost is a significant factor for the client company.

TABLE 3 Checklist of Pharmacokinetic Study Requirements that Should Be Included in the RFP

	Check (✓)
Pharmacokinetic analyses	Noncompartmental
	Compartmental modeling
Specific software requirements	SAS
	WinNonlin
	Other (Specify)
Bioequivalence analysis	Average BE
	Population BE
	Individual BE
The number of analytes and matrices (e.g., parent drug only in plasma vs. parent plus three metabolites in plasma and urine)	Enter the number of plasma analytes
	Enter the number of urine analytes
	Enter the number of analytes in "other" matrix and identify
Pharmacokineticist responsible to evaluate bioanalytical data for aberrant values	CRO
	Client
Analytical and data base file formats	CRO
	Client
Timelines (i.e., expedited turnaround within 1–2 days may be a significant cost variable for the CRO)	Normal
	Expedited
	Other (define)
Format requirement of pharmacokinetic tables and graphs	CRO
	Client

- The number of unique tables, listings, and graphs will affect the cost.
- The complexity of the statistical analyses will affect the cost.

5. PROPOSAL REVIEW

Once the RFP has been compiled and submitted, each CRO will provide a detailed proposal. These proposals should be carefully evaluated to assure that each CRO used the same set of assumptions. This is especially important when the company has submitted an RFP with only minimal information or with information that could be subject to interpretation. When comparing the resulting proposals, it is important to make sure that all of the pharmaceutical company's criteria are met.

Often, study costs contained in proposals from different CROs may be substantially different. These differences may be explained by additional assumptions contained within the proposal. For example, one CRO may have assumed a larger dropout rate (due to adverse events) based on previous experience with the drug. In order to meet the expected timeline, the CRO may require (1) a larger stipend and (2) to dose a larger number of volunteers in order to complete the required number of subjects. A different CRO may not have had experience with the drug product and would have based their proposal on dosing and completing the same number of subjects in the RFP while providing a stipend that would be appropriate for drug studies which have little or no adverse events. Thus, it is obvious that a simple comparison of cost alone is not sufficient when evaluating the proposals.

A number of case examples are provided below which some of the proposal differences in BA and BE studies are demonstrated. These cases were selected since they illustrate the dependency of cost on the complexity of the data management, pharmacokinetics, statistics, and final report.

5.1. Generic BE Studies

A Generic Manufacturer wishes to outsource a BE study (or studies) intended to establish the bioequivalence of their generic formulation with that of the reference listed product. The goal of this program, then, is to provide a final written report containing all BE data required by Office of Generic Drugs (OGD), in a format acceptable to OGD. In this case, the CRO should bid on either one or two studies (a fasting and perhaps a fed study (5), depending on the FDA requirement for the food effect study for this particular drug product). Since OGD does not require a comprehensive clinical database, it is not necessary for the CRO to include a database in the proposal. Also, since the client is only submitting the application to the OGD, a fully integrated/ICH-formatted report is not necessary. Thus the proposal should reflect costs for one or two BE clinical studies, bioanalytical services (including report), and a final pharmacokinetic report (with minimal statistics) which provides confidence intervals for C_{max} and AUC.

5.2. Generic Scale-up and Post-Approval BE Studies

A Generic Manufacturer wishes to outsource the BE study intended to support the BE of a reformulated solid oral dosage form that is the subject of an approved ANDA. Since the FDA does not require a comprehensive safety database, the CRO should base their costs on a relatively simple BE trial and pharmacokinetic report that establishes the bioequivalence of the reformulated drug product (with the reference listed product).

5.3. BA or BE Study for a New Chemical Entity

A pharmaceutical company is developing an NCE (new chemical entity) for marketing approval in the United States and Europe. This company is outsourcing a bioavailability study comparing the bioavailability of a tablet (to be used in Phase II and III clinical trials) to that of a solution. This client has determined that they need an ICH compliant report and a clinical database that can be integrated into their overall NDA safety database. In this case, the CRO's proposal should encompass much more than that in Cases 1 and 2. In addition to clinical and bioanalytical services, the proposal should also include data management, biostatistics, pharmacokinetics, and medical writing.

5.4. Drug Interaction Study (BA); Short Turnaround Time from RFP to Proposal

An international pharmaceutical company is developing an NCE for marketing approval in the United States and Europe. This company is outsourcing a drug interaction study; the RFP is based on a draft protocol and the proposal had to be received within 3 days. This client specified that they needed an ICH compliant report and a clinical database for integration into the NDA safety database.

In this case, one CRO based their costs on the information contained in the summary sections (a single analyte in plasma and a simple statistical analysis) while another CRO based their costs on a more in-depth analysis of the protocol. Unfortunately, since the protocol was a draft, it provided contradictory specifications. The second CRO provided a budget based on additional data that required pharmacokinetic and statistical analyses on the parent drug and three metabolites in plasma and urine. Additionally, this CRO included a more comprehensive statistical analysis and, obviously, their proposal was significantly more expensive than that of the first CRO. If the company bases their CRO choice on price alone, then the project would be awarded to the first CRO. Also, if the company did require the more complex analyses, then this CRO will ask for an out-of-scope increase in budget (and could be accused of a "bait and switch"). It is clear that these parties (the client company and both CROs) failed to communicate their assumptions. However, this is a common event when proposals need to be delivered within a short timeframe.

As can be seen with these case examples, it is critical that the CRO and company fully understand the objectives of the clinical trial and the specifications of the deliverables. If the expectations are not clear, then it is incumbent on both parties to communicate, understand, and discuss/confirm all requirements.

6. CONTRACTUAL OBLIGATIONS BETWEEN CROS AND SPONSORS

Contract terms and conditions provide the best controls that both the company and CRO have with each other. However, in the rush to get a study initiated, contract considerations are often overlooked. These controls are necessary since the FDA holds the company (not the CRO) responsible for any contractor failures. A good contract provides the company with control and remedies in the event of poor contractor performance.

When drafting a contract, the following areas need to be considered:

- Do the individuals, responsible for drafting the contract, understand the objectives and details of the clinical trial?
- Is the contract specific as to the duties?
- Is the scope adequately defined?
- Is there a legal review by both the company and CRO?
- Are there acceptable objective performance standards? What standards are used to assess performance?
- Is a schedule for critical tasks included? A detailed description of tasks should include monitoring, audits, data handling, and timing of the clinical, bioanalytical, and final report.
- Any contract modifications should include protocol amendments.
- The contract should provide details of mutual responsibilities.
- The contract should provide remedy for contract breech or substandard performance. These remedies include discussion/mediation, arbitration, and refund/rework if performance does not meet contract specifications.
- Does the contract provide for disclosure of FDA inspections and/or inquiries?
- The contract should address intellectual property (e.g., patents, copyrights, trade secrets) and use and disclosure of company technology, data, and publicity.

Master Service Agreements (MSAs) are becoming popular with many pharmaceutical firms. These agreements enable companies to work under a single agreement; individual projects are appended as attachments (sometimes called work orders) to the MSA. It is important that each amendment contain precise specifications, timelines, and any terms that may be different from the MSA. The MSA is a useful concept when it is necessary to quickly begin a study. Since most of the legal wording has already been approved, it is usually easier to append the work order and initiate the project.

7. PROJECT MANAGEMENT AND TIMELINES

It is important that the CROs appoint a project manager who will be assigned for the duration of the project and will serve as the central contact person. The Project Manager's responsibilities will include managing the technical and administrative aspects of the study as defined by the company. The project manager will also coordinate the organization, implementation, and management of the study. In addition, the Project Manager will interact directly with the Clinical Project Director, Medical Director, Project CRA and Compliance, Data Management, Biostatistics, Pharmacokinetic, and Medical Writing personnel to ensure the effective and timely completion of the study.

7.1. The CRO/Client Project Team

Although the goal of outsourcing is to minimize the amount of effort that a company is required to perform, it is still incumbent on the firm to invest resources into study management, and to develop the optimal relationship that will drive the program to success.

7.1.1. Project Team for NDA BA/BE Studies

Those companies that outsource NDA BA or BE studies need to assemble a project team that includes individuals from both the client company as well as the CRO. In addition to the Project Manager, and in order to facilitate communication of all deliverables and expectations to the CRO, the client company should include representatives from Contracts, Pharmacokinetics (and Clinical Pharmacology if these are different departments), and Biostatistics. As mentioned earlier, although they are not part of the project team, both the CRO and company should identify individuals responsible for finance and legal issues.

7.1.2. Project Team for ANDA BE Studies

ANDA BE studies are often outsourced using very little client company participation. Most services are generally assigned to the CRO. The CRO project team should include the clinical and bioanalytical project managers, a pharmacokineticist, and a statistician.

7.2. CRO/Client Team Meetings and Communications

For programs involving multiple studies, a "kick-off" or initiation meeting between the combined project team should be held. This should be a "face-to-face" meeting at a client or CRO facility. To encourage open and frequent communication, regular team meetings should be held via teleconference. The frequency of these meetings should be specified in the project or program proposal.

8. RUNNING THE STUDY—THE DELIVERABLES

8.1. Prestudy Activities

8.1.1. Regulatory Documentation

Prior to drug shipment, the sponsor should collect, review, and approve all regulatory documents required under the United States Code of Federal Regulations (CFR) from the clinical site. Some of the more critical documents include the following:

- Protocol: Signed by the Principle Investigator and approved by the IRB.
- IRB approval letter together with a list of IRB members.
- Copy of the IRB-approved informed consent form to be used in the study.
- Signed FDA Form 1572 and curriculum vitae for the principal and sub-investigators.
- Laboratory certification and normal values.

Regulatory packets containing this information should be assembled and delivered to the pharmaceutical firm prior to shipment of drug supplies. Timely collection of these documents is critical to ensure timely shipment of the study drug to the study site. For most studies, it is expected that the client will submit the regulatory packet to the FDA as part of an IND or ANDA.

8.1.2. Management of the Test and Reference Formulations

It is important for the pharmaceutical company to understand that the reference and test products must be at the clinical site with sufficient lead-time to inventory and repackage according to the randomization. Usually, the sponsor provides all drug products that are to be used in the BA or BE trial. However, some sponsors request the CRO to purchase (through a local retail pharmacy) the reference product for BE studies. It is critical that the sponsor ensures that the CRO will purchase a sufficient amount (determined by the sponsor) of a single lot number and with an expiration date that will cover the duration of the study. Note that for ANDA BE studies, the sponsor must test the reference product for potency and dissolution.

If the CRO is responsible for repackaging the study drug products (into unit doses for each volunteer) prior to dosing, then the materials must be compatible with the drug products. This is especially important with labile drug products that may be repackaged days or weeks prior to dosing. Some clinical units dispense each subject's dose into small paper envelopes. This type of packaging may have an impact on the performance of a labile or hygroscopic dosage form. It is best for the sponsor to provide containers (bottles) that the CRO can use for repackaging the drug products.

8.1.3. Prestudy Monitoring

Many smaller firms often disregard the need for clinical monitoring. However, some monitoring is needed to ensure that all regulatory procedures are being met and that the study is conducted according to the protocol. The following areas should be reviewed with site personnel during the initiation visit:

- Background information, including the Investigator Brochure for the study drug and/or the product package insert(s).
- Protocol, study procedures, and associated forms.
- Regulatory requirements.
- Personnel training records.
- Ensure appropriate signed informed consent exists for each study participant.
- Review investigator study files for completeness.

8.1.4. The Project Initiation Meeting

Prior to study conduct, the CRO should hold a kick-off meeting that includes all departments (e.g., clinical, analytical, PK, data management, biostatistics, medical writing) and the client. If more than one CRO is involved, then representatives from each CRO should be in attendance. The following areas should be reviewed:

- Provide contact information for all project team members (including the client project team members).
- Background information, including the Investigator Brochure for the study drug and/or the product package insert(s).
- All study procedures within the protocol.
- Case report forms.
- Monitoring visit schedule.

- Regulatory requirements.
- The statistical analysis plan.
- Handoffs to other departments/CROs:
  - Shipment of specimens for bioanalysis.
  - Data transfers (including case report forms, data base, bioanalytical data, statistical, and pharmacokinetic data).
- Timelines.

8.2. Conduct of the Clinical Trial

Assuming that the protocol was clearly written, most outstanding clinical questions should have been addressed during the kick-off meeting and the clinical portion of the study should run with minimal sponsor input. However, the sponsor should not become completely complacent. It is advisable to visit the clinic at least once to monitor the first dose of the study. Ideally, this visit should begin the day before dosing in order to review regulatory compliance and to physically observe dosing and execution of the protocol procedures (which often begin by 7:00 am).

8.2.1. Clinical Monitoring

If the sponsor does not have in-house clinical monitoring capabilities, this task can be assigned to the CRO. If this is the case, the monitor should be independent of the clinic in order to prevent any possible conflict of interest.

Concurrent Monitoring. Concurrent monitoring (especially monitoring the first dose) allows the sponsor to assure that the protocol is being conducted as according to the written specifications. The tasks that need to be completed at this time include the following:

- Ensure appropriate signed informed consent exists for all study participants.
- Review investigator study files for completeness.
- Ensure investigator compliance to the study protocol.
- Tracking protocol violations and/or protocol deviations.
- Review source documents for serious adverse events.
- Review drug records.
- Provide written site monitoring reports.

The clinical monitor should provide written site monitoring reports. Because of the relatively short study duration, most BA/BE studies require minimal monitoring. For example, the monitor could observe the dosing procedures in the first study period and return for a close-out visit after study completion. Additional monitoring during the study can be accomplished via telephone. Items that should be covered in these calls include verification of patient/volunteer enrollment status, review study progress, answer protocol questions, discuss CRF completion, and ensure the study proceeds in a timely manner. The sponsor/monitor should document (in writing) these site contacts, including any relevant observations, discussions, questions, and commitments.

Study Close-Out Monitoring. A final close-out visit should be conducted after all subjects have completed. This visit should include:

- Compare 100% of the CRFs to the source documents.
- Review the CRFs and source documents for serious adverse events.
- Resolve CRF queries.
- Review drug accountability.
- Review investigator study files for completeness.
- Ensure investigator compliance to the study protocol.
- Review of record retention per FDA requirements.
- Review drug product accountability and reconcile number of dosage units for FDA Compliance.

8.2.2. Clinical Review of CRFs and Query Resolution

The Clinical Project Manager and Investigator should review all case report forms. These individuals should evaluate the following elements:

- Accurate transcription of data from source documents to the CRF.
- Accurate and appropriate documentation of adverse events.
- Overall study conduct and protocol compliance.
- Identification and documentation of potential protocol deviations or violations.
- Appropriate use of medical terminology.
- Correlation of all clinical information.

8.3. Data Management

8.3.1. Data Management for ANDA-Track Studies

The Office of Generic Drugs does not require an electronic database containing all CRF data for BE trials. However, they do require that the "paper" CRFs be submitted with the final report. The complex data management tasks (necessary for many NDA-track programs) are not necessary for ANDA studies. It is often sufficient for the clinical CRO to provide a clinical report that includes demographics, adverse events, and blood sampling time deviations. These data will be used in the pharmacokinetic/statistical calculations and in the completion of the final study report.

8.3.2. Data Management for NDA-Track Studies

With the advent of electronic data capture, many clinical CROs do not require the data management function needed for NDA trials which utilize paper CRFs. However, a number of pharmaceutical companies still require completion of paper CRFs that are specifically formatted for that organization. These organizations will require a significant data management component for the study conduct. For these studies, a Clinical Data Management (CDM) Project Manager compiles a data management plan that describes the processes and specifications to be used in the project. This plan includes documentation, logic and processes for data review and validation, critical timelines and milestones and timing and types of management reports. The client company should carefully review this plan in order to assure that the database will integrate with the overall NDA safety database.

8.4. Statistical Analysis of Safety Data

As mentioned earlier for Data Management, the Office of Generic Drugs does not require statistical analysis of safety data for ANDA BE studies. However, many sponsors still require that NDA BA studies include these analyses. The statistical analysis of the study "safety data" is usually conducted in parallel (at the same time) with the blood/plasma bioanalysis.

When statistical analyses of safety data are required, the CRO should develop detailed specifications for the statistical analyses and tables' production. Generally, the programming is done within SAS®, a statistical package (acceptable to FDA), which is used to provide the final tables, graphs, and statistical analyses. The CRO should provide a detailed analysis plan with examples of the statistical output (including the tables, listings, and graphs). Any programs or macros used should be fully validated (and not just quality controlled for accuracy). This statistical output is made available to the project team and the client company and is used as the basis for writing the integrated safety report.

8.5. Bioanalytical Data

The bioanalytical work is usually straightforward, assuming that both the laboratory and the method were fully evaluated prior to dosing. Although this proactive due diligence is a necessary first step in assuring that this phase of the study will go smoothly, it should not be the only contact that the CRO has with the laboratory.

One critical area is the shipment of samples from the clinic to the laboratory. Whether the clinic is in another building at the CRO or whether the samples are being shipped to another location, nationally or internationally, it is imperative that the samples arrive at the analytical laboratory intact and frozen. Prior to any analyses, the CRO should conduct a detailed inspection and inventory of all samples. The samples should then be placed in a suitable freezer for storage until analysis takes place.

Study timelines are affected by the CRO's experience with the drug and/or metabolite and the ruggedness of the analytical method. In fact, outside of clinical recruitment and dosing, the bioanalytical phase of BA/BE studies often becomes the rate-limiting factor in the CRO's timeline. For this reason, it is usually essential that the analytical method be developed and validated prior to dosing. The unpredictability of assay development and validation timelines can have an adverse effect on the overall timeline if samples arrive at the laboratory prior to validation. However, some companies will evaluate the benefit/risk ratio before dosing without analytical validation. Their decision is based on their past experience with the CRO, the anticipated complexity of the assay, and the potential for shortening the time to get their product to market. Generic companies will carry a substantial risk when working with a CRO that has not fully developed the analytical method. However, for paragraph IV submissions, the benefit of being the first generic to submit an ANDA can outweigh this risk.

With the advent of high throughput LC/MS/MS assays, the time required for bioanalysis can be substantially shortened. Although this is generally regarded positively, it can also have a negative impact (especially for those studies with limited sample volumes) if a problem goes undetected. Therefore, it is wise to reassess the sensitivity (LOQ), specificity, and standard curve range after the first couple of analytical runs:

- Are all pre-dose sample concentration values reported as "BLQ", i.e., below the lower limit of quantitation (LOQ)?
- Is the chromatography "clean" and free of interfering peaks?
- For mass spectrometry assays, is there any indication of suppression?
- For single dose studies, do the concentrations decrease to BLQ and remain undetectable or do the concentrations fluctuate between BLQ and measurable values?
- The calibration range should be reassessed:

    - Is the LOQ too high or low?
    - Is the top end of the range sufficiently high enough so that samples do not require dilution? Some CROs charge

additional fees for diluting and reassaying samples exceeding the range of the calibration curve.

- Is the top end of the range too high? Perhaps the method was originally set up for a parenteral dosage form or for higher doses that might be needed for toxicokinetic studies. FDA reviewers have been known to question studies in which the majority of the sample concentrations fall within only the lower quarter to third of the calibration range.

Once this assessment is complete, the remaining samples can be assayed. Upon completion of the entire data set, these data should again be evaluated for "aberrant data", i.e., data that are pharmacokinetically uncharacteristic of the drug. The chromatography of these samples should be closely inspected. It is important to note that FDA has stated that samples should not be reanalyzed without objective written criteria (2).

8.6. Pharmacokinetic Analyses

As mentioned earlier, once the project specifications are known and the client has approved the proposal, the CRO should provide a detailed analysis plan. This detailed plan is generally unnecessary for a generic BE study because the analyses and report formats are straightforward and similar for most conventional BE study designs. For NDA-track BA studies, the analysis plan is relevant and it is important to have input from both the project pharmacokineticist and statistician. For these studies, the analysis plan provides details of the pharmacokinetic analyses and the statistical analyses of the safety data.

Pharmacokinetic analyses are usually conducted in accordance with CRO SOPs unless previously arranged by the client. This is important to note that some pharmaceutical companies insist that the CROs use their company's SOPs for pharmacokinetic analyses.

Noncompartmental pharmacokinetic parameters should be calculated (using validated programs) based on final (QA-approved) bioanalytical data and actual sampling times. If interim pharmacokinetic analyses are necessary, it is usually adequate to conduct these analyses using preliminary analytical data and nominal sampling times.

8.7. Preparation and Review of the Final Report

The content and format of the final report was previously included in the overall project specifications. For example, the number and layout of in-text tables and graphs and the graphics software must be identified early and must be compatible with any client-specific report template.

When the data become available, the CRO team (consisting of the pharmacokineticist, statistician, and medical writer for NDA-track programs or only the pharmacokineticist for ANDA-track programs) and the client team should meet to discuss the study results. Usually, a teleconference will suffice. It is useful to include the client's project manager, pharmacokineticist, and statistician in these team meetings. This meeting provides an opportunity for the CRO to present and discuss any unusual observations (pharmacokinetic or statistical) that should be addressed in the report and it allows early input from the client team. Early client input allows for a consensus as to the clinical relevance of the pharmacokinetic results. The CRO can then use this discussion as a basis for writing the final report.

When reviewing integrated or pharmacokinetic reports, it is good practice for sponsors to consolidate all "internal" comments from each of their (the client's) reviewers. This consolidation is necessary because multiple client reviewers can (and often do) disagree on interpretation, format, and style. Timelines can be delayed if the CRO medical writer is required to negotiate changes across departments within the client organization.

9. EVALUATION OF THE DELIVERABLES

Once a study has been successfully concluded, the CRO will produce an integrated or pharmacokinetic report. If the CRO services were contracted to multiple CROs, then the sponsor (or one of the CROs) will need to integrate information from as many as three different reports or areas:

- A bioanalytical report that provides all details of the analytical method, validation, and the complete bioanalytical results including calibrators, QC values, and appropriate chromatograms.
- A clinical report that provides the details of the clinical conduct and protocol deviations.
- A final report (often a pharmacokinetic report) that integrates the clinical conduct, bioanalysis, pharmacokinetics, and statistics of the study into a concise report in a format suitable for submission to FDA.

9.1. Bioanalytical Report Checklist

The bioanalytical report should be assessed to confirm that it provides the required information on validation. Each analyte in each biological matrix must be validated with respect to sensitivity, selectivity, accuracy, precision, reproducibility, and stability. Table 4 provides a checklist that can be used to assist with this assessment.

TABLE 4 Bioanalytical Validation and Report Assessment Checklist

Critical area	Specific area to review	Check (✓)
Sensitivity	The validation report should define and validate the lower limit of quantification (LLOQ). Chromatography should be reviewed for potential interfering substances in a biological matrix and include endogenous matrix components, metabolites and decomposition products that can affect the LLOQ.	
Selectivity	Selectivity is the ability of an analytical method to differentiate and quantify the analyte in the presence of other components in the sample. If more than one analyte is required, then each analyte should be tested (in the presence of the others) to ensure that there is no interference. Assay selectivity in the presence of any concomitant medications should be assessed.	
Accuracy	Accuracy should be measured using a minimum of five determinations per concentration. The mean value should be within 15% of the actual value except at LLOQ, where it should not deviate by more than 20%.	
Precision	Does the report include data on the precision of the analytical method (describes the closeness of individual measures of an analyte when the procedure is applied repeatedly)? Generally, the precision determined at each concentration level should be less than or equal to 15% (CV) except for the LLOQ, where it should not exceed 20% (CV). If not, is justification provided?	
Reproducibility	Does the report establish the relationship between concentration and response of the analytical method? Is it linear? Does the report demonstrate that the relationship between response and concentration is continuous and reproducible?	
Stability	Has freeze/thaw stability been assessed for at least three cycles? Has short-term temperature stability been assessed at room temperature for 4–24 h? Has long-term stability been assessed? The long-term	

(*Continued*)

Table 4 (*Continued*)

Critical area	Specific area to review	Check (✓)
	stability duration should exceed the storage time between the date of first sample collection and the date of last sample analysis. Does the report document stock solution stability? This is the stability of drug and the internal standard stock solutions that should be evaluated at room temperature for at least 6 h. Has the post-preparative stability been assessed? This is the stability of processed samples, including the resident time in the autosampler.	
Additional supportive data	The report should include separate tables summarizing calibrators and QC values collected during the analysis of the study samples. The report should include a table summarizing all repeat analyses with explanations. The report should include example chromatograms. FDA OGD requires 20% of the standard curve, QCs and study samples to be submitted.	

9.2. Clinical Report Checklist

The clinical report should be assessed to confirm that it provides all of the information required by FDA and the sponsoring company. Table 5 provides a checklist that can be used to assist with this assessment.

9.3. Integrated Pharmacokinetic Report Checklist

The integrated pharmacokinetic report (i.e., the final report) should be assessed to confirm that it provides all of the information required by FDA and the sponsoring company. Table 6 provides a checklist that can be used to assist with this assessment.

10. WORKING TOGETHER WHEN A STUDY GIVES UNEXPECTED RESULTS

Because BA and BE studies include complex processes, it is not unusual for unanticipated "problems" to arise. However, clear and effective

TABLE 5 Clinical Study Report Checklist

Specific area to review	Check (✓)
Were there any protocol deviations?	
Did all subjects meet inclusion/exclusion criteria?	
If not, were the deviations clinically significant and did the principle investigator and client approve all deviations?	
Did the study recruit and dose the number of subjects required by the protocol?	
Were the appropriate number of men and women (where applicable) dosed?	
If not, are the reasons identified in the clinical report?	
Did all subjects complete all phases of the study?	
Are dropouts described?	
Was the study dosed as a single group?	
If not, are the reasons discussed in the report and did the client approve multiple dosing groups?	
Does the report include a demographics table identifying subject number, age, gender, weight, height, frame size, and smoker/non-smoker status?	
Are all adverse events summarized in the report?	
Were any adverse events classified as serious and unexpected?	
Were these reported to FDA within the required time interval?	
Did any subjects vomit at any time during the treatment phases?	
If so, are the dates and times relative to dosing recorded?	
Were all blood (and urine when appropriate) samples collected?	
Were all samples collected on time?	
If not, does the report identify missing samples (with reasons) and late/early blood and urine collections?	
Does the report include a physical description of the drug products, lot numbers and expiration dates?	
Were the drug products administered in the fasting state (except for food effect studies) with 240 mL (8 oz.) of water?	
If not, is justification included in the report or protocol?	
Were subjects allowed to have water (ad lib) except for one hour before and after drug administration?	
Was the washout period identical for all subjects (and groups, where applicable)?	
Were standardized meals provided no less than four hours after drug administration?	
Were meals identical in each phase of the study?	
Did the subjects abstain from alcohol for 24 h prior to each study period and until after the last sample from each period was collected?	

(Continued)

Table 5 (*Continued*)

Specific area to review	Check (✓)
Does the report provide a summary of dosing and the randomization (subject, sequence, period, treatment)?	

communications, appropriate planning and willingness of both parties to identify and fix the problem can prevent most of these problems or issues. These problems can be as "simple" as missing expected timelines to as complex as failure to establish bioequivalence in a BE study. A number of issues and problems are discussed in the following sections.

10.1. Clinical

10.1.1. Recruitment Issues Delayed Study Timelines

Recruitment issues can lead to delayed clinical timelines and may result in analytical delays that can cause the overall study timeline to increase. Sponsors and CROs need to pay special attention to any protocol design issue that may affect the ability to recruit the target population. For example, if the sponsor insists on an exact 50/50 mix of males and females, then the CRO could have difficulty in recruiting the study as a single dosing group. As another example, recruitment could be an issue if a sponsor places a very narrow age range on an elderly subject population. In these cases, it is prudent for the client and CRO to discuss any recruitment issues early and to work closely during the "recruitment" phase so that there are no surprises.

10.1.2. Clinical Dropouts and Clinical "No-Shows"

Clinical dropouts and no-shows can affect the clinical completion date. The number of dropouts and no-shows should be anticipated by the CRO. Given this information (based on past studies) the CRO and sponsor should agree to recruit and dose additional subjects so that the required number to complete can be met. As above, the sponsor and CRO should stay in close communication during the planning phases to allow for this potential (but predictable) problem.

The clinical dropouts and no-shows can also have a significant effect on the outcome and validity of the study. It is critical that the protocol includes information as to the statistical treatment of data due to dropouts, the use of replacement and/or reserve subjects, the bioanalysis of samples from dropouts, replacement and/or reserve subjects. Several examples/issues follow.

TABLE 6   Integrated Pharmacokinetic Report Checklist

	Check (✓)

Is the study design appropriate?

Does the PK report provide lot numbers, expiration dates, and
potency values?

Did the test and reference product potencies differ by no more
than 5%?

Were the appropriate moieties (analytes) measured
  (as defined in section IV.B of the general BA/BE guidance)?
    Parent drug and major active metabolites for NDA BA
      studies
    Parent only for BE studies, unless the metabolite is formed
      as a result of gut wall or other presystemic metabolism

Was blood sampling adequate to define the PK of the drug
  (and active metabolites)?
    Twelve to eighteen samples including pre-dose
    C_{max} should not be the first point
    Three to four samples should be obtained during the
      terminal log-linear phase

Was the washout period adequate (≥ 5 times the half-life)?

Were all pre-dose values $< LOQ$?
    If not, were all pre-dose values $\leq 5\%$ of each respective
      C_{max} value?
    Were all subjects with pre-dose values $\geq 5\%$ of
      C_{max} dropped from all BE study calculations?

First-point C_{max}: Do any of the concentrations vs. time profiles
  exhibit first-point C_{max} (i.e., the first sample collected is the
  C_{max} value)?
    If so, were 3–5 samples collected within the firsthour and
      was one of these collected between 5 and 15 min
      post-dose?
    If these early samples were collected, no change indata
      analysis is warranted.
    If these early samples were not collected, then those
      subjects with first point C_{max} values should be
      dropped from the primary statistical analysis

Did any adverse events (e.g., emesis) occur that would alter
  the drug pharmacokinetics?
    For IR products, did any subject vomit at or before the
      median T_{max}? If so, were these subjects dropped from
      the analyses?
    For MR products, did any subject vomit at anytime during
      the labeled dosing interval? If so, were these subjects
      dropped?

(Continued)

Table 6 (*Continued*)

	Check (✓)
Does the PK report provide the following information?	
Plasma concentrations and actual sampling time points	
Identification of subject, period, sequence, and treatment assignments	
Values for AUC_{0-t}, $AUC_{0-\infty}$, C_{max}, T_{max}, Kel and half-life	
Subject by formulation interaction variance component (for individual bioequivalence {replicate design} studies)	
For steady-state studies: C_{min}, C_{ave}, degree of fluctuation, Partial AUC, and % Swing for drug products in which early exposure is important	
Geometric and arithmetic means, ratio of the means, and confidence intervals on log-transformed AUC and C_{max}	
Do confidence intervals fall between 80.00% and 125.00%?	

A common result of a protocol that does not allow for the replacement of dropouts is a statistically nonbalanced study. Small differences in the number of subjects in each treatment (i.e., 1 or 2 out of a group of 12–18) will not usually have a statistically significant effect on a two period (two treatment) BE study. This study design is usually robust enough to handle small differences in group sizes. However, larger numbers of dropouts can cause a significant sequence or subject-by-sequence effect. A statistically significant effect (due to an unbalanced design) can result in a "nonapprovable" BE study.

Protocols that allow replacement of dropouts can experience another problem that can potentially invalidate a biostudy. Some protocol designs allow "make-up" groups to be dosed if an insufficient number of subjects do not report for any one dosing period. The use of make-up groups can have disastrous consequences for a BE or BA study. As mentioned earlier, a statistical test for pool-ability of the data from these groups is required. If these make-up groups are unbalanced, or small in number, then it is difficult to statistically prove pool-ability. If this occurs, then the data cannot be pooled and the result is often (or usually) an inability to establish bioequivalence.

The bioanalysis of samples from dropout subjects becomes a dilemma if not addressed in the protocol. Many companies specify (in the protocol) that only samples from subjects completing both (or all) periods of a study will be analyzed. The analysis of samples from "incomplete subjects" usually will not affect the statistical outcome of a study. However, an unbalanced study may affect the arithmetic mean data. Also, since the unbalanced data are of no use in establishing bioequivalence, it is not cost-effective to analyze these samples. Unfortunately, and unless stated in the protocol, FDA generally expects to see all data generated from samples obtained in clinical trials.

A similar problem is encountered when dosing "reserve" subjects to assure completion of a minimum number of completers. If 28 subjects are dosed to complete 24 and all 28 complete both periods, then the company/CRO must "decide" which subjects (or how many subjects) to assay. This problem is alleviated if the protocol specifically addresses which subjects will have samples assayed (for example, the first 12 subjects from each dosing sequence who complete both periods).

Dropout and/or replacement subjects can cause a number of potential problems; some of these problems can be trivial while others can cause a study to "fail" FDA criteria. It is important to address these issues within the protocol otherwise the company/CRO will have to live with the consequences. While addressing these problems during the protocol development phase of the study, the company will need to come to terms with the financial implications of dosing replacement/reserve subjects (including the bioanalytical costs) as well as the ethical implications of exposing more human subjects to an experimental drug and possibly discarding data from those subjects.

10.1.3. Unanticipated Adverse Events

Unanticipated adverse events, or a larger than expected number of adverse events, can affect the completion date for those studies that require a fixed number of subjects to complete all treatments. The sponsor and CRO should discuss the effect of adverse events (based on the drug class if there is no experience) on the dropout rate for the study. Although, unanticipated adverse events are difficult to estimate, it is prudent to develop protocols that overestimate the dropout rate so that a sufficient number of subjects complete.

10.1.4. Dosing Errors

Dosing errors should not occur if the protocol is clearly written and the clinic follows the instructions. If dosing errors do occur, the credibility of the CRO clinic comes into question. The CRO should provide the results of an in-depth investigation together with a procedure to insure that the problem would not be repeated. If the problem was due to vague protocol instructions, then the CRO should address any questions prior to dosing.

10.1.5.   Blood Collection Errors

Blood collection errors involving collection of the wrong time points or collection of blood using the wrong anticoagulant can occur. Analytical methods are usually developed for a particular matrix and additional validation may be required for matrix changes (e.g., plasma to serum, heparinized plasma vs. EDTA plasma). Although, blood collection errors do occasionally occur, the problem may be due to conflicting instructions within the protocol. It is incumbent on the CRO to thoroughly read all sections of the protocol and to identify any discrepancies prior to clinical conduct.

10.2.   Bioanalytical Issues

Most of these bioanalytical "problems" can be avoided if appropriate due diligence is provided prior to awarding the study or at least prior to dosing.

10.2.1.   Validated Methods not Reproducible Under Clinical Conditions

Bioanalytical methods are usually validated using five or six sources of "control" matrix (serum, plasma, etc.). However, this is often not sufficient to provide assurance that the assay will be sufficiently rugged to measure concentrations from 24 or more subjects. Sponsors should be cautious when awarding studies to a CRO with an "untested" or unvalidated analytical method. Experience is the key; unless timing is an issue, sponsors should thoroughly assess validation packages and the CRO's experience.

10.2.2.   Excessive Number of Rejected Runs

This becomes a problem when an excessive number of rejected runs affects analytical timelines. This problem is often indicative of an assay that is not rugged and has not been developed for studies with large numbers of samples. As above, lack of experience with the method should have indicated that the CRO might have a difficult time in meeting aggressive timelines. Sponsors should carefully assess the validation package for ruggedness and should include additional analytical time for those methods without a high experience level.

10.2.3.   Number of Reassays Exceeds Freeze–Thaw Validation Cycles

Occasionally, the number of times that some samples are reassayed exceeds the number of freeze–thaw cycles included in the validation package. This is another indicator that an assay was not sufficiently rugged for routine clinical studies. If a CRO has to reassay samples several times (perhaps due to rejected runs), then the FDA will question the validity of the analytical method. Close communication between the sponsor and the CRO is required in this situation; the CRO should not finalize the analytical report until the validation report is supplemented to contain data that will support the additional freeze–thaw cycles.

10.2.4.   Clinical Samples Arrive at Laboratory Prior
          to Assay Validation

Study delays occur when clinical samples arrive at the laboratory prior to completion of assay development or validation. This is a problem that occurs most often when a sponsor is on a tight timeline and has provided a "dosing date" to their management. It is unwise and risky to begin dosing a study while assay development or validation is still ongoing. It is usually best to delay dosing until the assay has been fully developed and validated.

10.2.5.   Insufficient Long-Term Frozen Stability Data

Delays in assay validation can have additional trickle-down effects on the conduct of BA/BE studies. This can result in a report that provides insufficient long-term stability data necessary to support clinical trial sample stability. FDA's bioanalytical guidance requires that drug companies and CROs include, in each report, long-term stability data that should exceed the time between the date of first sample collection and the date of last sample analysis. Clinical study delays may lengthen the storage time to beyond that in the validation report. However, most CROs will ship "spiked frozen controls" to the clinical site prior to dosing. These samples are stored with the samples from the clinical trial and are shipped back to the analytical laboratory upon completion of the trial. Assay of these control samples will provide the necessary long-term stability needed for FDA approval. If these control samples were not prepared proactively, then the sponsor will have to accept a delayed timeline since the analytical report is not considered complete without these additional data.

10.2.6.   Clinical Sample Matrix Different from Validated Matrix

This problem sometimes occurs when clinical protocols are not written specifically with regard to the anticoagulant. For example, a protocol may specify EDTA as the anticoagulant but the laboratory has validated the analytical method for heparinized plasma (using sodium heparin), then the laboratory will be required to conduct a "cross-validation" to establish that there is no matrix effect. This situation may occur when multiple CROs are involved in a single study. It is incumbent on the client to assure that the protocol contains the necessary collection and storage conditions that match the analytical validation.

10.2.7.   Limit of Quantification (LOQ) Set Too High/Calibration Curve Range not Appropriate

The LOQ is sometimes set inappropriately based on experience with alternative dosage strengths, dosage forms or even based on preclinical experience. Similarly, the validated calibration range may be based on experience with higher doses. This problem can usually be avoided by obtaining advice from a pharmacokineticist from either the client company or the CRO.

10.2.8.   Specificity not Adequately Established

FDA expects specificity to be established in the presence of metabolites and concomitant medications. All analytical methods should be validated in the presence of all known, major metabolites. Often, the metabolites are unknown during early phase I studies on new chemical entities. However, once the metabolites are identified, the validation should be amended to contain the additional specificity data. Also, analytical methods should be validated in the presence of known OTC drugs. Usually, this is accomplished by testing a "cocktail" or mixture during validation. This is usually done as a precaution since BE studies should be conducted in volunteers and in the absence of any concomitant medications. However, it is not unusual for one or two volunteers in a study to take an OTC drug product (e.g., ibuprofen or acetominophen for headache relief). Once a clinical study is completed, the clinic should report all concomitant medications to the laboratory. The laboratory should include additional assay specificity data in the final analytical report.

10.3.   Statistical (When a Study Fails)

10.3.1.   Insufficient Subjects Due to Adverse Events

Adverse events (such as emesis) can alter the number of subjects that can be included in the pharmacokinetic and statistical analysis. The FDA general BA/BE guidance is quite specific on how these events should be handled. It is extremely important that the project pharmacokineticist, clinical, and analytical project managers and the client discuss the impact of these adverse events prior to completing the clinical conduct and/or the bioanalytical analyses. If these adverse events alter the number of "pharmacokinetically evaluable" subjects, then consideration should be given to amending the protocol (prior to assaying samples) to ensure that an adequate number of evaluable subjects (to yield statistical power) will complete the clinical phase of the study.

10.3.2. Statistical Issues: Power and Failed BE Study

It is important to maintain the statistical power of a study by ensuring that the required numbers of subjects complete the study. Often, though, statistical power is a secondary consideration. However, for generic BE studies, it is critical that an adequate number of subjects be dosed in order to meet the confidence interval criteria for bioequivalence. The inability to prove BE may be due to dosing too few subjects or to a true formulation difference. If the ratio of the means (for AUC or C_{max}) is close to unity, but the confidence intervals do not include the goalposts (usually 80%–125%), then the solution may be to dose a new study with more subjects. However, if the ratio of the means is substantially different from 1.00, then the test formulation may indeed be bioinequivalent. At this point, the client should discuss these data with their drug product formulators.

10.3.3. Statistical Issues: Group Effects

Group effects are relevant only when a study is unable to dose as a single group. For example, if a CRO enrolls only 16 subjects (from a 24 subject study), then a "makeup group" is required. However, FDA now requires that "pool-ability" be tested. A significant group effect often means that a BE study may fail to establish bioequivalence since the data from the two groups cannot be pooled and must be evaluated separately. The best solution is to avoid using multiple groups within BE studies by recruiting and dosing an adequate number of subjects to complete as a single dosing group.

10.4. FDA Preapproval Inspection of the CRO and FDA Form 483

It is not unusual for FDA's Office of Compliance to "inspect" the clinical and analytical conduct of most generic BE studies for ANDA applications and to issue an FDA Form 483. This form provides a listing of observations that are to be corrected. These observations can range from relatively minor observations to significant cGLP or cGCP violations. However, serious FDA 483's can usually be avoided by conducting a thorough due diligence assessment of the CRO prior to study assignment.

In the past, only major problems were listed on an FDA 483; however, today, even minor observations are being recorded. One of the keys to a successful study is to provide an acceptable and timely response to the Agency. The CRO should notify the client company of any FDA inspection at the time of the inspection and should provide a copy of the 483 to the client company. The CRO response to the 483 should be discussed with the client company prior to submitting the response to the Agency. Finally, when the response is submitted to FDA, a copy should be provided to the client company.

11. SUMMARY

This chapter has provided a process for working with CROs to conduct BA or BE studies. The process began with an assessment of a number of CROs (and their capabilities) and included a due diligence inspection. It is critical to the process of working effectively with CROs that client companies (and the CRO) precisely define deliverables and expectations, assign a qualified project team and develop communication systems that work for both the CRO and client company. If the client and CRO team members monitor and review deliverables and timelines, then there should be no surprises with regard to the timeliness and quality of the final deliverables.

Finally, it is worth emphasizing that the success of an outsourced clinical study is dependent on close collaboration and seamless communication between their organizations. This collaboration (partnership) requires open communication, sensitivity to project requirements and timelines and flexibility on the part of both the CRO and client company that are necessary to achieve study success.

REFERENCES

1. Shah VP, Midha KK, Findlay JWA, Hill HM, Hulse JD, McGilveray IJ, McKay G, Miller KJ, Patnaik RN, Powell ML, Tonelli A, Viswanathan CT, Yacobi A. Bioanalytical method validation—a revisit with a decade of progress. Pharma Res 2000; 17(12):1551–1557.
2. Guidance for Industry: Bioanalytical Method Validation. US Department of Health and Human Services, Food and Drug Administration, Center for Drug Evaluation and Research (CDER), Center for Veterinary Medicine (CVM), May 2001. http://www.fda.gov/cder/guidance/4252fnl.pdf.
3. Guidance for Industry: Bioavailability and Bioequivalence Studies for Orally Administered Drug Products—General Considerations. US Department of Health and Human Services, Food and Drug Administration, Center for Drug Evaluation and Research (CDER), October 2000. http://www.fda.gov/cder/guidance/3615fnl.pdf.
4. Approved Drug Products with Therapeutic Equivalence Evaluations. 21st ed. Department of Health and Human Services, Public Health Service, Food and Drug Administration, Center for Drug Evaluation and Research, Office of Information Technology, Division of Data Management and Services, 2001. http://www.fda.gov/cder/ob.
5. Guidance for Industry: Food-Effect Bioavailability and Bioequivalence Studies, Draft Guidance. US Department of Health and Human Services, Food and Drug

Administration, Center for Drug Evaluation and Research (CDER), October 1997. http://www.fda.gov/cder/guidance/1719dft.pdf.

6. Guidance for Industry: Preparing Data for Electronic Submission in ANDAs. US Department of Health and Human Services, Food and Drug Administration, Center for Drug Evaluation and Research (CDER), OGD, September 1999. http://www.fda.gov/cder/guidance/3223fnl.pdf.

14

Legal and Legislative Hurdles to Generic Drug Development, Approval, and Marketing

Arthur Y. Tsien

Olsson, Frank and Weeda, P.C., Washington, DC, USA

1. INTRODUCTION

The preceding chapters have discussed a variety of scientific, technical, and regulatory considerations related to the development and approval of generic drug products. To compliment that discussion, this chapter is written from the perspective of a lawyer specializing in the drug regulatory process. This chapter discusses a variety of legal and legislative considerations, as well as some miscellaneous regulatory considerations. There are, of course, no clear lines dividing the "scientific," "regulatory," and "legal" arenas in the context of generic drug development and approval. While some of the disputes discussed in this chapter have a "scientific" underpinning, the matters have often presented themselves in the litigation context.

As of this writing, there is litigation in progress that affects, in particular, Orange Book patent listings. This and other areas discussed in this chapter are in a state of flux. Thus, a prudent prospective ANDA sponsor that does not have the requisite in-house resources would be well advised to consult with competent regulatory consultants or legal counsel on these issues during the business decision-making, drug development, and drug approval processes.

Some of the examples described in this chapter do not involve solid oral dosage forms. These examples have nevertheless been included because similar situations could arise in the context of an ANDA for a solid oral dosage form.

2. CITIZEN PETITIONS AND LEGAL CHALLENGES TO ANDA APPROVALS

Not surprisingly, innovator drug sponsors have mounted a number of challenges to FDA approval decisions, or anticipated approval decisions, for generic versions of their drug products. Frequently, innovator firms have filed citizen petitions with FDA, raising reasons why FDA should not grant an anticipated approval of a generic version of their products.

By way of background, a citizen petition is nothing more than the formal procedural mechanism for any individual or entity to ask FDA to take, or refrain from taking, some specified agency action. The requirements for citizen petitions are set forth in FDA regulations (1). Citizen petitions can also be filed by generic firms for a wide variety of purposes. For example, they include ANDA suitability petitions (discussed in Section 4.1 below).

The submission of a citizen petition to FDA by an innovator firm seeking to block the approval of generic products serves several purposes. First, it is possible that FDA may grant the requested relief. (FDA has not done so except on very rare occasions.) Second, even if FDA does not grant the requested relief, its consideration of a citizen petition can be a lengthy process that may delay the approval of the generic product. Third, and perhaps most importantly, the submission of a citizen petition helps counter the argument frequently made by FDA (and other government agencies) that a person challenging an agency action in court has not first "exhausted" all available administrative remedies. The reason that courts may apply the "exhaustion" requirement is to help conserve judicial resources, by ensuring that courts are not asked to address situations that might have been resolved had relief been sought from the administrative agency in the first instance.

At the present time, FDA accepts citizen petitions on any topic, without limit. In 1999, FDA published a proposed rule that would reform its citizen petition process, so that FDA would no longer accept citizen petitions regarding specific products that are pending approval (2). FDA stated its tentative view that issues regarding pending products should be raised less formally, such as by letter. To date, FDA has not finalized its proposal. Even if finalized, it is not apparent to this author that there will be any meaningful benefit to the generic drug industry.

On a number of occasions, adversely affected innovator drug sponsors have sought judicial review of FDA's ANDA approval decisions. In some cases, FDA has denied a relevant citizen petition contemporaneously with an ANDA approval; in other cases, FDA did not act on the petition despite the granting of the challenged ANDA approval, and the innovator firm regarded FDA's ANDA approval as tantamount to denial of its petition. Generally, the innovator firm has sued FDA, to block approval of the generic product. Typically, the generic firm or firms involved have been allowed to intervene in the lawsuit to protect their economic interests in their ANDA approvals. ANDA sponsors have intervened to bring to the court's attention the economic consequences of granting or blocking ANDA approval, a topic that FDA routinely ignores.

In a number of situations involving disputes over 180-day generic drug exclusivity, an adversely affected ANDA sponsor has sued FDA regarding a 180-day exclusivity decision. As with challenges brought by innovator drug sponsors, those challenges are often preceded by the submission of a citizen petition to FDA. In these disputes, it has been commonplace for other affected ANDA sponsors—and sometimes the sponsor of the innovator product—to be allowed to intervene in the lawsuit to protect their rights (3).

The substance of various legal challenges to ANDA approvals is discussed in the subsections below.

3. EXCLUSIVITY ISSUES

3.1. Five-Year New Chemical Entity Exclusivity

The Hatch–Waxman Amendments grant the sponsor of an NDA for a drug product containing what is commonly referred to as a "new chemical entity" or "NCE," i.e., an active ingredient that was not previously used in an approved drug product, a five-year period, which starts running with the date of NDA approval, during which FDA cannot accept any ANDAs for review (4). However, if the ANDA sponsor challenges an Orange Book patent on the innovator product by submitting a Paragraph IV certification (which contends that the patent is invalid or not infringed), the ANDA may be submitted four years after the date of initial NDA approval, thereby potentially saving the ANDA sponsor one year.

Hatch–Waxman exclusivity operates independently of any patents that protect the active ingredients or other aspects of the innovator product. In most (but not all) cases, the innovator product is protected by one or more "blocking" patents (on the active ingredient itself, the use of the active ingredient, or both) until well after the expiration of the five-year new chemical entity exclusivity. Because challenges to these "blocking" patents usually do not succeed, five-year exclusivity is generally not a determinative factor in when generic competition will begin.

3.2. Three-Year Exclusivity for Product "Improvements"

The Hatch–Waxman Amendments also provide NDA sponsors with a three-year period free from generic competition for the approval of an NDA or supplemental NDA for a drug product containing a previously approved active ingredient, when the approval is supported by new clinical studies (other than bioavailability studies) essential to the approval (5). Unlike five-year new chemical entity exclusivity, three-year exclusivity does not bar the submission of ANDAs to FDA; it only prohibits final approval of an ANDA.

When FDA grants three-year exclusivity for the approval of a new drug product or new form of an approved drug product containing a previously approved active ingredient, generic competition is effectively blocked for three years with little recourse to an ANDA sponsor. While an ANDA sponsor could challenge FDA's determination that a particular clinical study is essential to support the approval, such a challenge is unlikely to prevail. In an analogous situation involving Rogaine® (minoxidil), the NDA sponsor challenged FDA's decision to deny three-year exclusivity, because FDA had concluded that the sponsor's clinical study was not essential to support the approval. The court rejected the challenge, noting that FDA's evaluation of clinical trials and related determinations are within its area of expertise and that the courts must grant wide deference to these determinations (6).

A situation that is of far greater practical significance to the generic industry is three-year exclusivity granted for the approval of a supplemental NDA that provides for revised labeling. In general, FDA has interpreted three-year exclusivity narrowly in this situation. In the case of FDA approval of a new (additional) indication, FDA allows the generic sponsor to seek ANDA approval based on the "old" labeling, "carving out" or deleting the newly approved, additional indication (7). This practice has been upheld in a judicial challenge (8).

The situation becomes more problematic where the NDA sponsor obtains three-year exclusivity for revised labeling that provides for replacement of certain aspects of the previously approved labeling. For example, a titration-dosing requirement may be eliminated or the duration of an infusion schedule may be entirely changed. As of this writing, FDA has issued a draft guidance and has tentatively determined that it will permit ANDA approvals based on the former labeling, if the ANDA sponsor petitions FDA to determine that the "old" labeling was not withdrawn for safety or effectiveness reasons and the agency makes such a finding (9). However, FDA has not issued any final ANDA approvals using the rationale set forth in the draft guidance. It remains to be seen how FDA will ultimately handle this situation. Further litigation to define the extent of approvals based upon "old" labeling is a definite possibility.

A particularly thorny situation involved the grant of three-year exclusivity to an NDA sponsor for labeling information regarding pediatric use of the product. As the result of a 1994 rulemaking, FDA regulations require all drug labels to include pediatric use information, based on the premise that pediatric use information is necessary for the safe and effective use of drug products (10). Based on that regulation, the innovator industry took the position that FDA could not approve generic versions of innovator products with the pediatric use labeling information "carved out". Congress addressed this situation in late 2001 by amending the Hatch–Waxman Amendments so that the omission of pediatric use labeling information would not make an ANDA ineligible for final approval. FDA is authorized to require the labeling of the generic product to include appropriate pediatric contraindications, warnings, or precautions, as well as a statement that the drug product is not labeled for pediatric use (11). Based on this statutory change, FDA started granting ANDA approvals without exclusivity-protected pediatric use labeling information in early 2002.

3.3. 180-Day Generic Drug Exclusivity

The Hatch–Waxman Amendments provide for a 180-day period of exclusivity, where the first Paragraph IV ANDA sponsor (which challenges an Orange Book patent on the innovator product being copied) is entitled to a 180-day period during which it is the only generic product on the marketplace (12). This provision has been the source of much litigation in recent years, with a number of unresolved issues. In 1999, FDA proposed a major revision of its 180-day exclusivity regulations (13), but the proposal has been withdrawn because of several court decisions (14).

As currently interpreted by the courts and FDA, 180-day exclusivity is available to the sponsor of the first substantially complete Paragraph IV ANDA, regardless of whether it prevails in patent litigation (15) or is even sued for patent infringement at all (16). The availability of 180-day exclusivity where the first Paragraph IV ANDA sponsor loses its patent infringement litigation, or discontinues its patent challenge in a settlement with the innovator drug sponsor and patent holder, is unsettled (17). It appears to be FDA's view that an ANDA sponsor that settles Hatch–Waxman patent infringement litigation—even by conceding patent validity or patent infringement—and as part of the settlement obtains a patent license, is entitled to maintain its Paragraph IV certification and, therefore, its eligibility for 180-day exclusivity. If the patent license is only effective at a future date, the net result is the entire generic market is blocked.

An ANDA sponsor's 180-day exclusivity is "triggered", or starts running, with the earlier of two events: the date that ANDA sponsor begins commercial marketing, or the date of a "court decision" finding the patent in question invalid or not infringed (18). As interpreted by the courts and FDA, the court decision of invalidity or non-infringement is the first court decision involving that patent and any ANDA sponsor; it need not involve the ANDA sponsor entitled to exclusivity (19). By guidance document, FDA finally acquiesced in a number of district court decisions that the "court decision" can be the decision of a district court (20). However, FDA's guidance takes the position that the new interpretation will only be applied prospectively; that position appears vulnerable to challenge in an appropriate case.

For 180-day exclusivity purposes, each strength or form of an innovator drug product is treated separately. Thus, a court decision involving one strength will not serve as the "court decision trigger" for a different strength (21).

Under the current judicial and FDA interpretations of 180-day exclusivity, 180-day exclusivity is available in connection with every innovator product where a Paragraph IV ANDA is filed. This exclusivity has become an important business consideration for ANDA sponsors. Without doubt, 180-day exclusivity is highly valuable, as the first firm to enter the generic marketplace can often "fill the pipeline" and derive a long-term benefit from its 180-day head start. Unfortunately, business planning in this important area is stifled by FDA's refusal to disclose whether a firm is entitled to 180-day exclusivity before its ANDA is ready for final approval. As of this writing, FDA's website (22) only discloses whether a Paragraph IV ANDA has been submitted in connection with a particular innovator drug product; no additional details are provided. In some cases, ANDA sponsors can draw reasonable inferences about their actual entitlement to 180-day exclusivity from publicly available information in patent infringement litigation, or even from publicly available information about ANDA reference numbers of tentatively approved ANDAs. However, this information is not always available (for example, some or all of Paragraph IV ANDA applicants may not be sued) and may not be reliable in all regards.

FDA recognizes that 180-day exclusivity is a valuable property right that can be sold or traded. This recognition provides a valuable opportunity for an ANDA sponsor entitled to 180-day exclusivity that is, for whatever reason, not positioned to receive meaningful benefit from its exclusivity. (For example, that sponsor is unable to obtain final ANDA approval.) FDA permits exclusivity to be "selectively waived" in favor of another ANDA sponsor otherwise eligible for final approval, but only if the exclusivity has been "triggered" and is then running (23). If the exclusivity has not been "triggered", FDA only permits it to be "relinquished" in its entirety, permitting all otherwise eligible ANDA sponsors to receive final approval. In a particular situation, there may be no meaningful difference between a "selective waiver" and a complete "relinquishment" of 180-day exclusivity.

In some situations, the entire generic market can be blocked because of the existence of 180-day exclusivity. This situation can occur if no Paragraph IV ANDA applicant is sued for patent infringement (so the "court decision trigger" is never activated), and the first Paragraph IV ANDA applicant (entitled to 180-day exclusivity) is not able to begin commercial marketing (because it is unable to obtain final approval or, for example, supply problems keep it from beginning manufacture even if it has received final approval). It can also happen if the first Paragraph IV ANDA sponsor settles patent litigation in exchange for a patent license that starts on a future date. One possibility is for a subsequent Paragraph IV ANDA applicant to file a declaratory judgment lawsuit against the patent holder, seeking a declaration that the patent is invalid or not infringed. If obtained, such a declaratory judgment will serve as the "court decision trigger" that starts the running of the 180-day exclusivity period.

The problem with this declaratory judgment approach is that the patent holder will typically take the position that it has no plans to sue the ANDA sponsor for patent infringement. As a result, there will be no actual "case or controversy," a constitutional pre-requisite for litigation in federal court. Although one judicial decision concluded that the patent holder's statements that it would not sue for patent infringement, coupled with the resulting dismissal of the declaratory judgment lawsuit, would serve as the "court decision trigger" for starting 180-day exclusivity, that decision appears to have depended on the particular form of the documents involved (24). Thus, there can be no guarantee that the dismissal of a declaratory judgment lawsuit would necessarily serve as the "court decision trigger" in a different case. From a business perspective, the filing of a declaratory judgment lawsuit is undercut by the fact that a favorable decision benefits all generic sponsors, not just the company that bears the burden and cost of initiating the lawsuit.

FDA states that it is regulating "directly from the statute" in the area of 180-day exclusivity (25). Because of the ambiguous statutory language, some situations are unresolved. One unresolved situation is the availability of 180-day exclusivity when multiple Paragraph IV certifications to different Orange Book patents are involved. FDA's proposed (now withdrawn) rule on 180-day exclusivity would have made 180-day exclusivity available only in connection with the first Paragraph IV certification to an Orange Book patent (26). Regulating "directly from the statute", it is FDA's position that a separate 180-day exclusivity period is potentially available in connection with each Orange Book patent.

Thus, in one 1999 situation involving generic versions of Platinol® (cisplatin injection), two ANDA sponsors were each the first to file a Paragraph IV certification on a different Orange Book patent. One patent expired before the 180-day period associated with that patent had been triggered. FDA concluded that that patent and its associated 180-day exclusivity period were of no continuing relevance, and did not prevent a 180-day exclusivity period in favor of the first Paragraph IV applicant on the later expiring Orange Book patent (27).

In 2002, FDA invoked the concept of "shared exclusivity" in connection with generic versions of Prilosec® (omeprazole delayed release capsules) (28). Two ANDA sponsors, each of whom was the first to file a Paragraph IV certification to a different Orange Book patent, were allowed to share a single 180-day exclusivity period. The exclusivity period would begin running with the earlier of onset of commercial marketing by either of the two firms sharing exclusivity or a court decision involving either Orange Book patent. Absent this pragmatic solution, the two firms would have had overlapping and conflicting 180-day exclusivity periods. Litigation in this area is in progress as of the time of this writing (29).

3.4. Six-Month Pediatric Labeling Exclusivity

An innovator drug sponsor is entitled to an additional six months of exclusivity if it conducts a clinical study to study the safety or effectiveness of its drug product in a pediatric population. The additional six months is added to the term of an unexpired Orange Book patent or three-year or five-year non-patent exclusivity (30). FDA cannot grant final approval to an ANDA until the expiration of the six-month period. Six-month pediatric labeling exclusivity appears to be easy for innovator firms to obtain; the key statutory elements are that FDA issue a "written request" for a pediatric study and the drug sponsor submit a study that "fairly responds" to FDA's written request.

When engaging in business planning, many generic drug sponsors assume that FDA will grant pediatric labeling exclusivity, even if only at the last moment. In one recent situation, FDA denied the innovator firm's request for pediatric exclusivity on the day of patent expiration and issued final approvals for several ANDAs. After the innovator firm challenged FDA's denial of pediatric exclusivity for Mevacor® (lovastatin), the court concluded that FDA had applied an overly stringent standard in reviewing the study. Thereafter, FDA agreed to re-evaluate the study, and subsequently concluded that the innovator drug sponsor was in fact entitled to pediatric exclusivity (31). While the overall effect was a six-month delay in generic competition, there were differing effects on different generic drug sponsors.

The several firms that had received final approvals and were ready to begin product distribution before the grant of pediatric exclusivity lost the benefit of being early entrants in the generic market. In comparison, those firms that did not expect to receive final approvals until later or were not prepared to launch upon original patent expiration apparently benefited from the delay of generic competition.

One issue that was the subject of considerable recent attention was the interplay between 180-day exclusivity and six-month pediatric labeling exclusivity. In early 2002, a statutory change clarified the situation by providing that any portion of the 180-day period lost due to "overlap" with 6-month pediatric exclusivity will be restored (32).

4. DIFFERENCES BETWEEN INNOVATOR AND GENERIC PRODUCTS

4.1. ANDA Suitability Petitions

The Hatch–Waxman Amendments permit a generic drug product to differ from its brand name counterpart in one of four regards if the difference is petitioned for and approved before ANDA submission (33). These petitions, commonly known as ANDA suitability petitions, are submitted to FDA using the format for a citizen petition and are, upon filing, in the public domain. For this reason, many prospective ANDA sponsors prefer to have petitions submitted for them by a consultant or law firm, on a "blind" basis. In this way, the identity of a firm that intends to file an ANDA for a modified form of an innovator product is not publicly disclosed.

The Hatch–Waxman Amendments permit ANDA suitability petitions for only four types of changes: dosage form, strength, route of administration, or active ingredient in a combination product. To date, over 800 ANDA suitability petitions have been submitted to FDA (34). The great majority of ANDA suitability petitions have sought changes in dosage form or strength. If properly prepared, these petitions are routinely granted. About 70 petitions have sought permission to file an ANDA for a new combination. In FDA's view, these petitions are appropriate only if the proposed change of active ingredient is the substitution of one active ingredient for another in the same pharmacological or therapeutic class, such as the substitution of aspirin for acetaminophen in a combination product. A substantial percentage of ANDA suitability petitions seeking a change in active ingredients have been denied, on the basis that the proposed change cannot be adequately evaluated in the context of an ANDA. Very few ANDA suitability petitions have been submitted seeking a new route of administration; most of these have been denied.

FDA is required by the Hatch–Waxman Amendments to approve or disapprove an ANDA suitability petition within 90 days (35). In practice, while FDA has generally not met that deadline, its decisions have typically not taken more than six months.

A generic drug product authorized by an ANDA suitability petition will not be rated as therapeutically equivalent to the innovator product upon which it is based in FDA's Orange Book. Thus, under the pharmacy laws of the great majority of states, no substitution at the pharmacy level is permitted. The lack of substitution at the pharmacy level may pose new sales and marketing challenges for many generic drug firms, as the new product will have to be "detailed" to physicians.

FDA's pediatric use information regulation may create an obstacle to obtaining approval of new dosage forms. This regulation requires, in relevant part, the sponsor of an application seeking approval for a new form of an approved drug product to provide data regarding the safety and effectiveness of the proposed drug product in pediatric sub-populations (36). The pediatric studies requirement can be waived by FDA, in whole or in part, if the proposed drug product does not represent a meaningful therapeutic benefit over existing treatments for pediatric patients and is not likely to be used in a substantial number of pediatric patients. While the rule is likely to be applied by FDA in situations where the proposed new dosage form is particularly amenable to pediatric use (e.g., proposed generic drug product in liquid form, where the innovator drug product is a solid oral dosage form), its applicability is not necessarily so limited. Thus, prospective ANDA sponsors—which typically may have very little or no experience in conducting clinical trials—may find themselves having to conduct a clinical trial to support ANDA approval, even though the approval of the innovator product is not supported by comparable clinical trials in a pediatric population. As of this writing, the pediatric studies regulation has been declared invalid by a federal district court; FDA's response is not known (37). Legislation is possible (38).

4.2. "Same" Active Ingredient

Except for the limited changes authorized by an ANDA suitability petition, the Hatch–Waxman Amendments require a generic product to have the "same" active ingredient as the innovator product upon which it is based. While the "sameness" of the active ingredient has generally not been a concern for chemically synthesized active ingredients, several challenges have been raised in connection with drug products of natural origin.

In an important decision for the generic drug industry, the United States Court of Appeals for the District of Columbia Circuit concluded that

FDA has the scientific expertise and discretion to determine "sameness" for ANDA approval purposes; exact chemical identity is not required (39). That case involved a challenge to FDA's approval of a generic version of Pergonal® (menotropins for injection), a fertility drug. Rather than being chemically synthesized, the active ingredient of the product is derived from natural sources; natural variations lead to slightly different chemical side chains in different batches of the active ingredient. Based on these natural variations, the sponsor of the innovator product challenged FDA's ANDA approval decision, contending that the active ingredient in the generic product was not the "same" as the active ingredient in its product. That challenge was rejected.

A noteworthy administrative challenge to a proposed generic product on the basis that its active ingredients are not the "same" as the innovator product involved Premarin® (conjugated estrogens tablets), for treating the symptoms of menopause and preventing osteoporosis. As Premarin is derived from natural sources, not all active constituents have been fully characterized. Ultimately, FDA decided that it could not approve any generic version of Premarin using chemically synthesized active ingredients until the active constituents of Premarin have been better characterized and more information is available about them (40). Thus, even though Premarin has been marketed for two generations and relevant patents are long expired, it is not readily available for generic copying because the innovator drug sponsor has not sufficiently characterized its active constituents.

At some levels, FDA's decisions on Pergonal and Premarin seem inconsistent. FDA's administrative decision on generic versions of Premarin was not challenged in court. Had it been challenged, presumably FDA would have received substantial deference from the court on the agency's scientific and medical decisions, just as the agency received in connection with a generic version of Pergonal.

4.3. "Same" Dosage Form

Except for changes authorized by the granting of an ANDA suitability petition, the Hatch–Waxman Amendments require a generic product to be in the "same" dosage form as the innovator product upon which it is based. While several innovator firms have challenged ANDA approval decisions on the basis of apparent distinctions between dosage forms, FDA and the courts have had little difficulty disposing of these challenges. FDA's decision that a generic product using conventional extended release tablet technology was the "same" dosage form as the innovator product using patented osmotic pump extended release tablet technology (Procardia XL®, nifedipine) for ANDA approval purposes has been upheld (41). Similarly, the courts have upheld FDA's determination that a generic drug product described as a tablet inside a gelatin capsule was the "same" dosage form as the innovator's capsule (Dilantin®, phenytoin sodium) (42).

4.4. "Same" Labeling and Inactive Ingredient Differences

Except for differences related to the identification of the different firms involved or changes authorized by the granting of an ANDA suitability petition, the Hatch–Waxman Amendments require the labeling of the proposed generic product to be the "same" as the labeling of the innovator product (43).

FDA's decision to approve a generic version of a parenteral innovator product, Diprivan® (propofol), with a different preservative and slightly different labeling, was upheld in a judicial challenge. In this case, the innovator product contained the preservative disodium edentate (EDTA) to prevent microbial contamination. FDA approved a generic version of the product with sulfite as the preservative rather than EDTA. Because some individuals are allergic to sulfite, the labeling of the generic product included a sulfite warning. The innovator firm challenged the ANDA approval, on the basis that the generic product did not have the "same" labeling as the innovator. The court rejected that contention, ruling that FDA's decision to allow the sulfite warning was entitled to substantial deference (44).

4.5. Bioequivalency

Although the Hatch–Waxman Amendments define bioequivalency solely in terms of the rate and extent of absorption of the innovator and proposed generic products (45), FDA has long taken the view that alternative ways of establishing bioequivalence may be warranted (46). FDA's waiver of in vivo bioequivalency for generic versions of a non-systemically absorbed drug (Intal NebSol, cromolyn sodium for inhalation using a nebulizer) has been upheld (47). Similarly, a court rejected a challenge to an FDA guidance that allowed the use of in vitro testing to establish bioequivalence for generic versions of Questran® (cholestyramine) (48). A court rejected a judicial challenge that contended that the statutory definition of bioequivalence was the only acceptable measure of bioequivalence, in a case involving generic versions of non-systemically absorbed inhalation (Proventil®, albuterol) and topical anti-fungal (Lotrimin®, clotrimazole) drug products (49). In upholding FDA's decision to rely on an assay for the metabolite rather than the parent drug itself in assessing bioequivalency for generic versions of Eldepryl® (selegiline hydrochloride), one court concluded that the appropriate method to be used for determining bioequivalency is a matter of scientific judgment, squarely within FDA's discretion (50). With this history of judicial deference to FDA's interpretation of bioequivalence, it seems unlikely that a successful challenge will be mounted in the future.

4.6.   OTC Switches

The innovator sponsor's decision to switch its drug product from prescription to over-the-counter status could present additional obstacles to generic firms. If the supplemental NDA providing for OTC labeling is supported by clinical studies, the innovator firm is entitled to three years of exclusivity during which no ANDA could be approved. Moreover, under FDA policy, an ANDA could no longer be approved based on the previously approved prescription labeling (51). Even if the innovator is not entitled to exclusivity, a prescription to OTC switch near the end of the innovator's patent expiration is likely to cause some delays in ANDA approvals, as generic firms would be required to create, and obtain FDA approval for, new labeling and packaging. If the innovator product is switched to OTC status after final ANDA approval, FDA would presumably give the ANDA sponsor a reasonable length of time to supplement its approved ANDA to provide for an OTC product. However, if the innovator firm received three-year exclusivity, the generic firm would be forced off the market until exclusivity expiration, despite having an approved ANDA for a prescription product. Finally, the marketing and distribution of an OTC product could present new challenges for many generic firms that have no experience competing in this market, which is dominated by private label products marketed by large retail pharmacy chains.

5.   PATENT-RELATED ISSUES

5.1.   Scope of Hatch–Waxman Patent Listing Provisions

The Hatch–Waxman Amendments require the NDA sponsor to submit for Orange Book listing "any patent which claims the drug for which the applicant submitted the application or which claims a method of using such drug and with respect to which a claim of patent infringement could reasonably be asserted if a person not licensed by the owner engaged in the manufacture, use, or sale of the drug" (52). If such a patent issues after the NDA is approved, patent information must be submitted to FDA within 30 days after patent issuance (53). The scope of these provisions has been the subject of much controversy, which continues as of the date of this writing.

In its implementing regulation, FDA interpreted these provisions to provide for the listing of drug substance (ingredient) patents, drug product (formulation and composition) patents, and method of use patents. Drug substance patents are eligible for listing only if they claim a "component" of the approved drug product, and drug product patents are eligible for listing only if they claim an approved drug product. Method of use patents are eligible for Orange Book listing only if they claim approved indications or other conditions of use. Process patents are not eligible for Orange Book listing (54). In connection with each formulation, composition, or method of use patent submitted for Orange Book listing—but not for drug substance patents—the NDA sponsor must submit a declaration, that the patent "covers the formulation, composition, and/or method of use" of the drug product for which approval is being sought or which has been approved (55).

Considerable controversy has surrounded the appropriate interpretation of FDA's patent listing regulation. Innovator drug firms have increasingly interpreted FDA's patent listing regulation to their benefit.

The general approach of FDA's implementing regulation—that product patents are eligible for listing only if they claim an approved drug product—has been upheld. In one suit against FDA, a district court rejected the innovator's argument that any product patent related to the active ingredient in an approved drug product is eligible for Orange Book listing (56). In that situation, the patent claimed a drug product in tablet form, whereas the approved drug product (Procardia®, nifedipine) was in capsule form.

In a handful of cases, an ANDA sponsor has sued the sponsor of the NDA product to compel the "delisting" of an Orange Book patent. In one case, the active ingredient in the approved drug product (Hytrin®, terazosin hydrochloride) was in dihydrate form; the NDA sponsor submitted a patent claiming the active ingredient in anhydrous form for Orange Book listing. An ANDA sponsor, which had filed an ANDA using the anhydrous form of the active ingredient, sued the NDA sponsor to compel delisting. Under FDA policy, different waters of hydration are generally regarded as the "same" active ingredient for ANDA approval purposes. The district court held that the patent was properly listed, because different waters of hydration are the "same" active ingredient for ANDA purposes (57). In another case involving differing waters of hydration, the active ingredient in the approved drug product (Aredia®, pamidronate disodium) was in lyophilized form, with no water of hydration. The innovator drug sponsor listed a patent for the active ingredient in pentahydrate form. An ANDA sponsor sued to compel delisting, on the theory that a drug substance must actually be present in the finished product before a patent is eligible for Orange Book listing. The district court rejected that argument, holding that the patent was properly listed because the pentahydrate form had been used as a "component" in the manufacturing process, consistent with FDA's regulation (58).

In another controversy, the NDA sponsor obtained a method of use patent that claims a method of using a metabolite of the active ingredient in the approved drug product (Buspar®, buspirone). The patent was submitted to FDA for Orange Book listing, on the rationale that it claimed a method of using the approved drug product for all approved indications. After some hesitancy, FDA listed the patent. A district court considered in detail the prosecution history of the patent in question before the Patent and Trademark Office, and concluded that the particular claims in question had been abandoned. On this basis, that district court concluded that the patent was not eligible for Orange Book listing (59).

The decision of the US Court of Appeals for the Federal Circuit on appeal of this case was a major setback for the generic industry. The Federal Circuit decided that an ANDA sponsor cannot sue an NDA sponsor seeking the delisting of an Orange Book patent (60). Thus, at this time there is no meaningful direct remedy for an ANDA sponsor to challenge the innovator drug sponsor's decision to list a patent in the Orange Book.

FDA has long taken the position that its role in the listing of Orange Book patents is strictly ministerial, and that it will not become involved in disputes between NDA sponsors and others (61). In a lawsuit against FDA, one district court concluded that FDA was entitled to accept the patent listing declaration at face value and the court would not second guess FDA's decision (62). Recently, however, FDA has shown at least a little willingness to play some role in determining whether patents are in fact appropriate for Orange Book listing. As noted above, FDA delayed listing the method of use patent that claimed a metabolite of the active ingredient in the approved drug product. In a different lawsuit involving a generic version of Tiazac™ (diltiazem hydrochloride), FDA filed a document in district court in which it tentatively took the view that the challenged Orange Book patent listing was not in fact eligible for Orange Book listing because the innovator drug sponsor's own court briefs showed that the formulation patent did not claim an approved drug product (63).

There is pending litigation against FDA, asserting interpretations of the Hatch–Waxman Amendments that would impose limitations on the listing of patents in the Orange Book, and the corresponding need to certify to the patents. The impetus for this lawsuit is patents that issue well after initial FDA approval of the innovator product, and typically during the time that ANDAs are pending before FDA. In that case, it has been posited that only patents that claim the drug product as initially approved in the NDA, and not product improvements approved in supplements to the NDA, are eligible for Orange Book listing; that an ANDA sponsor is not required to certify to any patents that are first listed in the Orange Book after the time of initial ANDA submission; and that patents that issue after initial NDA approval can be listed in the Orange Book only if there is no patent available for Orange Book listing at the time of initial ANDA approval. As of the time of this writing, these arguments have been rejected by a federal district court; an appeal is pending (64). Previously, the US Court of Appeals for the Federal Circuit had recognized that these arguments are judicially cognizable, under the usual standards that apply to challenges to federal agency decision making (65).

In October 2002, FDA proposed to revise its regulations with new interpretations of the Hatch–Waxman patent listing provisions. If adopted as a final rule, an innovator company would be required to list patents claiming those chemically different forms of the active ingredient or ingredients in its approved drug product that are regarded as the "same" active ingredient for ANDA purposes (66). Typically, this would include patents claiming different waters of hydration and different polymorphs. FDA also proposed that patents claiming intermediates or metabolites of the approved drug product would not be eligible for Orange Book listing. FDA clarified that product by process patents are eligible for Orange Book listing. FDA proposed to adopt a more detailed declaration to be used as a "checklist" by innovator sponsors submitting patent information, to ensure that only appropriate patents are listed in the Orange Book. FDA proposed that its new interpretations would be prospective in operation. The provisions of FDA's proposed rule are unquestionably controversial. In this author's opinion, it remains to be seen when, or if, the proposed requirements will be finalized. Moreover, a final rule could be challenged by an innovator firm, a generic firm, or very possibly by both.

5.2. Thirty-Month Delay of ANDA Final Approval

The Hatch–Waxman Amendments provide that ANDA final approval is automatically delayed by 30 months following a Paragraph IV certification to an Orange Book patent, notice of the certification to the NDA sponsor and patent holder, and the timely filing of a Hatch–Waxman patent infringement lawsuit. The 30-month period can the lengthened or shortened by the court hearing the patent case "because either party to the action failed to reasonably cooperate in expediting the action" (67).

One district court's decision to shorten the 30 months, based on what it viewed as the NDA sponsor's improper conduct before FDA in connection with the listing of the patent, was rejected on appeal by the Federal Circuit. The Federal Circuit concluded that the 30-month period could be shortened based only on delay related to the particular infringement lawsuit (68).

At the time of this writing, ANDA sponsors are asserting in several pending lawsuits that the Hatch–Waxman Amendments only permit a single 30-month delay of ANDA approval for each ANDA, not successive

30-month delays. In one pending lawsuit, the District Court ruled against the plaintiff ANDA sponsor without expressly reaching the single 30-month delay argument; the case is on appeal (69).

In October 2002, FDA proposed to adopt a regulation that would change its longstanding interpretation of the 30-month delay requirement (70). If FDA's proposal is adopted as a final rule, there would be a maximum of one 30-month delay period imposed for each ANDA. An ANDA applicant would still be required to certify to any relevant patents that are listed in the Orange Book after ANDA submission, but would not be required to give notice of its Paragraph IV certification to such a patent. As the 30-month delay is tied to the receipt of notice of a Paragraph IV certification, there would be no additional 30-month delay periods in connection with these subsequently listed patents. If adopted, FDA's new interpretation would be prospective in operation. As previously noted, the provisions of FDA's proposed rule are unquestionably controversial. In this author's opinion, it remains to be seen when, or if, the proposed requirements will be finalized; litigation is a distinct possibility.

5.3. Hatch–Waxman Patent Infringement Litigation

Under the current interpretation of 180-day generic drug exclusivity, 180-day exclusivity is available whenever a Paragraph IV ANDA is filed. While a discussion of patent infringement litigation is beyond the scope of this book, two brief points are worthy of note.

First, the sponsor of a Paragraph IV ANDA always stands a reasonably likelihood of being sued for patent infringement in the Hatch–Waxman 45-day window. While ANDA sponsors may, as a matter of business tactics, want to be aggressive in filing Paragraph IV ANDAs and pursuing patent challenges, the merit—or lack of merit—of any particular challenge should be viewed objectively. In one recent case, the Paragraph IV ANDA applicant was liable for the NDA sponsor's and patent holder's attorneys' fees for pursuing what the court characterized as a baseless patent challenge (71). In such cases, attorneys' fees often amount to several million dollars or more.

Second, in some cases Paragraph IV ANDA applicants have been sued, within the Hatch–Waxman 45-day window, for infringement of patents not listed in the Orange Book. The US Court of Appeals for the Federal Circuit ruled that the patent holder can seek a declaratory judgment that its process patent (which is not eligible for Orange Book listing) will be infringed by the ANDA sponsor (72). In other cases, Paragraph IV ANDA applicants were sued, again within the 45-day Hatch–Waxman window, for alleged inducement to infringe an Orange Book method of use patent for an unapproved use. Whether a patent holder can bring such a lawsuit before commercial marketing of the generic product is pending before the Federal Circuit (73). The relevant point is that a Paragraph IV ANDA applicant may be inviting more patent infringement litigation than anticipated.

5.4. Bolar-Type Considerations

The Hatch–Waxman Amendments permit an ANDA sponsor or prospective sponsor to engage in activities reasonably related to seeking government approval for its generic drug, without infringing any patents covering the innovator drug (74). This provision is commonly known as the Bolar provision. Because FDA requires validation data from three commercial size manufacturing batches as a condition of ANDA approval, the Hatch–Waxman Bolar provision effectively permits an ANDA sponsor to stockpile reasonable quantities of product for product launch in anticipation of ANDA final approval. However, it does not provide a safe harbor from infringement for any additional product manufactured before ANDA approval. To the extent that an ANDA sponsor's product is manufactured in a foreign country, differing patent laws will apply and there may be no safe harbor for commercial production before ANDA approval.

6. AMENABILITY TO ANDA SUBMISSION

6.1. ANDA Vs. 505(b)(2) NDA

Section 505(b)(2) of the FDC Act, added as part of the Hatch–Waxman Amendments, authorizes an NDA where some of the safety or effectiveness investigations required to support NDA approval were not conducted for the applicant, and for which the applicant has not obtained a right of reference or use (75). In the interest of simplicity, 505(b)(2) NDAs have generally not been discussed elsewhere in this chapter.

A 505(b)(2) NDA sponsor must certify to any patents listed in the Orange Book on the innovator product on which the 505(b)(2) application is based, and the effective date of approval may be delayed, just as with an ANDA (76). The effective date of approval of a 505(b)(2) may also be delayed by five-year or three-year non-patent exclusivity for the innovator product upon which it is based, or by six-month pediatric labeling exclusivity (77). Unlike an ANDA, a 505(b)(2) NDA is not eligible for, and not affected by, 180-day exclusivity.

A 505(b)(2) NDA sponsor is eligible for its own three-year exclusivity if its application is supported by a clinical study essential to the approval; this exclusivity would delay by three years the effective date of approval of another 505(b)(2) application or ANDA based on the 505(b)(2) sponsor's drug product (78).

A 505(b)(2) NDA may be suited for modified "generic" versions of innovator products, such as extended or delayed release versions of regular release innovator products. It may also be appropriate for drug products that present bioequivalence difficulties, where it may be easier to conduct a clinical trial to assess product comparability rather than a traditional bioequivalence trial. Although FDA's regulations provide that the agency may refuse to accept a 505(b)(2) application where the product may be addressed through an ANDA (79), FDA has not strictly enforced this requirement.

A 505(b)(2) application is appropriate for changes from an innovator product that are not permitted to be addressed through an ANDA. These situations include different salts or esters of the active ingredient in the innovator product and different indications and conditions for use, neither of which can be addressed through the ANDA suitability petition process.

Although, in theory, an ANDA can be based on any innovator product that was approved under an NDA, special hurdles exist for biological-type drug products. These problems stem from the inherently variable nature of biological-type products. Recombinant protein products, such as human growth hormone and insulin, are regulated as drugs under the NDA provisions of the FDC Act. However, FDA has to date taken the position that it will not approve an ANDA for a generic version of these products. FDA's view appears to be that it is not able to evaluate these products under the Hatch–Waxman ANDA provisions; however, a 505(b)(2) NDA may be appropriate. As noted above, at this time, FDA will not approve synthetic conjugated estrogens tablets drug product using the ANDA route, on the basis that the active constituents of the innovator product have not been sufficiently characterized. However, a synthetic version of the innovator product has been approved through a 505(b)(2) NDA (Cenestin®, synthetic conjugated estrogens A). That synthetic product is not rated as therapeutically equivalent to Premarin in the Orange Book.

A drug product approved through a 505(b)(2) NDA is not automatically rated as therapeutically equivalent to its brand name counterpart, and thus could not be substituted for the innovator product by a pharmacist under typical state pharmacy laws. It may be necessary to "detail" such a product to physicians, thereby creating new marketing hurdles for some generic firms. However, where the innovator and 505(b)(2) products are regarded by FDA as pharmaceutically equivalent, it may be possible to conduct additional testing to demonstrate bioequivalence and therapeutic equivalence with the innovator product.

6.2. Withdrawal of Approval of Innovator Drug

The Hatch–Waxman Amendments provide that an ANDA may be based on an innovator drug that is no longer marketed, provided the innovator drug was not withdrawn from sale for safety or effectiveness reasons (80). An ANDA sponsor that wants to base its product on a discontinued innovator drug must petition FDA to make a determination that the product was not discontinued for safety or effectiveness reasons (81). In addition, an ANDA may not be based on an innovator product for which FDA has begun the formal administrative process to withdraw NDA approval for safety or effectiveness reasons (82).

The withdrawal of approval of the innovator product upon which an ANDA is based can present special obstacles. In one case, the approved innovator product was in tablet form (Eldepryl®, selegiline hydrochloride). Less than one month before the expiration of non-patent exclusivity on the innovator product, the innovator firm obtained FDA approval for a capsule form of its drug product. It then discontinued the tablet form, and attempted to attribute a safety reason for this decision: prevention of counterfeit versions of its tablet product and the elimination of mix-ups of the tablet product with other, similar appearing drug products. Thereafter, FDA determined that the innovator tablet product had not been withdrawn for safety or effectiveness reasons. This determination allowed ANDA sponsors to seek approval for generic version of the tablet product, even though the innovator tablet product was no longer being marketed. When the innovator firm challenged that FDA decision, FDA's decision was upheld, with the court stating that the determination that the withdrawal was not for safety or effectiveness reasons was, in the first instance, within FDA's discretion (83).

7. COMPLIANCE ISSUES

7.1. In General

Regulatory compliance issues may pose a hurdle to approval of an ANDA in the first instance, to approval of supplements to an approved ANDA seeking permission to change the formulation or manufacturing process or make other product improvements, or to the continued manufacture and distribution of an approved drug product. These issues generally first come to light during FDA inspections. FDA may conduct inspections as part of its statutory obligation to inspect all drug manufacturers once every two years (84), the agency's investigation of complaints or other reports about product failures, or pre-approval inspections.

If an FDA investigator observes what he or she views as significant problems, particularly in the area of current good manufacturing practices, the investigator is likely to leave a Form FDA-483 listing "Inspectional Observations" at the close of the inspection. Depending on the seriousness of the perceived deviations, FDA may send the inspected firm a Warning Letter, which is a cease-and-desist letter. While a further discussion of compliance issues is beyond the scope of this book, it should be noted that a "483" or Warning Letter should be taken seriously and responded to in an appropriate fashion. Firms that do not have the requisite in-house resources should consult with knowledgeable technical, regulatory, and legal personnel, as appropriate.

If a drug manufacturer fails to resolve alleged violations that are addressed in the Warning Letter, and particularly if the alleged violations continue over a series of inspections, federal court legal action may result. By going to federal court, where FDA is represented by the US Department of Justice, the government can seek to seize and condemn violative products, enjoin a firm and its employees from continued violations of the law, and impose criminal sanctions against a firm and its management (85).

The approvability of an ANDA or supplemental ANDA may be affected not only by the compliance status of the sponsor's own facilities, but also by the regulatory status of active pharmaceutical ingredient (API) suppliers, clinical research organizations, testing laboratories, and other firms referenced in the ANDA that have a role in the development and production of the generic drug product. This situation is complicated by the fact that, under typical commercial arrangements, the ANDA sponsor has no direct access to its suppliers' internal procedures and similar documents, which are typically made available to FDA in the form of a drug master file (DMF) that the ANDA sponsor has the right to reference but not actually review. Similarly, correspondence between FDA and a supplier may not be available to the ANDA sponsor. Thus, the ANDA sponsor may be at the mercy of others, without having any ability to resolve the compliance issues, or even find out about them.

7.2. Recalls

Problems uncovered during FDA inspections, as well as problems uncovered by a manufacturer itself, can lead to product recalls. In general, FDA has no legal authority to compel a firm to conduct a recall; thus, recalls are nominally "voluntary." As a practical matter, however, firms often have no alternative but to conduct a recall of product that violates legal and regulatory requirements in some manner. The factors that support a decision to conduct a "voluntary" recall include FDA's ability to issue adverse publicity about the firm, the threat of legal action, and mitigation of product liability exposure. FDA has issued recall "guidelines," and strongly prefers that firms conducting a recall follow the guidelines (86).

While a discussion of the conduct of a recall is beyond the scope of this book, it should be noted that every drug manufacturer should have contingency plans for conducting a recall. If properly handled, the impact of a recall can be minimized. A firm's recall plan should address assessing the health hazard associated with a product problem; contacting regulatory authorities; contacting customers; public relations; handling physician, pharmacist, and consumer inquiries; and collecting and handling returned product. Of course, in any particular situation, some of these steps may not be necessary, depending on the nature of the product and a firm's operations. A firm that does not have the requisite in-house expertise should seek the assistance of qualified outside help in this area, preferably before the need arises.

Recalls are commonplace and affect all drug firms ranging from multinational innovator companies to small niche generic firms. In a typical year, approximately 500 recalls of drug products are reported by FDA. The great majority of these recalls involve the failure of a product to comply with its specifications in some manner, such as dissolution problems or subpotency near the end of the product's shelf life. For the most part, these recalls present technical violations that present either no or minor public health issues.

7.3. "Fraud Policy"

In response to widespread problems involving the submission and review of ANDAs in the late 1980s and early 1990s, FDA adopted its application integrity policy, commonly known as the "fraud policy," in 1991 (87). The fraud policy is triggered if FDA concludes that the sponsor of an ANDA (or other pre-market approval application) has committed fraud, bribery, illegal gratuities, or other unlawful acts that call into question the integrity of data supporting the sponsor's application. The policy can also be triggered by a pattern of material errors due to sloppiness and similar causes. If FDA notifies a firm that the fraud policy is applicable, FDA will stop reviewing the firm's applications until the firm has rehabilitated itself. Rehabilitation consists of removal of all individuals who were associated with the improper acts, followed by a validity assessment to determine the reliability of data in the firm's applications. Validity assessments are typically conducted by independent consultants, retained at the firm's expense, followed by FDA spot-checking of data. FDA's decision to invoke the fraud policy with respect to an ANDA sponsor, or even a contract manufacturer with a significant role in preparation of an ANDA, could result in delays of one to a number of years in ANDA approval.

7.4. Debarment

In response to irregularities in the generic drug industry, the Federal Food, Drug, and Cosmetic Act (FDC Act) was amended in 1992 to include debarment provisions (88). Both individuals and business entities can be debarred if convicted of certain crimes associated with a lack of trustworthiness (e.g., fraud, perjury, obstruction of justice); a high managerial agent can also be debarred if he or she had knowledge of such activity and failed to take remedial action. An ANDA is required to include a certification that the sponsor did not use and will not use in any capacity the services of a debarred person in connection with the application. Thus, ANDA sponsors have an obligation to ensure that they do not employ debarred individuals and do not use the services of a company that has been debarred.

8. LEGISLATIVE ISSUES—HATCH–WAXMAN REFORM

As of this writing, reform of some of the Hatch–Waxman provisions adopted in 1984 within the next several years is a definite possibility (e.g.) (89). In particular, from the generic industry's perspective, provisions that have been widely discussed as in need of revision include the patent listing provisions for NDA sponsors, the automatic 30-month delay of ANDA final approval, and 180-day exclusivity. Any reform will undoubtedly involve trade-offs between the rights and obligations of the innovator and generic drug industries. For the benefit of the innovator side, possible trade-offs include enhancements to the exclusivity and patent term restoration provisions of the Hatch–Waxman Amendments.

As enacted in 1984, the abbreviated approval and non-patent exclusivity provisions of the Hatch–Waxman Amendments do not apply to biological products licensed by FDA under the Public Health Service Act. (However, biological products are within the scope of the patent term restoration provisions of Title II of the Hatch–Waxman Amendments (90).) Some generic drug firms have advanced the notion of extending the ANDA-type abbreviated approval mechanism to generic versions of biological products. While such an extension is likely to receive serious consideration, there is at this time no agreement on the underlying scientific standard for assessing comparability or equivalence.

9. MISCELLANEOUS

9.1. "Moving Target" and Disagreements with FDA

A longstanding industry complaint with the FDA pre-market approval process (not limited to generic drugs, by any means) is the so-called "moving target," in which product sponsors satisfy what they believe were the applicable requirements, only to be told that the requirements have changed or that additional requirements are now applicable. In an effort to address this longstanding concern, the FDC Act was amended in 1997 to provide for a binding ANDA pre-submission conference. Assuming written agreement is reached, the agreement is not to be changed after testing begins, except with the sponsor's consent or based upon an FDA determination that a new, substantial scientific issue essential to the safety or effectiveness of the drug has been identified (91). In practice, the provision has been of limited use. By its terms, it applies only to agreements on the design and size of bioavailability and bioequivalence studies. Even within that limited scope, very few prospective ANDA sponsors have reached written agreements with FDA regarding study design.

To reduce the "moving target" problem to the maximum extent possible, prudent ANDA sponsors should attempt to get written confirmation whenever possible from FDA regarding any understandings reached. If that is not possible, the sponsor should memorialize the understanding reached at a meeting or during a telephone conference, send a copy of the document to FDA, and ask that it be reviewed and any inaccuracies be brought to the attention of the firm as soon as possible.

Disagreements with FDA staff over scientific or technical issues can be appealed up through the chain of command (92). If a disputed technical issue cannot be resolved through the appeals process, judicial review is probably not a realistic option. Before seeking judicial review, a drug sponsor generally must seek a formal evidentiary hearing on whether its application should be approved. This procedure calls for a formal evidentiary hearing before FDA's Administrative Law Judge (ALJ), an initial decision by the ALJ, and a final agency decision by the FDA Commissioner or his delegate. Only then is judicial review available (93). Unfortunately for industry, this administrative process is unlikely to result in a satisfactory decision on the merits for the drug sponsor. Moreover, it is very time consuming and is likely to take a number of years to run its course. Thus, as a practical matter, it has very seldom been used by industry. In some cases, it may be possible to characterize an ANDA dispute in legal terms, thereby increasing the chance of obtaining judicial review without first resorting to the administrative hearing process.

9.2. ANDA Approval Delays

Although Hatch–Waxman Amendments provide that FDA will approve or disapprove an ANDA within 180 days (94), the median ANDA approval time is, as of this writing, approximately 18 months. While there have been substantial improvements in recent years in ANDA review and approval times, these times are still far longer than the statutory timeframes. One court challenge to compel FDA to review a sponsor's ANDA in timely fashion was rejected (95).

Much of the delay in reviewing and approving ANDAs can be attributed to the successful Prescription Drug User Fee Act, which requires drug sponsors to pay user fees in connection with NDAs for prescription drugs (96). The user fee legislation includes a commitment by FDA that it will review and take action on 90% of all complete NDAs within 12 months, and FDA has done so. The user fee legislation has had the practical effect of diverting agency resources that would otherwise have been used for the review of ANDAs to the innovator product side of FDA's Center for Drug Evaluation and Research.

Delay is a particular problem for those ANDAs that require a "consult" opinion from the corresponding new drug review division. Examples of such ANDAs include sustained release products with complex bioequivalency issues and non-systemically absorbed drug products where a small clinical trial is used to assess bioequivalency. These "consults" are typically assigned a low priority by the new drug review division because they do not count against FDA's user fee deadlines and quotas. In appropriate situations, a 505(b)(2) NDA may be preferable to an ANDA, as the 505(b)(2) application will get the benefit of the user fee time commitments.

9.3. State Formulary Issues

Under most state pharmacy laws, a pharmacist may (or must) substitute a generic version of an innovator product when the physician prescribes the innovator product by brand name, unless the physician or patient objects to substitution. The substitution provisions of most state pharmacy laws cover all ANDA products that have been approved by FDA as therapeutically equivalent to their brand name counterparts. However, in a small number of states, state formulary boards may conduct their own review of the information and data submitted to FDA to support an ANDA approval, and may make their own decisions on product substitutability within that state. Although senior FDA officials are on record as stating that there is no evidence that an FDA-approved generic product cannot be safely and effectively substituted for its brand name counterpart, these states that engage in making their own drug substitution decisions provide another opportunity for innovator drug sponsors to block substitution. Most recently, these efforts have focused on so-called "narrow therapeutic index" drugs, such as Coumadin® (warfarin sodium).

9.4. Copyrighted Labeling

One innovator drug manufacturer attempted to block generic competition by copyrighting portions of its FDA-approved labeling, and then seeking an injunction under federal copyright law against the ANDA sponsor on the basis that its copyright was being infringed. The court ultimately rejected this argument, concluding that the Hatch–Waxman requirement for the "same" labeling takes precedence over copyright law. However, that court recognized that use of the copyrighted materials in a context other than labeling (such as advertising) could well constitute copyright infringement (97).

9.5. Anti-trust Considerations

Agreements between competitors or potential competitors that have the effect of restricting competition may run afoul of federal and state antitrust laws and similar laws. Particularly noteworthy in this respect are agreements between the innovator drug sponsor and the ANDA sponsor entitled to 180-day exclusivity to settle Hatch–Waxman patent infringement litigation in a way that blocks or significantly delays the entire market for generic versions of the innovator product. These arrangements have led to enforcement action by the Federal Trade Commission (FTC) (which with the Department of Justice is charged with enforcing federal anti-trust statutes) e.g., (98), as well as lawsuits seeking damages filed by state governments, health care insurers, and consumer groups. The FTC has studied these agreements (99), which may result in additional investigations. Exclusive supply arrangements between an ANDA sponsor and the API supplier are also suspect, particularly if no other sources of the API are available.

The actions of innovator companies that have the effect of delaying all generic competition are also under FTC scrutiny and the subject of private anti-trust lawsuits see for, e.g., (100). A major concern in this area is the listing of patents in the Orange Book that may not meet the statutory and regulatory criteria for listing.

10. CONCLUSION

In addition to the technical hurdles that a prospective generic drug sponsor must overcome, there are a number of obstacles that many would characterize as being of a legal nature. Uncertainties about how FDA is implementing and interpreting some statutory provisions, such as 180-day generic drug exclusivity, along with the possibility of litigation, complicate business planning in some cases. A prospective ANDA sponsor facing a situation that could pose hurdles of this type would be well advised to seek appropriate regulatory and legal advice.

REFERENCES

1. 21 C.F.R. section 10.30.
2. 64 Fed. Reg. 66,822 (Nov. 30, 1999).
3. See Mova Pharmaceutical Corp. v. Shalala, 140 F.3d 1060 (D.C. Cir. 1998).
4. 21 U.S.C. section 355(j)(5)(D)(ii).
5. 21 U.S.C. section 355(j)(5)(D)(iii) and (iv).
6. Upjohn Co. v. Kessler, 938 F. Supp. 439 (W.D. Mich. 1996).
7. 21 C.F.R. section 314.94(a)(8)(iv).
8. Bristol-Myers Squibb Company v. Shalala, 91 F.3d 1493 (D.C. Cir. 1996).
9. 65 Fed. Reg. 64,225 (Oct. 26, 2000).
10. 21 C.F.R. section 201.57(f)(9).
11. 21 U.S.C. section 355a(o)(added by the Best Pharmaceuticals for Children Act, Pub. L. No. 107-109).
12. 21 U.S.C. section 355(j)(5)(B)(iv).
13. 64 Fed. Reg. 42,873 (Aug. 6, 1999).
14. 67 Fed. Reg. 66,593 (Nov. 1, 2002).
15. Mova Pharmaceutical Corp. v. Shalala, 140 F.3d 1060 (D.C. Cir. 1998).
16. Purepac Pharmaceutical Co. v. Friedman, 162 F.3d 1201 (D.C. Cir. 1998).
17. See Mylan Pharmaceuticals, Inc. v. Henney, 94 F. Supp.2d 36 (D.D.C. 2000), vacated sub nom., Pharmachemie B.V. v. Barr Laboratories, Inc., 276 F.3d 627 (D.C. Cir. 2002); Mova Pharmaceutical Corp. v. Shalala, 140 F.3d 1060, 1071 (D.C. Cir. 1998).
18. 21 U.S.C. section 355(j)(5)(B)(iv).
19. Granutec Inc. v. Shalala, 1998 WL 153410 (4th Cir. Apr. 3, 1998) (unpublished opinion); 139 F. 3d 889 (4th Cir. 1998) (table).
20. 65 Fed. Reg. 16,922 (Mar. 30, 2000).
21. Apotex, Inc. v. Shalala, 53 F. Supp. 2d 454 (D.D.C. 1999), summary affirmance, 1999 WL 956686 (D.C. Cir. 1999).
22. www.fda.gov/cder/ogd/ppiv.htm (accessed November 2002).
23. Boehringer Ingelheim Corporation v. Shalala , 993 F.Supp.1 (D.D.C. 1997).
24. Teva Pharmaceuticals USA, Inc. v. FDA, 182 F.3d 1003 (D.C. Cir. 1999); on remand, 1999 U.S. Dist. LEXIS 14,575 (D.D.C. Aug. 18, 1999) (unpublished decision); affirmed, 2000 U.S. App. LEXIS 38,667, 254 F.3d 316 (D.C. Cir. Nov. 15, 2000) (table, unpublished decision).
25. 67 Fed. Reg. 66,593 (Nov. 1, 2002).
26. 64 Fed. Reg. 42,873 (Aug. 6, 1999).
27. FDA letter dated Aug. 2, 1999, Docket No. 99P-1271, available at www.fda.gov/ohrms/dockets/dailys/080699/pdn0001.pdf (accessed November 2002).
28. FDA letter dated Nov. 16, 2001, ANDA 75–347, available at www.fda.gov/cder/ogd/shared_exclusivity.htm (accessed November 2002).
29. Dr. Reddy's Laboratories, Inc. v. Thompson, Nos. 02–452 and 02–1769 (D. N.J.).
30. 21 U.S.C. section 355a.
31. Merck & Co., Inc. v. FDA, 148 F. Supp.2d 27 (D.D.C. 2001).

32. 21 U.S.C. section 355a(n) (added by the Best Pharmaceuticals for Children Act, Pub. L. No. 107-109).
33. 21 U.S.C. section 355(j)(2)(C); 21 C.F.R. section 314.93.
34. ANDA suitability petitions and their status are summarized in a chart on FDA's website, www.fda.gov/cder/ogd/suitabil.htm (accessed November 2002).
35. 21 U.S.C. section 355(j)(2)(C).
36. 21 C.F.R. section 314.55.
37. Association of American Physicians and Surgeons, Inc. v. U.S. Food and Drug Administration, _ F. Supp.2d _, 2002 U.S. Dist. LEXIS 19689 (D.D.C. Oct. 17, 2002).
38. S. 2394 (2002); H.R. 5594 (2002).
39. Serono Laboratories, Inc. v. Shalala, 158 F.3d 1313, 1320 (D.C. Cir. 1998).
40. 62 Fed. Reg. 42,562 (Aug. 7, 1997).
41. Pfizer Inc. v. Shalala, 182 F.3d 975 (D.C. Cir. 1999).
42. Warner-Lambert Company v. Shalala, 202 F.3d 326 (D.C. Cir. 2000).
43. 21 U.S.C. section 355(j)(2)(A)(v).
44. Zeneca, Inc. v. Shalala, 213 F.3d 161 (4th Cir. 2000).
45. 21 U.S.C. section 355(j)(8).
46. 21 C.F.R. Part 320.
47. Fisons Corporation v. Shalala, 860 F. Supp. 859 (D.D.C. 1994).
48. Bristol-Myers Squibb Company v. Shalala, 923 F. Supp. 212 (D.D.C. 1996).
49. Schering Corp. v. Food and Drug Administration, 51 F.3d 390 (3rd Cir. 1995).
50. Somerset Pharmaceuticals, Inc. v. Shalala, 973 F. Supp. 443, 453 (D. Del 1997).
51. 21 C.F.R. section 310.200(d).
52. 21 U.S.C. section 355(b)(1).
53. 21 U.S.C. section 355(c)(2).
54. 21 C.F.R. section 314.53(b).
55. 21 C.F.R. section 314.53(c)(2).
56. Pfizer, Inc. v. Food and Drug Administration, 753 F. Supp. 171 (D. Md. 1990).
57. Zenith Laboratories, Inc. v. Abbott Laboratories, 1997 U.S. Dist. LEXIS 23954 (D.N.J. Oct. 1, 1997) (unpublished decision).
58. Ben Venue Laboratories, Inc. v. Novartis Pharmaceutical Corp., 10 F. Supp.2d 446 (D.N.J. 1998).
59. Mylan Pharmaceuticals, Inc. v. Thompson, 139 F.Supp.2d 1 (D.D.C. 2001), reversed on other grounds, 268 F.3d 1323 (Fed. Cir. 2001).
60. Mylan Pharmaceuticals, Inc. v. Thompson, 268 F.3d 1323 (Fed. Cir. 2001).
61. See 21 C.F.R. section 314.53(f) and section 314.94(a)(12)(vii).
62. Watson Pharmaceuticals, Inc. v. Henney, 2001 U.S. Dist. LEXIS 2477 (D. Md. Jan. 18, 2001)(unpublished decision), appeal pending, No. 01-1285 (Fed. Cir.).
63. Andrx Pharmaceuticals, Inc. v. Biovail Corporation, 276 F.3d 1368 (Fed. Cir. 2002).
64. Apotex, Inc. v. Thompson, slip op., No. 00-0729 (D.D.C. Feb. 7, 2002), appeal pending (Fed. Cir. No. 02-1295).
65. Andrx Pharmaceuticals, Inc. v. Biovail Corporation, 276 F.3d 1368 (Fed. Cir. 2002).

66. 67 Fed. Reg. 65,448 (October 24, 2002).
67. 21 U.S.C. section 355(j)(5)(B)(iii).
68. Andrx Pharmaceuticals, Inc. v. Biovail Corp., 276 F.2d 1368 (Fed. Cir. 2002).
69. Apotex, Inc. v. Thompson, slip op., No. 00–0729 (D.D.C. Feb. 7, 2002), appeal pending (Fed. Cir. No. 02-1295).
70. 67 Fed. Reg. 65,448 (October 24, 2002).
71. Yamanouchi Pharmaceutical Co., Ltd. v. Danbury Pharmacal, Inc., 2000 U.S. App. Lexis 27455, *20-*21 (Fed. Cir. Nov. 3, 2000).
72. Glaxo, Inc. v. Novopharm, Ltd., 110 F.3d 1562 (Fed. Cir. 1997).
73. Warner-Lambert Company v. Apotex Corp., 2001 U.S. Dist. LEXIS 14592 (N.D. Ill. Sept. 13, 2001) (unpublished decision), appeal pending (Fed. Cir., No. 02–1073); Allergan, Inc. v. Alcon Laboratories, Inc., 200 F. Supp.2d 1219 (C.D. Cal. 2002), appeal pending (Fed. Cir., No. 02-1449).
74. 35 U.S.C. section 271(e)(1).
75. 21 U.S.C. section 355(b)(2).
76. 21 U.S.C. section 355(c)(3)(A)–(C).
77. 21 U.S.C. section 355(c)(3)(D); section 355a.
78. 21 U.S.C. section 355(c)(3)(D) and (j)(5)(D).
79. 21 C.F.R. section 314.101(d)(9).
80. 21 U.S.C. section 355(j)(4)(I).
81. 21 C.F.R. section 314.122.
82. 21 U.S.C. section 355(j)(4)(I).
83. Somerset Pharmaceuticals, Inc. v. Shalala, 973 F. Supp. 443, 453 (D. Del. 1997).
84. 21 U.S.C. section 360(h).
85. 21 U.S.C. section 334, 332, and 333, respectively.
86. 21 C.F.R. section 7.40–7.59.
87. 56 Fed. Reg. 46,191 (Sept. 10, 1991).
88. 21 U.S.C. section 335a.
89. S. 812 (2002); H.R. 5272 (2002); H.R. 5311 (2002).
90. 35 U.S.C. section 156.
91. 21 U.S.C. section 355(j)(3).
92. 21 U.S.C. section 360bbb-1; 21 C.F.R. section 10.75.
93. 21 U.S.C. section 355(j)(5)(C) and (h).
94. 21 U.S.C. section 355(j)(5)(A).
95. In re Barr Laboratories, Inc., 930 F.2d. 72 (D.C. Cir. 1991).
96. 21 U.S.C. section 379g and section 379h.
97. SmithKline Beecham Consumer Health Care, L.P. v. Watson Pharmaceuticals, Inc., 211 F. 3d 21 (2d Cir. 2000).
98. 67 Fed. Reg. 44,606 (July 3, 2002).
99. "Generic Drug Entry Prior to Patent Expiration: An FTC Study," July 2002, available at www.ftc.gov/opa/2002/07/genericdrugstudy.htm (accessed November 2002).
100. In Re Buspirone Patent and Antitrust Litigation, 185 F. Supp.2d 340 (S.D. N.Y. 2002).

Glossary

Abbreviation	Definition
AB Rating	Products listed in the 'Orange Book' that meetnecessary bioequivalence requirements.
ADME	Absorption, Distribution, Metabolism and Excretion
ADR	Adverse Drug Reaction
AE	Adverse Event
Agency	The United States Food and Drug Administration
ANDA	Abbreviated New Drug Application
ANOVA	Analysis of variances
API	Active Pharmaceutical Ingredient (see Drug Substance)
AUC	Area Under the Curve (an expression of exposure or extent of systemic drug absorption)
BA	Bioavailability
BACPAC	Bulk Actives Post-Approval Changes
Batch	A specific quantity of a drug substance or drug product intended to have uniform character and quality, within specified limits, and produced according to a single manufacturing order during the same cycle or manufacture (see also Biobatch)
BCS	Biopharmaceutics Classification System
BE	Bioequivalence
Biobatch	The lot of drug product formulated for purposes of pharmacokinetic evaluation in a bioavailability/bioequivalence study.
Biostudy	An in vivo BA or BE study

Biowaiver	A request to the FDA to waive the requirements for an in vivo bioequivalence study. Biowaivers are often requested for lower dosage strengths whose formulations are dose proportional to the dosage strength used in a bioequivalence study.
BLA	Biologics License Application
CANDA	Computer Assisted New Drug Application
CBE	Changes Being Effected
CBE-30	Changes Being Effected—30 days
CBER	Center for Biologics Evaluation and Research (www.fda.gov/cber)
CDER	Center for Drug Evaluation and Research (www.fda.gov/cder)
CDMA	Canadian Drug Manufacturers Association (www.cdma-acfpp.org)
CFR	Code of Federal Regulations—Comprehensive drug regulations are found in Title 21 of the Code of Federal Regulations Part 300, Subchapter D: Drugs for Human Use (21 CFR Part 300)
Critical Manufacturing Variable	Includes those manufacturing materials, methods, equipment, and processes that significantly affect drug release from the formulation (e.g., coating thickness, particle size, crystal form, excipient type, and tablet hardness)
Critical Processing Variable	A specific step, unit process, or condition of a unit process that can affect a specific performance variable critical to the ultimate and predictable performance of the dosage form and the drug substance.
cGMP	Current Good Manufacturing Practices
CMC	Chemistry and Manufacturing Controls
CMCCC	Chemistry and Manufacturing Controls Coordinating Committee (CDER)
COSTART	Coding Symbols for Thesaurus of Adverse Reaction Terms
CRO	Contract Research Organization
DEA	Drug Enforcement Administration (www.usdoj.gov/dea)
DMF	Drug Master File
Drug Product	A finished dosage form (e.g., tablet, capsule, or solution) that contains a drug substance generally,

	but not necessarily, in association with one or more other ingredients.
Drug Substance	An active ingredient that is intended to furnish pharmacological activity or other direct effect in the diagnosis, cure, mitigation, treatment, or prevention of disease or to affect the structure or any function of the human body, but does not include intermediates used in the synthesis of such an ingredient. (Also considered as the active pharmaceutical ingredient.)
EFPIA	European Federation of Pharmaceutical Industries Associations
EIR	Establishment Inspection Report
EMEA	European Agency for the Evaluation of Medicinal Products (www.emea.eu.int)
EPA	Environmental Protection Agency (www.epa.gov)
EU	European Union
FDA	United States Food and Drug Administration (www.fda.gov)
FDA Form 483	FD-483 is the written notice of objectionable practices or deviations from the regulations that are prepared by the FDA inspector at the end of an investigation.
FD&C Act	Federal Food, Drug, and Cosmetic Act
FOI	Freedom of Information (www.fda.gov/foi/foia2.htm)
FR	Federal Register—the Federal Register is the official daily publication for Rules, Proposed Rules, and Notices of Federal agencies and organizations, as well as Executive Orders and other Presidential Documents (www.access.gpo.gov/su_docs/aces/aces140.html)
FTC	Federal Trade Commission (www.ftc.gov)
GGPs	Good Guidance Practices. GGPs define how the FDA develops and uses guidance documents
GLP	Good Laboratory Practices
GMP	Good Manufacturing Practices
GPA	Generic Pharmaceutical Association (www.gphaonline.org)
GRAS	Generally Recognized as Safe

Guidance	A guidance refers to any written communication that explains the FDA policy or procedure. The term guidance generally refers to guidance for industry. Guidances are prepared to establish clarity and consistency in FDA policies and in inspection and enforcement procedures. Guidances reflect FDA's current thinking on an issue. Guidance documents contain recommendations about how best to do things, but do not legally bind the FDA or the public.
Hatch–Waxman	Drug Price and Patent Restoration Act of 1984
HFD	Routing code for mail to CDER
HPB	Health Protection Branch (Canada's equivalent to the FDA, www.hc-sc.gc.ca/english/protection/index.html)
IBE	Individual Bioequivalence
ICH	International Conference on Harmonization of Technical Requirements for Registration of Pharmaceuticals for Human Use (www.ifpma.org/ich1.html)
IFPMA	International Federation of Pharmaceutical Manufacturers Associations (www.ifpma.org)
Impurity	Any component of a drug substance that is not the entity defined as the drug substance.
IND	Investigational New Drug
Installation Qualification (IQ)	The documented verification that all key aspects of the equipment and ancillary systems installations adhere to the approved design intentions (plans) and the recommendations of the manufacturer are suitably considered.
In Vitro–In Vivo Correlation (IVIVC)	A predictive mathematical model describing the relationship between an in vitro property of an oral dosage form (usually the rate or extent of drug dissolution/release) and a relevant in vivo response (e.g., plasma drug concentration or percentage of drug absorbed)
IRB	Institutional Review Board (ethics committee that reviews biostudies)
MAPP	Manual of Policy and Procedures
NCE	New Chemical Entity
NDA	New Drug Application

NME	New Molecular Entity
NTI	Narrow Therapeutic Index or Narrow Therapeutic Range Drugs
OGD	Office of Generic Drugs (http://www.fda.gov/cder/ogd)
Operational Qualification (OQ)	The documented verification that the equipment and ancillary systems perform as intended throughout anticipated operating ranges.
Orange Book	Approved Drug Products with Therapeutic Equivalence Evaluations (www.fda.gov/cder/ob/default.htm)
PAI	Pre-approval Inspection
PD	Pharmacodynamics
Pilot Scale	The manufacture of a drug substance or drug product on a reduced scale by processes representative of and simulating that to be applied on a larger commercial manufacturing scale.
PDR	Physician's Desk Reference, Medical Economics Company, Montvale, NJ (published annually)
PDUFA	Prescription Drug User Fee Act of 1992
PRMA	Pharmaceutical Research and Manufacturers of America (www.phrma.org)
PK	Pharmacokinetics
PQRI	Product Quality Research Institute (www.pqri.org)
Process validation	Establishing documented evidence that provides a high degree of assurance that a specific process will consistently produce a product meeting its predetermined specification and quality characteristics.
QA	Quality Assurance
QC	Quality Control
RLD	Reference Listed Drug
RTF	Refuse To File, the decision by the FDA to refuse to file an application
Specifications	A set of criteria to which a drug substance or drug product should conform to be considered acceptable for its intended use.
SUPAC	Scale-Up and Post-Approval Changes
TPD	Therapeutics Products Directorate (part of Canada's Health Protection Branch)
USAN	United States Adopted Name (www.usp.org)

| USP-NF | United States Pharmacopeia—National Formulary (http://www.usp.org) |
| WHO | World Health Organization (www.who.int/home-page) |

Index